Challenging Concepts in Emergency Medicine

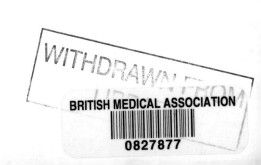

Published and forthcoming titles in the Challenging Concepts in series

Anaesthesia (Edited by Dr Phoebe Syme, Dr Robert Jackson, and Professor Tim Cook)

Cardiovascular Medicine (Edited by Dr Aung Myat, Dr Shouvik Haldar, and Professor Simon Redwood)

Emergency Medicine (Edited by Dr Sam Thenabadu, Dr Fleur Cantle, and Dr Chris Lacy)

Infectious Disease and Clinical Microbiology (Edited by Dr Amber Arnold and Professor George Griffin)

Interventional Radiology (Edited by Dr Irfan Ahmed, Dr Miltiadis Krokidis, and Dr Tarun Sabharwal)

Neurology (Edited by Dr Krishna Chinthapalli, Dr Nadia Magdalinou, and Professor Nicholas Wood)

Neurosurgery (Edited by Mr Robin Bhatia and Mr Ian Sabin)

Obstetrics and Gynaecology (Edited by Dr Natasha Hezelgrave, Dr Danielle Abbott, and Professor Andrew Shennan)

Oncology (Edited by Dr Madhumita Bhattacharyya, Dr Sarah Payne, and Professor Iain McNeish)

Oral and Maxillofacial Surgery (Edited by Mr Matthew Idle and Dr Andrew Monaghan)

Respiratory Medicine (Edited by Dr Lucy Schomberg and Dr Elizabeth Sage)

Challenging Concepts in Emergency Medicine:
Cases with Expert Commentary

Edited by

Dr Sam Thenabadu
Consultant Adult & Paediatric Emergency Medicine, Princess Royal University Hospital, King's College Hospital NHS Foundation Trust Kent, UK

Dr Fleur Cantle
Consultant in Adult and Paediatric Emergency Medicine, King's College Hospital NHS Foundation Trust, London, UK

Dr Chris Lacy
Consultant Emergency Medicine, King's College Hospital, London, UK

Series editors

Dr Aung Myat BSc (Hons) MBBS MRCP
BHF Clinical Research Training Fellow, King's College London British Heart Foundation Centre of Research Excellence, Cardiovascular Division, St Thomas' Hospital, London, UK

Dr Shouvik Haldar MBBS MRCP
Electrophysiology Research Fellow & Cardiology SpR, Heart Rhythm Centre, NIHR Cardiovascular Biomedical Research Unit, Royal Brompton & Harefield NHS Foundation Trust, Imperial College London, London

Professor Simon Redwood MD FRCP
Professor of Interventional Cardiology and Honorary Consultant Cardiologist, King's College London British Heart Foundation Centre of Research Excellence, Cardiovascular Division and Guy's and St Thomas' NHS Foundation Trust, St Thomas' Hospital, London, UK

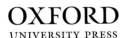

OXFORD
UNIVERSITY PRESS

UNIVERSITY PRESS

Great Clarendon Street, Oxford, OX2 6DP,
United Kingdom

Oxford University Press is a department of the University of Oxford.
It furthers the University's objective of excellence in research, scholarship,
and education by publishing worldwide. Oxford is a registered trade mark of
Oxford University Press in the UK and in certain other countries

Published in the United States of America by Oxford University Press
198 Madison Avenue, New York, NY 10016, United States of America

British Library Cataloguing in Publication Data

Data available

Library of Congress Control Number: 2014947263

ISBN 978-0-19-965409-3

Printed in Great Britain by
Ashford Colour Press Ltd, Gosport, Hampshire

For Richard, Martha and Barnaby
Fleur Cantle

For Molly and Reuben
Sam Thenabadu

FOREWORD

The publication of this book is a timely reminder of the maturity of the specialty of emergency medicine. The chapters, each written by an experienced EM physician and added to by renowned national and international experts, explore in depth the clinical challenges and conundrums that begin each chapter.

The diligent reference to key studies, not just via a simple citation but by use of a brief summary of the relevant findings, ensures that the reader is not only informed by the text but achieves a level of familiarity with a good deal of the academic literature.

The reader is guided through a series of questions and answers as the clinical path of each patient progresses and this interaction greatly increases the readability of the text. The other engaging feature is the inclusion of expert comments and opinions at various points in each chapter. The effect created is similar to that experienced in a small tutorial group overseen by a learned and experienced mentor. Key learning points assist in emphasizing the issues most relevant to patient outcomes. Finally each chapter concludes with an extensive and up to date reference list to ensure ease of access to the source literature.

For those EM physicians who are increasingly familiar with the use of ultrasound in the ED there are numerous excellent sonographic examples of key anatomy and pathophysiology.

This is not a traditional textbook, nor does it purport to cover any specific curriculum; instead this is a book that engages the reader, seeks to challenge and educate the EM physician and will do so whether they are recently qualified or an established consultant.

The book covers a wide range of conditions and any shift worked in the ED will include many of the patients and challenges so authoritatively covered by this text. The result is, in effect, a single volume approach to CPD. Those who read and note its contents will be better clinicians, better teachers, and better prepared to challenge concepts in emergency medicine.

Dr Clifford Mann FRCP FCEM
President of the College of Emergency Medicine

ACKNOWLEDGEMENTS

Emergency Medicine is a flourishing specialty, and the chance to coordinate bringing together a textbook by enthusiastic and inspiring EM colleagues was a real labour of love. The chapters truly emphasise the challenging grey cases seen in the ED and the expertise that the specialty has. I hope that the evidence based medicine described and the pragmatic expert opinions offered, will form a text that can be applied to both day to day ED scenarios, as well as an aide for exams.

It is essential to thank all the authors and experts that have produced great chapters and tolerated our relentless emails and phone calls. It is equally if not more important to thank Fleur as my fellow editor for her tireless energy, organisational skills and constant positivity to make this book a success despite being one of the busiest people I know. I shall never forget the colour coded excel charts!

Finally I must thank my parents for their lifelong support and encouragement, but most of all my biggest thank you is to my wonderful understanding, patient and unrelentingly supportive wife Molly and son Reuben – you are my constant inspirations.

Sam Thenabadu

CONTENTS

CONTRIBUTORS

Dr Olumayowa Adenugba
Consultant Emergency Medicine
Queen Elizabeth Hospital
Lewisham and Greenwich NHS Trust
Woolwich, London

Dr Harith Al-Rawi
Consultant Adult and Paediatric
Emergency Medicine
Guys and St Thomas' NHS Foundation Trust
St Thomas' Hospital
London, UK

Dr Meng Aw-Yong
Medical Director and Forensic Medical Examiner
Metropolitan Police Service
Empress State Building,
London, UK
Associate Specialist Emergency Medicine
Hillingdon Hospital
Middlesex, UK

Dr Mike Beckett
Consultant in Emergency Medicine
West Middlesex University Hospital
London, UK

Mr Duncan Bew
Consultant Trauma and Emergency Surgeon
Clinical Director for Trauma Surgery
King's College Hospital NHS Trust
London, UK

Dr Rhys Beynon
Consultant in Adult and Paediatric Emergency
Medicine
St George's Healthcare NHS Trust
London, UK

Dr Neel Bhanderi
Pre-Hospital and Emergency Physician
Kent, Surrey and Sussex Air Ambulance
Marden, Kent, UK

Dr Sunil Bhatia
Consultant Maxillofacial Surgeon
Royal Shrewsbury Hospital
Royal Shrewsbury and Telford NHS Trust,
Shrewsbury, UK

Dr Lisa Black
ST6 Emergency Medicine
Greater Glasgow and Clyde Health Board,
Royal Alexandra Hospital
Paisley, UK

Dr Duncan Bootland
Consultant in Emergency Medicine
Royal Sussex County Hospital
Brighton & Sussex University Hospital Trust
Brighton, UK

Dr Fleur Cantle
Consultant in Adult & Paediatric
Emergency Medicine
King's College Hospital NHS Foundation Trust
London, UK

Professor Douglas Chamberlain, CBE
Brighton
Honorary Professor of Cardiology,
Brighton and Sussex Medical School.
University of Sussex

Beth Christian
Consultant in Emergency Medicine
St. Thomas' Hospital
Guy's and St Thomas' NHS Foundation Trust
London, UK

Dr Evan Coughlan
Consultant in Emergency Medicine
Brighton & Sussex University NHS Trust
Royal Sussex County Hospital
Brighton, UK

Dr Sean Cross
Consultant Liaison Psychiatrist
South London and Maudsley NHS Foundation Trust
London, UK

Dr Paul Dargan
Consultant Physician and Clinical Toxicologist
Clinical Director and Reader in Toxicology
Guy's and St Thomas' NHS Foundation Trust
London, UK

Dr Rita Das
Consultant in Emergency Medicine
Whittington Health
London, UK

Dr Balj Dheansa
Consultant Burns & Plastic Surgeon
McIndoe Burns Centre
Queen Victoria Hospital
East Grinstead, UK

Dr Chidi Ejimofo
Consultant in Emergency Medicine
Lewisham and Greenwich NHS Trust
University Hospital Lewisham
London, UK

Dr Sarah Finlay
Consultant in Emergency Medicine
Chelsea and Westminster NHS Trust
London, UK

Dr Anna Forrest-Hay
Consultant in Adult and Paediatric Emergency
Medicine
Kingston Hospital NHS Foundation Trust
Kingston-upon-Thames, UK

Dr Anne Frampton
Consultant in Adult and Paediatric Emergency
Medicine
University Hospitals Bristol NHS Foundation Trust
Bristol, UK

Dr Robert Galloway
Consultant in Emergency Medicine
Brighton & Sussex NHS Trust
Brighton, UK

Dr Shweta Gidwani
Consultant in Emergency Medicine
Chelsea & Westminster Hospital NHS Trust
London, UK

Dr Ed Glucksman
Consultant in Emergency Medicine
King's College Hospital NHS Foundation Trust
London, UK

Professor Colin A Graham
Professor of Emergency Medicine
Chinese University of Hong Kong
Honorary Consultant in Emergency Medicine
Prince of Wales Hospital
Shatin New Territories, Hong Kong SAR

Dr Sara Hanna
Consultant in Paediatric Intensive Care
Evelina London Children's Hospital
Guy's and St Thomas' NHS Foundation Trust
London, UK

Professor Tim Harris
Professor of Emergency Medicine
Queen Mary University of London and Brats Health
London, UK

Mr Kambiz Hashemi
Consultant in Emergency Medicine
Croydon University Hospital
Croydon, UK

Dr Katherine Henderson
Consultant in Emergency Medicine
Guy's and St Thomas' NHS Foundation Trust
London, UK

Dr Geoff Hinchley
Consultant in Emergency Medicine
Barnet and Chase Farm Hospital
London, UK

Dr Andrew Hobart
Consultant in Emergency Medicine
Princess Royal University Hospital
Kings College Hospital NHS Foundation Trust
London, UK

Dr Anthony Hudson
Consultant in Emergency Medicine
St George's Hospital, London, UK
and
Kent, Surrey
Sussex Air Ambulance Trust
Marden, UK

Dr Anna Johnson
Consultant in Emergency Medicine
Medway Maritime NHS Foundation Trust
Gillingham, UK

Dr Jeff Keep
Consultant Emergency Medicine
King's College Hospital NHS Foundation Trust
London, UK

Dr Adham Khalek
Consultant in Emergency Medicine
John Radcliffe Hospital
Oxford University Hospital NHS Trust
Oxford, UK

Dr Lalarukh Khan
Consultant in Adult and Paediatric Emergency
Medicine
King's College Hospital NHS Foundation Trust
London, UK

Mr TJ Lasoye
Consultant and Honorary Senior Lecturer in
Emergency Medicine/Director of Medical Education
King's College Hospital NHS Foundation Trust
London, UK

Dr Ian Maconochie
Consultant in Paediatric Emergency Medicine
Imperial College Healthcare Trust
London, UK

Dr Katie Mcleod
Consultant in Adult & Paediatric Emergency Medicine
Princess Royal University Hospital, King's College
Hospital NHS Foundation Trust
London, UK

Dr Andrew Neill
Specialist Registrar in Emergency Medicine
Mater Misericordiae University Hospital
Dublin, Ireland

Dr Sophie Parker
Fellow in Intensive Care
Department of Intensive Care
Prince of Wales Hospital
South Eastern Sydney and Illawarra Area
Health Service
Sydney, Australia

Professor Sir Keith Porter
Professor of Clinical Traumatology
Queen Elizabeth Hospital Birmingham
University Hospital Birmingham NHS
Foundation Trust
Birmingham, UK

Dr Shwetha Rao
Consultant in Emergency Medicine,
King's College Hospital NHS Foundation trust
London, UK

Dr Anna Riddell
Consultant Paediatrician
Clinical Director for Children's Health
Barts Health NHS Trust
London, UK

Professor Emmanuel Rivers
Vice Chairman and Research Director
Department of Emergency Medicine
Attending Staff, Emergency Medicine and
Surgical Critical Care
Henry Ford Hospital
Clinical Professor, Wayne State University
Detroit, Michigan, USA

Professor John Ryan
Consultant in Emergency Medicine
St Vincent's University Hospital
Dublin 4
Ireland

Dr Samy Sadek
Consultant in Emergency Medicine
The Royal London Hospital Barts Health NHS Trust
London, UK

Tina Sajjanhar
Consultant in Paediatric Emergency Medicine
Lewisham and Greenwich NHS Trust
London, UK

Dr Jessica Spedding
Emergency Medicine SpR
The Royal London Hospital
London, UK

Dr Oliver Spencer
Consultant in Emergency Medicine
Croydon University Hospital
Croydon, UK

Dr Lindsey Stevens
Consultant in Emergency Medicine
Epsom and St Helier University NHS Trust
Surrey, UK
Honorary Senior Lecturer
St George's Hospital Medical School
London, UK

Michael Stone
Chief, Division of Emergency Ultrasound
Department of Emergency Medicine
Brigham & Women's Hospital
Assistant Professor of Medicine (Emergency Medicine)
Harvard Medical School
Boston, MA, USA

Dr Emer Sutherland
Consultant in Emergency Medicine
King's College Hospital NHS Foundation Trust
London, UK

Dr Sam Thenabadu
Consultant in Adult & Paediatric Emergency Medicine
Princess Royal University Hospital
King's College Hospital NHS Foundation Trust
Kent, UK

Dr Emma Townsend
Consultant in Emergency Medicine
Maidstone and Tunbridge Wells NHS Trust
Kent, UK

Dr Chetan Trivedy
National Institute for Health Research
Academic Clinical Lecturer in Emergency Medicine
Warwick Medical School
Warwick, UK

Dr André Vercueil
Consultant in Intensive Care Medicine and Anaesthesia
King's College Hospital NHS Foundation Trust
London, UK

Dr Simon Walsh
Consultant in Adult and Paediatric Emergency Medicine
The Royal London Hospital
Barts Health NHS Trust
London, UK

Dr Gavin Wilson
Consultant in Adult & Paediatric Emergency Medicine
Kingston Hospital
Kingston Hospital NHS Foundation Trust
Kingston upon Thames, UK

ABBREVIATIONS

AANA	American Association of Nurse Anesthetists
ABG	arterial blood gas
ACEP	American College of Emergency Physicians
ACPs	Advanced Care Paramedics
AHA	American Heart Association
ALS	advanced life support
ANC	absolute neutrophil count
ASA	American Association of Anaesthesiology
ASIS	anterior superior iliac spine
ATLS	advanced trauma life support
BDZ	benzodiazepine
CA	cardiac arrest
CBT	cognitive behavioural therapy
CDRs	clinical decision rules
CEM	College of Emergency Medicine
CES	Cauda equine syndrome
CESi	incomplete CES
CI	confidence interval
CNS	central nervous system
CPB	cardiopulmonary bypass
CPR	Cardiopulmonary resuscitation
CRP	C-reactive protein
CSE	convulsive status epilepticus
CSF	cerebrospinal fluid
CVP	central venous pressure
DV	domestic violence
DVT	deep vein thrombosis
EAC	exercise-associated collapse
ECMO	extra-corporeal membrane oxygenation
ECW	extracorporeal warming
ED	emergency department
eFAST	extendedFAST
EGDT	early goal-directed therapy
EHS	exertional heat stroke
ENP	emergency nurse practitioner
ENT	ear, nose, and throat
FACT	focused assessment by CT in Trauma
FAST	focused abdominal sonography in trauma
FIB	fascia iliaca block
FIC	fascia iliaca compartment
FNB	Femoral nerve block
FUO	fever of unknown origin
GCA	Glasgow Coma Scale
GTN	glyceryl trinitrate
HBSS	Hanks balanced salt solution
Hib	Haemophilus influenza type b
HMIC	Her Majesty's Inspector of Constabulary
HS	hypertonic saline
ICP	intracranial pressure
ICU	intensive care unit
IDDM	insulin-dependent diabetes mellitus
IFP	idiopathic facial paralysis
IL-6	Interleukin-6
ILE	intra lipid emulsion
IO	intra-osseous
IOFB	intraocular foreign bodies
IPCC	Independent Police Complaints Commission
ISS	injury severity score
ITU	intensive therapy unit
LA	local anaesthetic
LBP	lower back pain
LOC	loss of consciousness
LP	lumbar puncture
MAP	mean arterial blood pressure
MCA	Mental Capacity Act (2005)
MHA	Mental Health Act (1983)
NAI	non-accidental injury
NDTMS	National Drug Treatment Monitoring System
NMDA	N-methyl-D-aspartic acid
NNT	number needed to treat
NOF	neck of femur
NSM	neurogenic stunned myocardium
OOHCA	out-of-hospital cardiac arrest
OR	odds ratio
PCI	percutaneous coronary intervention
PCT	procalcitonin
PDL	periodontal ligament
PEA	pulseless electrical activity
PICU	paediatric intensive care unit

PUO	pyrexia of unknown origin		SSC	Surviving Sepsis campaign
QR	quantitative resuscitation		STEMI	ST elevation myocardial infarction
RBC	red blood cell		SUFE	slipped upper femoral epiphysis
RCT	randomized controlled trial		SVC	superior vena cava
RDT	rapid diagnostic testing		TCA	tricyclic antidepressant
RDTS	rapid diagnostic tests		TDI	traumatic dental injury
RLQ	right lower quadrant		TMJ	temporomandibular joint
ROSC	return of spontaneous circulation		TPO	telephone outpatient score
RROM	restricted range of movement		TS	transient synovitis
SA	septic arthritis		URTI	upper respiratory tract infection
SAH	subarachnoid haemorrhage		US	ultrasound scan
SCD	sickle cell disease		VA	visual acuity
$ScvO_2$	central venous oxygen saturation		VAS	visual analogue scale
SHEP	sonography of the hip joint by the emergency physician		VF	ventricular fibrilation
			VT	ventricular tachycardia
SIRS	systemic inflammatory response syndrome		WCC	white cell count

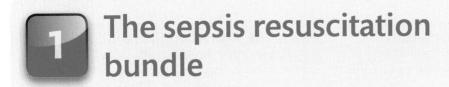

The sepsis resuscitation bundle

Adham Khalek

ⓘ **Expert Commentary** Jeff Keep and Emmanuel Rivers

Case history

A 48-year-old man is brought to the emergency department (ED) by his wife complaining of a 5-day history of worsening dyspnoea, chest pain, and fever. He has a history of hypertension for which he is on an ACE inhibitor, and diet-controlled diabetes. He has no allergies. He works in the financial industry and is normally well. He smokes 3–4 cigars a day.

On initial assessment, he is noted to be clammy and appears pale. He is short of breath at rest. Observations taken during triage are as follows: heart rate 118 regular, BP 96/49 mmHg, temperature 38.8 °C, respiratory rate 28 breaths per minute, oxygen saturation 87 % on room air.

The potential diagnosis of sepsis is recognized and he is moved to the resuscitation room for further assessment and interventions.

See Box 1.1 for a clinical summary of sepsis.

Box 1.1 Clinical summary of sepsis

- Sepsis describes a spectrum of illness, the severe end of which represents some of the sickest patients seen in the ED.
- It represents a growing problem; in the UK, cases of severe sepsis requiring admission to the intensive treatment care unit (ITU) have risen from 50 to 70 per 100 000 population per year over the last decade.
- 21 % of these patients are admitted from the ED and in-hospital mortality for these patients is over 35 %.[1]
- It is estimated that the UK spends £700 million per year treating severe infections in ITU patients.

⭐ **Learning point** Definitions

The definition of sepsis was produced by consensus in 1991.[2] The diagnosis requires the presence of the systemic inflammatory response syndrome and a suspected or confirmed source of microbiological infection. Additional definitions were produced at the time to further categorize sepsis into severe sepsis and septic shock (see Table 1.1).

Table 1.1 Consensus definition of SIRS and sepsis (2)

Systemic inflammatory response syndrome (SIRS)	At least 2 of the following: Temperature <36 °C or > 38.8 °C Heart rate > 90 Respiratory rate > 20 breaths/minute or PaCO2 <4.2 kPa White cell count < 4000 or >12 000 or > 10 % immature forms 7.7mmol/L (unless patient is diabetic) Acute confusion / reduced conscious level

(continued)

Sepsis	SIRS + confirmed or suspected infection
Severe sepsis	Sepsis + organ hypoperfusion or dysfunction
Septic shock	Sepsis with refractory hypotension or vasopressor-dependent after adequate volume resuscitation

Data from Bone RC, Balk RA, Cerra FB et al., 'Definitions for sepsis and organ failure and guidelines for the use of innovative therapies in sepsis', The ACCP/SCCM Consensus Conference Committee, American College of Chest Physicians/Society of Critical Care Medicine, Chest, 1992, 101, pp. 1644–1655.

Assessment of organ dysfunction should take place early when managing any patient with suspected sepsis in order to risk stratify their condition. Measurement of blood lactate provides objective evidence of hypoperfusion and can help to identify patients with severe sepsis or septic shock rapidly. Venous and arterial lactate have been shown to be closely correlated[3] and the relative ease with which the former can be tested can help reduce the delay in identifying this group of patients. Early measurement of blood lactate has been shown to be independently linked with mortality[4,5] and can help identify those who would benefit from more urgent intervention. A raised lactate in the presence of a normal blood pressure is known as 'cryptic shock' and suggests organ hypoperfusion in spite of haemodynamic compensation maintaining arterial pressure. Lactate levels over 4.0 mmol/L are associated with a significantly increased in-hospital mortality (LR+2.6, 95 % CI 1.9–3.7).[6]

✚ **Clinical tip** Signs associated with organ dysfunction

Organ system	Examples of dysfunction
Cardiovascular system	Systolic BP < 90 mmHg
	Decrease in systolic BP > 40 mmHg
	Mean arterial pressure < 65 mmHg
	Increased capillary refill time or mottling
Respiratory system	Increasing FiO_2 to maintain SaO_2
Renal system	Cr > 176.8 micomol/L
	Creatinine increase > 60 micromol/L from baseline
	Creatinine increase > 60 micromol/L in 24 hours
	Urine output < 0.5 ml/kg/hour for 2 hours despite fluid resuscitation
Coagulation	Activated partial thromboplastin time > 60 seconds
	International normalized ratio > 1.5
	Platelets < 100×10^9/L
Hepatic	Bilirubin > 34.2 micomol/L
Acid-base	Lactate > 2 mmol/L
Central nervous system	Confusion or decreased level of consciousness

Reproduced from AD Bersten and N Soni, Oh's Intensive Care Manual, Sixth Edition, p. 711, Copyright 2009, with permission from Elsevier.

Identification of septic patients in the ED remains a challenge. A recent audit of three EDs in the UK[8] found that only 17 % of patients were recognized as having severe sepsis or septic shock while they were in the ED.

Clinical question: Does the timing of antibiotics in sepsis have a significant effect on outcome?

The surviving sepsis campaign (SSC), launched in 2004 in response to the high mortality of sepsis, published international guidelines for the resuscitation and management of septic patients: they were revised in 2008 and 2013. The campaign recommends that patients should receive intravenous antibiotics within an hour of recognition of severe sepsis or septic shock.[9] Originally based largely on expert consensus, there are now compelling data to support this recommendation.

> ✅ **Evidence base** Early administration of antibiotics in sepsis
>
> **Kumar *et al.* (2006):**[10] performed a multi-centre retrospective cohort study on 2731 adult patients with septic shock in the ITU. 44.4% of patients had been admitted from the ED. Administration of an antimicrobial effective for isolated or suspected pathogens within the first hour of documented hypotension was associated with a survival rate of 79.9%. Each hour of delay was associated with an average decrease in survival of 7.6% (range 3.6–9.9%).
>
> **Puskarich *et al.* (2011):**[11] performed an analysis of a multi-centre randomized controlled trial of early sepsis resuscitation. 291 patients presenting to the ED with septic shock were included. Mortality was significantly increased in patients who received initial antibiotics after shock recognition compared with before shock recognition (OR 2.4; 1.1–4.5).[2]

Answer

Antibiotics should be given without delay upon recognition of severe sepsis or septic shock.

> ❝ **Expert comment**
>
> Early administration of antibiotics to the patient with severe sepsis/septic shock reduces mortality. This means that it is a time-critical illness similar to acute myocardial infarction, acute stroke, and trauma.
>
> As such, it is imperative to develop emergency systems to triage these patients. Like all time-critical illnesses there must be an acceptable level of false positives within the system making it highly sensitive in the early stages. Systems for a pre-hospital alert from the local ambulance service would be ideal, and indeed these are in various stages of development in the UK. Complementary to this, early recognition through education, triage, and/or a modified early warning score system using initial patient history and observations should be used. Pre-hospital development of early risk stratification and identification has been shown to improve outcomes.[3-5]
>
> A dedicated area within the ED with a more favourable staff to patient ratio, such as a resuscitation room, must be used. Point-of-care testing for serum lactate should be available. There should be clear local antibiotic guidelines available and all antibiotics mentioned therein should be available in the ED.
>
> Delays may occur when hypoperfusion and organ dysfunction are diagnosed on blood tests alone. Point-of-care testing for serum lactate analysis and blood culture bottles should be available. Local antibiotic guidelines must include guidance for sepsis of unknown aetiology (and variants for neutropaenia and nosocomial infections), and should be clearly available to all staff. These antibiotics must be adequately stocked in the ED and staff should be appropriately trained in their administration. Blood sampling and laboratory turnaround times are the major issues here. Above all else, staff education, clinical audit, and regular review of a 'whole systems' approach are the key to success.

Case progression

A focused history reveals no recent travel, a cough producing purulent green sputum and right-sided pleuritic chest pain. Sputum is obtained and sent for culture. Intravenous access is sited and blood is taken and sent for blood cultures, haematology and biochemistry. A 12-lead ECG shows a sinus tachycardia. An arterial blood gas (ABG) sample is taken on 40 % oxygen which shows the following (see Table 1.2):

Table 1.2 ABG on 40 % O_2

pH	7.32
pO_2	9.1 kPa
pCO_2	2.8 kPa
HCO_3	15 mmol/l
BE	−7 mmol/l
Lactate	5.1 mmol/l

Ostrosky-Zeichner L, Pappas PG. Invasive candidiasis in the intensive care unit. *Crit Care Med* 2006; 34:857–863.

A chest X-ray is taken which demonstrates right lower lobe consolidation with effusion.

A diagnosis of severe sepsis secondary to a community-acquired pneumonia is made. A 20 ml/kg fluid bolus is given at the same time as the first dose of antibiotics in accordance with the hospital antibiotic policy.

His initial blood tests demonstrate the following (see Table 1.3).

Table 1.3 Initial blood test results

Hb	14.1 g/dL	Sodium	148 mmol/L
WCC	18.2×10^9/L	Potassium	3.8 mmol/L
Neutrophils	17.8×10^9/L	Urea	16.5 mmol/L
Platelets	420×10^9/L	Creatinine	198 micromol/L
CRP	370 mg/L	Glucose	11.4 mmol/l

✚ **Clinical tip** Risk factors associated with invasive fungal infections

Risk factors associated with candidaemia

Immunosuppression
Renal failure
Severe liver failure
Antibiotic use
Intravenous catheters
Candida colonization
Oropharyngeal candidosis
Parenteral nutrition

Reproduced from L Ostrosky-Zeichner and PG Pappas, 'Invasive candidiasis in the intensive care unit', Critical Care Medicine, 34, pp. 857–863, Copyright 2006, with permission from Wolters Kluwer and the Society of Critical Care Medicine.

✪ **Learning point** Antibiotics in sepsis

Once severe sepsis has been identified, further investigations and treatment should be carried out concurrently as delays in initial therapy have been shown to worsen outcome.[10] The core elements of resuscitation of the septic patient are microbiological testing, appropriate antibiotics, and restoration of adequate tissue perfusion.

Broad-spectrum antibiotics should be given as soon as possible, within an hour of recognition of severe sepsis or septic shock. Blood cultures and other microbiological specimens taken before antibiotic administration are important and may later prove crucial to the care of the patient, but should never significantly delay (> 45 minutes) antibiotic administration.[9]

Antibiotic choice should be influenced by the suspected source of infection, hospital guidelines, and patterns of infection and resistance. Inappropriate initial antibiotics are associated with increased mortality,[10,12] and if the source is unclear, broad-spectrum agents should be used and rationalized when further microbiology results are available.

Certain patient groups are at increased risk of invasive fungal infections (see Table 1.3) and in these cases consideration should be given to co-treatment with an anti-fungal agent. If a fungal infection is suspected, commercially available antigen assays such as 1,3 β-D-glucan, mannan, and anti-mannan assays[13] can assist the early diagnosis and treatment of invasive candidiasis.

Surgically drainable sources of infection are unlikely to respond to antibiotics alone: examples of these include pelvic collections, infections surrounding foreign bodies and empyemas. In such cases, or with sepsis of unknown origin, further diagnostic imaging may be required to locate collections which could then be considered for surgical or percutaenous drainage.

Fluid resuscitation with the aim of restoring tissue perfusion should be given as soon as signs of hypoperfusion are recognized (see Table 1.2). Large volumes of crystalloid (20–40ml/kg) may be required initially. Albumin can be added to the fluid regimen if it is anticipated or known that the serum albumin is low.[15] Central venous catheters and arterial lines are usually required in patients with severe sepsis and are unavoidable in those with septic shock to assist administration and monitoring of resuscitative efforts.

The use of a quantitative resuscitation (QR) strategy can also help guide fluid and vasoactive agent administration. QR, a 'structured cardiovascular intervention with intravascular volume expansion and vasoactive agent support to achieve explicit, predefined end points'[16] was originally reported in surgical patients in 1988.[17] In 2001, a QR strategy for septic patients known as early goal-directed therapy (EGDT) was described by Rivers et al. The protocol structured the use of fluids and vasoactive agents in the initial resuscitation of septic patients. The three principal end-points targeted were:

- Central venous pressure (CVP) of between 8 and 12mmHg.
- Mean arterial pressure (MAP) of between 65 and 90mmHg.
- Central venous oxygen saturation ($ScvO_2$) of over 70%.

Lactate clearance is an alternative to $ScvO_2$ as a measure of tissue oxygen delivery,[18] and the aim of resuscitation should be to normalize lactate as rapidly as possible in those patients with a raised level.[9] One benefit of lactate clearance is that it does not require a central line to be inserted so it can be used on ward patients.

> **Expert comment**
>
> Regional rates of systemic fungal infections are variable and not insignificant—probably around 5%. The patient's risk factors should be assessed and the likelihood, investigations, and treatment options discussed with a microbiologist. Although empirical administration is not recommended, delays increase mortality. The risk of a fungal infection must be frequently considered and actively sought in all patients beyond the ED.

> **Expert comment**
>
> Caution is advised when using lactate clearance as a sole resuscitation target because a normal lactate (<2mmol/L) can be present in up to 50% of septic shock patients. These patients are prone to multi-system organ failure with a mortality of over 50%.[6–14] These observations indicate that using lactate and $ScvO_2$ are complementary endpoints and not mutually exclusive.
>
> Early involvement of critical care is essential to ensure adequate monitoring of the patient during resuscitation using central venous and arterial lines, and their placement (and by whom) is a resource-management issue that should be resolved in advance through protocol to ensure time-critical management. The ED must be adequately equipped in this respect and if it is not, as soon as possible the patient must be transferred to a facility that is.

Clinical question: Is the timing of goal directed therapy important at reducing mortality in septic patients?

In 2001, Rivers et al.[19] published the results of a landmark randomized controlled trial that described a significant reduction in mortality in ED patients with severe sepsis and septic shock treated with early (within 6 hours) goal-directed therapy

(EGDT). The results showed an absolute mortality reduction of 16 %. Critics of the trial stated that the presence of extra resources in the ED impacted on the external validity of the study.

Jones *et al.* (2008)[16] conducted a systematic review of randomized controlled trials comparing quantitative resuscitation with standard resuscitation in septic patients. All 9 studies were based in the ITU with the exception of the Rivers study. A clear mortality benefit was found when quantitative resuscitation was used at or near the time of recognition (OR 0.5; 95 % CI 0.37–0.69) that was completely lost if the intervention was initiated late (OR 1.16; 95 % CI 0.60–2.22).

Answer

Early goal-directed resuscitation reduces the mortality of patients with severe sepsis.

Case progression

Despite fluid resuscitation, his blood pressure is 87/44 mmHg. Intensive care is contacted and a review of the patient requested. Central venous, arterial, and urinary catheters are placed. Further fluid boluses are administered against his central venous pressure (CVP) up to a total of 40 ml/kg but he remains hypotensive. A noradrenaline infusion is started and titrated to maintain a mean arterial blood pressure (MAP) of greater than 65 mmHg. Over the next hour, he appears drowsier and a repeat ABG on 60 % oxygen at this point shows the following (see Table 1.4):

Table 1.4 Results at repeat ABG

pH	7.21
pO_2	10.1 kPa
pCO_2	6.1 kPa
HCO_3	15 mmol/L
BE	−6 mmol/L
Lactate	3.8 mmol/L

The patient undergoes a rapid sequence intubation and lung-protective mechanical ventilation is commenced. While waiting for transfer to the ITU, a sliding scale is commenced to maintain tight glycaemic control. Thromboprophylaxis and gastric protection are prescribed.

🔾 Expert comment

The 2013 SSC guidelines recommend (grade 1, the strongest) the protocolized resuscitation of a patient with sepsis-induced shock. It further recommends that it should start as soon as hypoperfusion is recognized and should not be delayed pending ITU admission. CVP, MAP, urine output, and $ScvO_2$ measurement are all listed as inclusions within the QR.[1]

➕ Clinical tip Noradrenaline in the ED

Patients with sepsis require noradrenaline if the MAP is < 65 mmHg despite adequate CVP post fluid resuscitation.[19]

The College of Emergency Medicine provides a noradrenaline infusion reference guide (available at <http://www.collemergencymed.ac.uk/Shop-Floor/Clinical%20Standards/Sepsis/>).

4 mg = 4 ml of 1:1000 noradrenaline

4 mls of 1:1000 noradrenaline should be added to 46 ml of 5 % dextrose making 50 mls and placed in a syringe driver.

The starting dose is 0.025 mcg/kg/minute (infusion table available on the CEM website).

⭐ Learning point Care bundles in sepsis

Sepsis is a complex systemic pathophysiological process and as such, it requires a complex multifaceted approach to treat it.

The optimal endpoints for resuscitation will evolve as the evidence base grows. The Surviving Sepsis campaign[9] recommends the following bundle of measures as seen in Box 1.2:

Taking blood cultures before administering antibiotics, commencing broad-spectrum antibiotics, and achieving tight blood glucose control are individual aspects of sepsis management that have a significant effect on mortality (OR 0.76, 0.86, 0.67 respectively, all $p < 0.0001$).[20] Optimal care therefore involves paying attention to all aspects of managing the critically ill septic patient once resuscitation has commenced. Liaison with intensive care, medicine, surgery, radiology, and microbiology may all be required prior to the patient leaving the ED.

(continued)

Box 1.2 To be completed within 3 hours:

1. Measure lactate level
2. Obtain blood cultures prior to administration of antibiotics
3. Administer broad spectrum antibiotics
4. Administer 30 mL/kg crystalloid for hypotension or lactate

---

Reproduced from R Dellinger et al., 'Surviving Sepsis Campaign: International Guidelines for Management of Severe Sepsis and Septic Shock', Critical Care Medicine, 41, 2, pp. 580–637, Copyright 2013, with permission from Wolters Kluwer and the Society of Critical Care Medicine.

Clinical question: Are care bundles effective in reducing mortality in septic patients?

The theory behind care bundles is that several evidence-based interventions, grouped or 'bundled' together, will improve overall outcome. The sepsis bundle was an idea first introduced by the Surviving Sepsis campaign in 2004.[10,17,18,20] Individual bundle components will have different levels of evidence behind them necessitating subjective application in certain circumstances.

✔ Evidence base Care bundles in sepsis

Nguyen et al. (2007)[21] published a prospective observational cohort study looking at the effects of implementing a bundle of measures in septic patients presenting to the ED. The study described the achievement of a bundle of 5 targets in 330 patients. In those patients in whom no aspect of the bundle were completed, in-hospital mortality was 39.5% which dropped to 20.8% ($p<0.01$) in those patients in whom all aspects of the bundle were competed.

Levy M et al. (2010)[22] published an analysis of the data on 15 022 subjects (over half from the ED) at 165 sites comparing surviving sepsis bundle compliance and hospital mortality over 3 years. Resuscitation bundle compliance increased from 10.9% initially to 31.3% ($p<0.0001$). Unadjusted in-hospital mortality over the same period decreased from 37% to 30.8% ($p=0.001$), the adjusted mortality reduction was 5.4% over 2 years (95% CI=2.5 – 8.4%).

Answer

Sepsis care bundles provide significant reductions in the mortality of septic patients attending the ED.

See Box 1.3 for future advances in sepsis care.

Box 1.3 Future advances

There are 3 separate randomized multi-centre trials on goal-directed resuscitation and protocolized sepsis care that are ongoing at the moment. PRoCESS in the US, ProMISE in the UK, and ARISE in Australasia[2] will all add significantly to the evidence base regarding EGDT and sepsis resuscitation in the ED and ITU settings.

Other areas of development include the use biomarkers of bacterial infection (such as procalcitonin) to rationalize the use of antibiotics in non-bacterial infections and help combat antibiotic resistance.

The VANISH trial aims to identify the best first-line vasopressor to use in septic shock by comparing vasopressin with noradrenaline in a randomized controlled trial.

A Final Word from the Expert

As sepsis becomes better understood, and as our management of it improves through further research, its place as a time-critical illness is likely only to become more firmly established. The role of the ED is crucial to decreasing mortality.

All aspects of the initial few hours of care are simple and effective and success depends upon early recognition and the activation of collaborative multidisciplinary processes. The results of the College of Emergency Medicine's national clinical audit in severe sepsis and septic shock showed that success is possible for all of these patients who present to the ED.

References

1. Harrison DA, Welch CA, Eddleston JM. The epidemiology of severe sepsis in England, Wales and Northern Ireland, 1996 to 2004: secondary analysis of a high quality clinical database, the ICNARC Case Mix Programme Database. *Crit Care* 2006; 10:R42.
2. Bone RC, Balk RA, Cerra FB, *et al*. Definitions for sepsis and organ failure and guidelines for the use of innovative therapies in sepsis. The ACCP/SCCM Consensus Conference Committee. American College of Chest Physicians/Society of Critical Care Medicine. *Chest* 1992; 101:1644–55.
3. Lavery RF, Livingston DH, Tortella BJ, *et al*. The utility of venous lactate to triage injured patients in the trauma center. *J Am Coll Surg* 2000; 190:656–64.
4. Cannon CM, Holthaus CV, Zubrow MT, *et al*. The GENESIS Project (GENeralized Early Sepsis Intervention Strategies): A Multicentre Quality Improvement Collaborative. *J Intensive Care Med* 2012; Epub
5. Mikkelsen ME, Miltiades AN, Gaieski DF, *et al*. Serum lactate is associated with mortality in severe sepsis independent of organ failure and shock. *Crit Care Med* 2009; 37:1670–77.
6. Trzeciak S, Dellinger RP, Chansky ME, *et al*. Serum lactate as a predictor of mortality in patients with infection. *Intensive Care Med* 2007; 33:970–7.
7. Gaudio ARD. Severe Sepsis. In: Bernstein AD, Soni N, eds. *Oh's Intensive Care Manual*. 2009. p. 711.
8. Cronshaw HL, Daniels R, Bleetman A, *et al*. Impact of the Surviving Sepsis Campaign on the recognition and management of severe sepsis in the emergency department: are we failing? *Emerg Med J* 2011; 28:670–5.
9. Dellinger RP, Levy MM, Rhodes A, *et al*. Surviving Sepsis Campaign: International Guidelines for Management of Severe Sepsis and Septic Shock: 2012. *Crit Care Med*. 2013; 41:580–637.
10. Kumar A, Roberts D, Wood KE, *et al*. Duration of hypotension before initiation of effective antimicrobial therapy is the critical determinant of survival in human septic shock. *Crit Care Med* 2006; 34:1589–96.
11. Puskarich MA, Trzeciak S, Shapiro NI, *et al*. Association between timing of antibiotic administration and mortality from septic shock in patients treated with a quantitative resuscitation protocol. *Crit Care Med* 2011; 39:2066–71.
12. Gaieski DF, Mikkelsen ME, Band RA, *et al*. Impact of time to antibiotics on survival in patients with severe sepsis or septic shock in whom early goal-directed therapy was initiated in the emergency department. *Crit Care Med* 2010; 38:104553.
13. Eggimann P, Bille J, Marchetti O. Diagnosis of invasive candidiasis in the ICU. *Ann Intensive Care* 2011; 1:37.
14. Ostrosky-Zeichner L, Pappas PG. Invasive candidiasis in the intensive care unit. *Crit Care Med* 2006; 34:857–63.

15. Group ESCIMSR. Albumin for fluid resuscitation. *Clinical Evidence in Intensive Care. Medizinisch Wissenschaftliche Verlagsgesellschact*; 2011. p. 278–82.

16. Jones AE, Brown MD, Trzeciak S, *et al*. The effect of a quantitative resuscitation strategy on mortality in patients with sepsis: a meta-analysis. *Crit Care Med* 2008; 36:2734–9.

17. WC S, PL A, HB K. Prospective trial of supranormal values of survivors as therapeutic goals in high-risk surgical patients. *Chest* 1988; 94:1176–86.

18. Jones AE, Shapiro NI, Trzeciak S, Arnold RC, Claremont HA, Kline JA. Lactate clearance vs central venous oxygen saturation as goals of early sepsis therapy: a randomized clinical trial. *JAMA* 2010; 303:739–46.

19. Rivers E, Nguyen B, Havstad S, *et al*. Early goal-directed therapy in the treatment of severe sepsis and septic shock. *N Engl J Med* 2001; 345:1368–77.

20. Townsend SR, Schorr C, Levy MM, Dellinger RP. Reducing mortality in severe sepsis: the Surviving Sepsis Campaign. *Clin Chest Med* 2008; 29:721–33, x.

21. Nguyen B, Corbett S, Steele R, *et al*. Implementation of a bundle of quality indicators for the early management of severe sepsis and septic shock is associated with decreased mortality. *Crit Care Med* 2007; 35:1105–12.

22. Levy M, Dellinger R, Townsend S, *et al*. The surviving sepsis campaign: Results of an international guideline-based performance improvement targeting severe sepsis. *Crit Care Med* 2010; 38:367–74.

Cardiopulmonary resuscitation for the twenty-first century

2

Robert Galloway

Expert commentary Douglas Chamberlain

Case history

A 50-year-old Asian male with a history of hypertension and hypercholesterolemia has become acutely unwell with central chest pain and shortness of breath whilst eating dinner at a nearby local restaurant. Bystander first aid had initially taken place but the patient has deteriorated to full cardiac arrest. The ambulance service is at the scene within 6 minutes and initiates advanced life support measures and obtains a return of spontaneous circulation.

They telephone the priority call for your department to receive this patient within the next few minutes. The 2 junior doctors on duty with you ask how the patient should best be managed both during and after the cardiac arrest.

See Box 2.1 for a clinical summary of cardiac arrest.

Box 2.1 Clinical summary of cardiac arrest

It is estimated that ambulance services treat approximately 37 patients per 100 000 population/year[1] with an out-of-hospital cardiac arrest (OOHCA). An appreciable number of these patients have a successful return of spontaneous circulation (ROSC) and are brought into the resuscitation room. Knowledge of how to manage these patients is clearly an essential prerequisite for any emergency medicine specialist.

The management of patients in cardiac arrest (CA) has undergone a revolution in the last few years.[2,3] In the not-too-distant past there was a general perception of pessimism about chances of survival following an out of hospital cardiac arrest. Attitudes have, however, thankfully now changed with recent remarkable improvements in survival rates abroad[4,5,6] and in the UK.[7]

A recent audit from 2011 by Fletcher *et al.*[7] showed survival rates to hospital discharge of 13% for all cardiac arrests and 30% for witnessed shockable (VF/VT) arrests.

Previous lack of interest shown in this area is now totally unacceptable with ever improving outcomes, and indeed the enthusiasm and research developments for optimizing our care for this cohort of patients have never been greater.[8]

A key reason for the improvement in outcomes after cardiac arrest is based on improvements in each of the links of the resuscitation chain: community response, ambulance service, emergency department, intensive care specialist, and cardiologists.

The days of just thinking about advanced life support (ALS) protocols and the 4Hs and 4Ts are also numbered. For optimal management one must now need to think about another paradigm—the 8Cs; *Choosing* wisely on whom it is appropriate to perform CPR; *Communication* and *Control* (leadership) of the arrest; the importance of *Compressions*; *Cutting* the time between last compression and shocking; *Cardiac* echo during pulse check, *Cooling* post ROSC; considering *Cardiac Catheterization* and *Critical* care management by protocol. The importance of the 9th C—cardiac arrest centres—is up for debate.

It is essential to remember that no resuscitation drugs or advanced airway interventions have been shown to increase survival to hospital discharge. However, 'basic skills' of compressions and defibrillation have. The temptation to use 'advanced skills', whilst not worrying about the life-preserving 'basic' skills, must always be resisted.

> ⭐ **Learning point**   The ALS (2010) changes
>
> The treatment options during ALS are limited. The recent updates however have further rationalized how, when and why we use the resources at hand:
>
> - Delivery of **drugs** via a tracheal tube is no longer recommended—if intravenous access cannot be obtained, drugs should be delivered by the intra-osseous (IO) route. Drugs can be given just as quickly and serum levels established just as rapidly by IO compared to a central line.[9]
> - Despite the lack of human data, the use of **adrenaline** is still recommended. This is based largely on animal data and increased short-term survival ROSC rates.[10,11] No certainty exists as to the optimal dose of adrenaline or exactly when to give it; however, expert consensus recommends its use directly after the third shock and after every other shock thereafter, or if in pulseless electrical activity (PEA) then straight away and after every other 2-minute cycle. The theoretical risks of giving adrenaline even if there is a ROSC after the third shock are minimal compared to the theoretical benefits.
> - **Amiodarone** should be given after the third shock and a further 150 mg if in refractory VF. It has been shown to improve short-term outcome of survival compared with placebo and Lignocaine in shock-resistant VF.[12,13]
> - Routine administration of **magnesium** in cardiac arrest does not increase survival[14] and it is not recommended unless Torsades de Pointes is suspected.
> - Routine administration of **sodium bicarbonate** during cardiac arrest and CPR or after ROSC is also not recommended. However, if cardiac arrest is associated with hyperkalaemia or tricyclic antidepressant overdose then administration is warranted.
> - **Atropine** is now out of the arrest algorithm as several studies have shown it to be ineffective[15-17]
> - Routine **fibrinolysis** is also not recommended,[18] although consider fibrinolytic therapy when cardiac arrest is thought to be due to an acute pulmonary embolus; just make sure that you are prepared to do prolonged CPR after you have given fibrinolysis—for up to an hour.[19,20]

> ➕ **Clinical tip**   Intubation during CPR
>
> Intubation is often a moot point during arrests. It is accepted that this is the optimal oxygen delivery system but also that intubation should not interrupt compressions, something that it does frustratingly often.[21] Common practice now exists that in the first couple of cycles intubation is deferred for risk of interfering with compressions. If there has been no ROSC within a couple of cycles, to then intubate, but by the most senior personnel available and only during the time needed for a pulse check. If unsuccessful or debatable whether the intubation was successful, then it is easier to go back to an 'I-GEL' supraglottic device and the patient oxygenated through that.

Clinical question: Does the quality of chest compressions affect the outcome of cardiac arrest?

The 2010 guidelines emphasize the key factors that improve chances of ROSC following a CA—good compressions and early defibrillation with minimal gap between CPR and defibrillation.[2] Although this statement may sound simple, this inevitably requires the cocoordinating skills of an organized and focused team leader.

Good chest compressions generate a small but significant amount of blood flow to the brain and myocardium and increase the likelihood of successful defibrillation. When compressing the chest think about rate (aim for 100/min, with a 30:2 ratio for breaths), depth (at least 5 cm) and allow the chest to completely recoil;[22,23] compressions should take the same amount of time as time for recoil.

The interposed abdominal compression technique uses compressions of the abdomen during relaxation phase of chest compressions to enhance venous return. However, there is conflicting evidence as to its benefit.[24–26]

Active compression–decompression CPR can also enhance venous return. It is a hand-held suction device that literally lifts the chest up during decompression. This creates a negative intrathoracic pressure during decompression and thus enhances venous return.[27–30]

Although the concept is promising, the reality is not as positive as the theory would suggest and results have been mixed. Some studies have shown improved haemodynamics,[28–31] but these surrogate markers haven't affected the clinical reality. A meta-analysis of 12 studies showed no improvement in outcomes using active compression–decompression vs standard CPR.[33]

The impedence threshold device should also theoretically improve outcome, and may therefore increase cardiac output. It is a valve that limits air entry into the lungs during active lung recoil between chest compressions. This decreased intrathoracic pressure increases venous return and thus may increase cardiac output. It is theoretically best used with an endotracheal tube, but it has been used with a face mask.[34]

Unfortunately a recent meta-analysis showed increased rates of ROSC but no improvement in rates of survival;[35] the Resuscitation Council thus does not currently recommend it. However, a high-quality RCT showing the use of both impedance threshold device and active compression–decompression, showed potential benefits.[36]

There are manual devices to help with compressions. Mechanical chest compressors theoretically should increase survival, by increasing cardiac output. There are two main systems on the market: the LUCAS, a gas-driven sternal compressing device that incorporates a suction cap for active decompression and the Autopulse, a constricting band and backboard which pneumatically constricts the chest.

Animal models have shown improved haemodynamics and short-term survival using the LUCAS vs standard CPR,[37,38] and also improved haemodynamics with the Autopulse.[39–41] However, RCTs have not shown an overall survival benefit with the use of devices.[42–45]

But, for prolonged CPR (e.g. whilst going to the catheter lab) following hypothermic arrest, overdoses, and thrombolysis following CPR, as well as prolonged ambulance journeys—especially where compressions in a moving vehicle are difficult and less effective—the use of such devices may facilitate CPR and they are starting to be used more frequently.[47]

The key to survival is 'simple' compressions. If done properly, manual compressions can be effective and life-saving; do not use the excuse of not having a mechanical compressor in the case of poor quality compressions. Unfortunately, the quality of chest compressions during in-hospital CPR is frequently sub-optimal.[48,49] To improve CPR quality during an arrest, it is imperative that metronomes are used to maintain the rate at 100/minute.[50] Feedback devices should be also used to make sure depth and recoil are adequate.

Many studies have shown that by 2 mins, chest compressions lose some of their effectiveness because of rescuer fatigue.[51] The role of the team leader is to ensure optimal compressions and that includes organizing the rotation of compressors.

Interruptions in external chest compression reduces the chances of successful defibrillation.[52] Procedures such as intubation and quick-look echo,[53] if required, should be done with the minimal interference in compressions and only done during the time needed for a pulse check. Even a 5–10 second delay will reduce the chances of the shock being successful.[52,54,55]

Although checking for safety is something that has been drummed into all of us, the risk of being hurt by a DC shock is negligible, especially if gloves are worn.[56] The best way to reduce the pre-shock pause thus remains to compress whilst charging, preferably using manual mode defibrillation. The person doing compressions should do a safety check whilst charging, and then he/she should press the defibrillate button. It is an effective way to keep the pause to a minimum and if a shock is delivered, he/she has no-one else to blame!

After a shock, you must restart CPR straight away without waiting for a pulse check. Even if the defibrillation was successful, it takes time until the post-shock circulation is established and it is also very unusual to feel a pulse immediately after successful defibrillation. Compressing even if you do have a ROSC it is unlikely to do any harm.[57–59] Not compressing whilst discussions continue and then realizing you do not have a ROSC will, however, cause harm so advice remains to go straight back to compressions after a shock.

The days of doing stacked shocks are long gone. Interruptions in external CPR reduce the chance of successful defibrillation[60] and stacked shocks helped create that delay. There is evidence that the single-shock protocol increases survival[61–63] so never be seduced by the temptation to administer more than one external shock.

Answer

Despite the panacea of advanced treatments, the multitudes of studies, and all the collected findings of resuscitation researchers, it is still the basics that improve survival; effective, interruption-free CPR and effective coordinated single-shock defibrillation.

❝ Expert comment

Few realize how poorly basic life support is generally performed. The universal errors are shown in any analysis of electronic downloads. It is salutary for those who have performed resuscitation attempts to see subsequently how they have performed. All must realize, however, that the procedure, conceptually simple as it is, is very hard to perform well in real emergencies. The key points have already been highlighted, but a few points are worth stressing. Intubation can be useful if performed by someone skilled in the procedure, but unfortunately all too often this leads to excessive number of ventilations at the expense of compressions. Ideally, no pause in compressions should ever exceed 10 seconds, again hard to achieve. As mentioned, the pause between the last compression and shock delivery is of particular importance, and with the use of manual defibrillation (as opposed to automated) this can be less than 3 seconds. The value of adrenaline in cardiac arrest is currently a hot topic. A recent large meta-analysis showed no survival (to discharge) benefit, even though there were increased rates of ROSC and increased survival-to-hospital rates.[64] Another observation study showed that adrenaline increased ROSC rates but caused a decrease in survival and survival with good neurological outcome.[65] But counter to this, an observational study in the BMJ in 2014 showed that the earlier adrenaline was delivered the better the outcome.[66] The conclusion is that we are not sure what to do! Use the latest Resuscitation Council guidelines but never let the use of drugs substitute the effectiveness of CPR and electricity.

> **⊕ Clinical tip** The role of ECHO in cardiac arrest
>
> No studies have shown that the use of echo improves the final outcome in cardiac arrest however it does help in ruling out reversible causes.[67] A subxiphoid position for the probe used during a pulse check is the ideal way to perform an echo during cardiac arrest.[68] The key is for the team leader to ensure that the use of echo does not interfere with compressions.
>
> Lack of any cardiac motion is highly predictive of death,[69-71] and so it may help in making the decision to stop in futile but emotionally charged, difficult circumstances. Paediatric cardiac arrest is inevitably one such occasion, and the use of an objective and visual marker such as echo can facilitate a timely and appropriate conclusion to resuscitation efforts.

Case progression

In the pre-hospital environment, the patient has an uncomplicated supraglottic airway placed and an intra-osseous line inserted into his right humeral head. The pre-hospital tem perform 2 cycles of CPR on the shockable algorithm with 2 asynchronous shocks. A three-point pulse check reveals a palpable pulse but no significant respiratory effort. The patient is stabilized and brought into hospital, but shows no signs of waking up or 'biting on the tube' so ongoing ventilation continues with a bag-valve mask.

Clinical question: should we be performing therapeutic hypothermia on all patients post ROSC regardless of initial rhythm?

There are strong theoretical arguments for the beneficial effects of therapeutic hypothermia, especially if applied early or even during cardiac arrest. During cardiac arrest there is interruption of cerebral blood flow and a cascade of ischaemic insults. Once cardiac output is restored, reperfusion injury compounds the deleterious effects of the original ischaemia. Mild hypothermia reduces cerebral metabolic rate, and reduces production of cytotoxic chemicals and free radicals.[74] Hypothermia also reduces cerebral blood flow during the reperfusion period thus decreasing the impact of the reperfusion injury.[74] A period of hyperthermia (hyperpyrexia) is common in the first 48 hrs after cardiac arrest and several studies have shown an association between post-cardiac-arrest pyrexia and poor outcomes.[72,73]

Over the last few years there has been an increasing amount of research into therapeutic hypothermia. Evidence has shown the benefits of therapeutic hypothermia (at least compared to no temperature control which is different to normothermia). It has become the treatment modality of choice, with good evidence for arrests of VF/VT origin and poorer quality evidence for non-shockable initial rhythms. It should be noted that there is only evidence for therapeutic hypothermia in patients who remain obtunded following return of spontaneous circulation. Those who are starting to wake should not be put back to sleep so as to cool down the brain, but allowed to wake up 'naturally' on a high-dependency unit.

Prior to 2013, there have been four RCTs[75-78] looking into therapeutic hypothermia post arrest of which one, the HACA trial[75] was of a high quality. However, the pooled data in the three meta-analyses[79-81] also showed an improved outcome with therapeutic hypothermia, with 6–7 patients treated per 1 survivor with a good quality of life.

Additionally, numerous observational studies[82–97] have shown the effectiveness of the therapy in real life, and not just the efficacy in studies. A meta-analysis[98] of these non-randomized data, including from PEA arrests, confirmed an odds ratio of 2.5 in favour of good neurological outcome after cooling. The registry data[99–101] also confirmed similar survival rates to those presented in the published RCTs.

There is a paucity of high-quality evidence for hypothermia in the management of post-ROSC PEA / asystolic arrests, and no RCTs looking into this. However, there is some low-quality evidence based on non-randomized trials, observational studies, and registry data to argue that it should be used. Added to the biological plausibility of the treatment in this group of patients, it is reasonable to strongly consider treatment in selected individuals, especially those with short ROSC times.[102]

In 2013, a landmark study confused what we all thought we knew.[103] There was no difference in outcome between patients cooled to 33 °C or 36 °C. Does this mean we should continue to cool to 33 °C or just cool between 33–36 °C? The jury is still out, but if the temperature is above 36 °C there is no question; make sure it is between 33–36 °C.

> ⊗ **Learning point** Initiation of cooling
>
> Evidence showing the correlation between time to start cooling and outcome is available, but this too is not of the best quality.[104] However, until new evidence comes to light, current recommendations are to be initiating cooling in the ED if not started pre-hospital and that clinicians should be following the protocols of the two main studies that have been shown to improve outcome. In those studies[75,-76] the cooling was pre-hospital or in the ED, where there was a median time of 105 mins from ROSC to commencement of cooling. Very few patients would get from ROSC to ITU in less than 105 mins and so it is imperative to start the cooling in the ED or earlier. However, a recent RCT showed no survival benefit in starting pre-hospital cooling with 2 litres of cold saline.[105] The inference we should take from this isn't that early cooling is ineffective, but that early cooling with 2 litres of normal saline is ineffective.

Although there have been excellent adoption rates of therapeutic hypothermia in ITU,[106,107] in 2009/2010 a telephone survey showed only 35 % of EDs started therapeutic hypothermia in the ED (120) and of those 55 % would cool only for VF/VT. This is clearly an area that ED physicians should be looking at improving. It is easy to start cooling in the ED with the easiest ways being the use ice bags placed around the major vessels, cold towels, and 30 ml/kg^{-1} of 4 °C saline or Hartmann's. A lack of financial resources for equipment can thus not be a credible excuse for ignoring this treatment modality, and EDs need to give the optimal care in the resuscitation room and not wait till they get to ITU.

Answer

The key to managing the post-arrest phase is pre-planning, a structured approach, and team work between the pre-hospital team, the ED, intensive care staff, and cardiologists.

> **🕐 Expert comment**
>
> Most agree that hypothermia is an important treatment modality after out-of-hospital cardiac arrest, but many years are likely to pass before we learn how to use the treatment to maximum effect. Whilst its use after non-shockable rhythms has not been proven beyond doubt, most accept it and act accordingly. However, we do not know how important it is to cool pre-hospital nor indeed whether cooling should ideally be started intra-arrest. Teamwork is important so that if pre-hospital hypothermia has been initiated, it should be continued in hospital. We lack evidence on whether we should aim to reach target temperature quickly, which in any case is not possible with most methods in common use. We can, however, be reassured that using the various conventional methods do provide overall benefit even though they may not be optimal.

Case progression

The ITU outreach team join you in the resuscitation room and agree to help to initiate the cooling measures required. Cooling packs are obtained and applied to the patient but the ITU team inform you that it will take at least an hour to free a bed in the critical care unit and request that you 'optimize' the patient as best as possible in the resus room setting.

Clinical question: What measures can be initiated in the post-ROSC phase to maximize the chance of return to baseline status?

Successful ROSC is not the end of the resuscitation process but just the start. Post-resuscitation care must start immediately *post resuscitation* (pre-hospital or in the ED) and not delayed till we get the patient into the intensive care. It is not fair on our patients to think that post-resuscitation care is the concern for the intensive care staff solely.

Some consider the post-cardiac arrest phase a syndrome comprising brain and myocardial dysfunction alongside a body-wide ischaemia/reperfusion injury. Generally the longer the down-time and the longer the duration of CPR, the worse the symptoms will be. Other factors exacerbate the symptoms; microcirculatory failure, impaired autoregulation, hypercarbia, hyperoxia, pyrexia, hyperglycaemia, and seizures. Minimizing these factors helps reduce the symptoms. Specific measures also improve outcome, such as therapeutic hypothermia. It must be remembered that in the first 48 hrs you cannot predict from initial neurology the final neurological outcome and so ongoing decisions with regard to whether the patient should go to ITU should not be based on initial neurological findings.

The post-arrest management proceeds along a step-by-step fashion. However alongside this, the appropriateness of post-arrest management to intensive care needs to be carefully assessed. If a 95-year-old with severe dementia from a nursing home has been brought in following a 'successful' post arrest, this does not mean that we need to continue inappropriate and undignified treatment. Extubation and tender loving care may well be in the patient's best interest and what we should do. What is appropriate is a consideration of the rationale as to why he/she was resuscitated in the first place and make sure that appropriate community systems are in place to prevent inappropriate attempts at CPR. Not only is it inhumane for the patient, it can inadvertently deter staff from being enthused to perform appropriate resuscitation attempts.

However, if it is appropriate to manage a patient in the intensive care unit, then they should have the most up-to-date, evidence-based treatment available.

If the patient is actively pulling at the endotracheal tube in a coherent way and is waking up appropriately, then it is sensible to extubate and send to a high-dependency ward. Otherwise, a critical care management bundle started in the ED and continued in the intensive care department should be used.

Make sure the airway is secure, use CO_2 monitoring and keep the patient sedated and initially muscle-blocked as required. Hypoxaemia and hypercarbia both can cause problems by increasing the likelihood of a further cardiac arrest and contributing to secondary brain injury. Clinical registry data has also shown an association between hyperoxaemia and poor outcome.[108]

As soon as a reliable saturation monitor is functioning, titrate the oxygen sats to 94–98 %. As soon as an arterial line has been placed aim for a normocapnia. This includes for transfer; the days of having an old-fashioned portable ventilator which only gives 'air mix' and 'no air mix' (100 % oxygen) must be resigned to the history books.

Once A and B are sorted, perform an ECG and aim to get the patient's blood pressure to a reasonable MAP which can perfuse brain and kidney. Post cardiac arrest, it is common to get myocardial dysfunction leading to low blood pressure and, more importantly, reduced cardiac output. If management of arrhythmias and simple fluids has not improved things, then insertion of a CVP line in the resuscitation room along with appropriate use of vasoactive agents is what is required. If this fails, consider cardiology review for an aortic pump and angiography.[109,110]

If the ECG shows ST elevation, then it is commonly accepted that the patient should undergo early coronary angiography and percutaneous coronary intervention (PCI). However, it is known that a lack of chest pain and/or lack of ST elevation does not indicate that the patient has not had acute coronary occlusion.[111] We must, therefore, ask the cardiologists to consider this intervention at the earliest possible opportunity in all post-cardiac-arrest patients who are suspected of having a cardiac arrest of cardiac origin, regardless of ECG findings.[109-118]

Recent guidelines say that all post-arrest patients of presumed cardiac origin should go immediately from the resuscitation room to the angiography suite. These guidelines have a good evidence base.[119]

Several studies have shown that the combination of therapeutic hypothermia and PCI is feasible and safe; if part of a predetermined management plan, excellent outcomes are obtained.[110-113]

There is no point to all this management if we produce patients with a poor quality of life. Therefore management interventions to preserve neurological function are of the highest priority. Seizures or myoclonus or both occur in 5–15 % of patients who achieve ROSC. Seizures show a threefold increase in cerebral metabolism and may cause cerebral injury; they therefore must be treated promptly with anti-epileptic medications. In practice this means adding in phenytoin and increasing the propafol infusion rate for comatosed intubated patients who are fitting.

Glucose control is very important. High blood glucose after resuscitation is associated with a poor neurological outcome. If BMs are high, start a sliding scale and aim for a blood glucose of $\leq 10\,mmoll^{-1}$ ($180\,mgdl^{-1}$). However, too strict glucose control should not be implemented because of the increased risk of hypoglycaemia.[121,122]

Answer

Post-resuscitation care is as essential as care during a cardiac arrest. It should start as soon as a pulse has been obtained and not wait until the patient is in the intensive care unit. The large variations of outcome need to be narrowed by routinely following post-arrest care bundles.

> ✚ **Clinical tip** Team leadership
>
> As a team leader awaiting a patient who has had a successful ROSC pre hospital, it is imperative that you plan for post-resuscitation care prior to the patient arriving. Arranging your team and planning for possible deteriorations is essential. The team leader should run through a checklist prior to the patient arriving so that all equipment is checked (including capnography) and all personnel know their role. Drugs should be readied to keep the patient sedated and ET tube secure (i.e. infusion of sedatives set up and neuromuscular junction blockers drawn up). Cooling equipment should be assembled and clear instructions given about whose role it is to start or continue this. Liaison with ITU and cardiologists should occur prior to the patient arriving.

> ✦ **Expert comment**
>
> Although none doubt the importance of good chest compressions, the details of post-resuscitation care are less well accepted and certainly poorly practised. The author has stressed measures that deserve careful attention from all in the field. The need for this is all too evident by comparing outcome ratios between hospitals for patients admitted with ROSC after an out-of-hospital cardiac arrest, but exactly the same considerations apply to those who arrest in hospital, especially if resuscitation was prolonged.

Future advances

How may the management of cardiac arrest and post-resuscitation care change?

When this type of question is asked people inevitably always look to new scientific advances. Greater improvements in outcome however may be achieved by focusing more on the areas that we know work, including improving community CPR and AED uptake as well as cardiac arrest prevention and appropriate post-arrest management and better education. In terms of education the future of improvement lies in learning from feedback of performance during the cardiac arrest and immediate aftermath, both of the technical quality of CPR and also the team dynamics.[123] An ideal world would allow us to have a team debrief after every arrest where we watch real-time video and analyse areas of potential improvement.

There are of course future scientific developments that we may yet see.

The actual way we do CPR may change. At best, standard manual CPR produces coronary and cerebral perfusion that is just 30 % of normal. Although manual chest compressions are often performed very poorly,[50,] adjuncts to CPR have never consistently been shown to be superior to conventional manual CPR in RCTs.

However in 2011, Aufderheide *et al.*[36] combined the use of a manual compressor and an impedance threshold device, a valve that limits air entry into the lungs during chest recoil thus decreasing intrathoracic pressure and increasing venous return to the heart. This showed an improvement—an odds ratio of 1.58 for the chances of survival with a good neurological outcome for all arrests of presumed cardiac origin.

A trial is currently underway into the role of cooling prior to obtaining ROSC[124] using an intranasal cooling system. The results are due January 2016.

It may soon be possible to predict how likely there will be successful defibrillation from the fibrillation waveforms. This may mean that in the future shock/CPR protocols will be more fluid and adapt to the clinical picture.

Finally, performing angiography on patients during CPR, may become more common.

A Final Word from the Expert

The days are long gone when it is sufficient only to know the ALS protocols in order to be a team leader. The role must now include coordinating the team, adapting the management to the specific situation, using feedback devices to optimize care, and most importantly, making sure that the basics are performed proficiently: good compressions, early defibrillation with the briefest possible interval between CPR and shock, along with optimal post-arrest care. These measures are the core strategies to achieve the best possible survival rate from cardiac arrest.

References

1. Atwood C, Eisenberg M, Herlitz J, *et al.* Incidence of EMS-treated out-of-hospital cardiac arrest in Europe. *Resuscitation* 2005; 67:75–80.
2. Nolan JP, Soar J, Zideman DA, *et al.* On behalf of the ERC Guidelines Writing Group. European Resuscitation Council Guidelines for Resuscitation 2010 Section 1. Executive summary. *Resuscitation* 2010; 81:1219–76.
3. Nolan JP, Standards for the management of patients after cardiac arrest. Intensive Care Society Publication. October 2008.
4. Nichol G, Thomas E, Callaway CW, *et al.* Regional variation in out-of-hospital cardiac arrest incidence and outcome. *JAMA* 2008; 300:1423–31.
5. Hollenberg J, Herlitz J, Lindqvist J, *et al.* Improved survival after out-of-hospital cardiac arrest is associated with an increase in proportion of emergency crew—witnessed cases and bystander cardiopulmonary resuscitation. *Circulation* 2008; 118:389–96.
6. Iwami T, Nichol G, Hiraide A, *et al.* Continuous improvements in 'chain of survival' increased survival after out-of-hospital cardiac arrests: a large-scale population-based study. *Circulation* 2009; 119:728–34.
7. Fletcher D, Chamberlain D, Handley A, *et al.* Utstein-style audit of protocol C: a non-standard resuscitation protocol for healthcare professionals. *Resuscitation* October 2011; 82
8. Nolan JP, Laver SR, Welch CA, *et al.* Outcome following admission to UK intensive care units after cardiac arrest: a secondary analysis of the ICNARC Case Mix Programme Database. *Anaesthesia* 2007; 62:1207–16.
9. Wenzel V, Lindner KH, Augenstein S, *et al.* Intraosseous vasopressin improves coronary perfusion pressure rapidly during cardiopulmonary resuscitation in pigs. *Crit Care Med* 1999; 27:1565–9.
10. Olasveengen TM, Sunde K, Brunborg C, *et al.* Intravenous drug administration during out-of-hospital cardiac arrest: a randomized trial. *JAMA* 2009; 302:2222–9.
11. Herlitz J, Ekstrom L, WennerblomB, *et al.* Adrenaline in out-of-hospital ventricular fibrillation. Does it make any difference? *Resuscitation* 1995; 29:195–201.
12. Kudenchuk PJ, Cobb LA, Copass MK, *et al.* Amiodarone for resuscitation after out-of hospital cardiac arrest due to ventricular fibrillation. *N Engl J Med* 1999; 341:871–8.
13. Dorian P, Cass D, Schwartz B, *et al.* Amiodarone as compared with lidocaine for shockresistant ventricular fibrillation. *N Engl J Med* 2002; 346:884–90.
14. Hassan TB, Jagger C, Barnett DB. A randomised trial to investigate the efficacy of magnesium sulphate for refractory ventricular fibrillation. *Emerg Med J* 2002; 19:57–62.
15. Stiell IG, Wells GA, Hebert PC, *et al.* Association of drug therapy with survival in cardiac arrest: limited role of advanced cardiac life support drugs. *Acad Emerg Med* 1995; 2:264–73.

16. Engdahl J, Bang A, Lindqvist J, *et al.* Can we define patients with no and those with some chance of survival when found in asystole out of hospital? *Am J Cardiol* 2000; 86:610–4.

17. Engdahl J, Bang A, Lindqvist J, *et al.* Factors affecting short- and long-term prognosis among 1069 patients with out-of-hospital cardiac arrest and pulseless electrical activity. *Resuscitation* 2001; 51:17–25.

18. Böttiger BW, Arntz HR, Chamberlain DA, *et al.* Thrombolysis during resuscitation for out-of-hospital cardiac arrest. *N Engl J Med* 2008; 359:2651–62.

19. Böttiger BW, Martin E. Thrombolytic therapy during cardiopulmonary resuscitation and the role of coagulation activation after cardiac arrest. *Curr Opin Crit Care* 2001; 7:176–83.

20. Spöhr F, Böttiger BW. Safety of thrombolysis during cardiopulmonary resuscitation. *Drug Saf* 2003; 26:367–79.

21. Wang HE, Simeone SJ, Weaver MD, *et al.* Interruptions in cardiopulmonary resuscitation from paramedic endotracheal intubation. *Ann Emerg Med* 2009; 54:645–52 e1.

22. Aufderheide TP, Pirrallo RG, Yannopoulos D, *et al.* Incomplete chest wall decompression: a clinical evaluation of CPR performance by EMS personnel and assessment of alternative manual chest compression-decompression techniques. *Resuscitation* 2005; 64:353–62.

23. Yannopoulos D, McKnite S, Aufderheide TP, *et al.* Effects of incomplete chest wall decompression during cardiopulmonary resuscitation on coronary and cerebral perfusion pressures in a porcine model of cardiac arrest. *Resuscitation* 2005; 64:363–72.

24. Sack JB, Kesselbrenner MB, Bregman D. Survival from in-hospital cardiac arrest with interposed abdominal counterpulsation during cardiopulmonary resus-citation. *JAMA* 1992; 267:379–85.

25. Sack JB, Kesselbrenner MB, Jarrad A. Interposed abdominal compression- cardiopul-monary resuscitation and resuscitation outcome during asystole and electromechanical dissociation. *Circulation* 1992; 86:1692–700.

26. Mateer JR, Stueven HA, Thompson BM, *et al.* Pre-hospital IAC-CPR versus standard CPR: paramedic resuscitation of cardiac arrests. *Am J Emerg Med* 1985; 3:143–6.

27. Lindner KH, Pfenninger EG, Lurie KG, *et al.* Effects of active compression-decompression resuscitation on myocardial and cerebral blood flow in pigs. *Circulation* 1993; 88:1254–63.

28. Shultz JJ, Coffeen P, Sweeney M, *et al.* Evaluation of standard and active compression-decompression CPR in an acute human model of ventricular fibrillation. *Circulation* 1994; 89:684–93.

29. Chang MW, Coffeen P, Lurie KG, *et al.* Active compression-decompression CPR improves vital organ perfusion in a dog model of ventricular fibrillation. *Chest* 1994; 106:1250–9.

30. Orliaguet GA, Carli PA, Rozenberg A, *et al.* End-tidal carbon dioxide during out-of-hos-pital cardiac arrest resuscitation: comparison of active compression-decompression and standard CPR. *Ann Emerg Med* 1995; 25:48–51.

31. Guly UM, Mitchell RG, Cook R, *et al.* Paramedics and technicians are equally successful at managing cardiac arrest outside hospital. *BMJ* 1995; 310:1091–4.

32. Tucker KJ, Galli F, Savitt MA, *et al.* Active compression-decompression resuscitation: effect on resuscitation success after in-hospital cardiac arrest. *J Am Coll Cardiol* 1994; 24:201–9.

33. Lafuente-Lafuente C, Melero-Bascones M. Active chest compression-decompression for cardiopulmonary resuscitation. *Cochrane Database Syst Rev* 2004:CD002751.

34. Aufderheide TP, Pirrallo RG, Provo TA, *et al.* Clinical evaluation of an inspiratory imped-ance threshold device during standard cardiopulmonary resuscitation in patients with out-of-hospital cardiac arrest. *Crit Care Med* 2005; 33:734–40.

35. Cabrini L, Beccaria P, Landoni G, *et al.* Impact of impedance threshold devices on cardio-pulmonary resuscitation: a systematic review and meta-analysis of randomized con-trolled studies. *Crit Care Med* 2008; 36:1625–32.

36. Aufderheide TP, Frascone RJ, Wayne MA, *et al.* Standard cardiopulmonary resuscita-tion versus active compression-decompression cardiopulmonary resuscitation with

augmentation of negative intrathoracic pressure for out-of-hospital cardiac arrest: a randomized trial. *Lancet* 2011; 377(9762):301–31.

37. Steen S, Liao Q, Pierre L, *et al.* Evaluation of LUCAS, a new device for automatic mechanical compression and active decompression resuscitation. *Resuscitation* 2002; 55:285–99.

38. Rubertsson S, Karlsten R. Increased cortical cerebral blood flow with LUCAS; a new device for mechanical chest compressions compared to standard external compressions during experimental cardiopulmonary resuscitation. *Resuscitation* 2005; 65:357–63.

39. Timerman S, Cardoso LF, Ramires JA, *et al.* Improved hemodynamic performance with a novel chest compression device during treatment of in- hospital cardiac arrest. *Resuscitation* 2004; 61:273–80.

40. Halperin H, Berger R, Chandra N, *et al.* Cardiopulmonary resuscitation with a hydraulicpneumatic band. *Crit Care Med* 2000; 28:N203–6.

41. Halperin HR, Paradis N, Ornato JP, *et al.* Cardiopulmonary resuscitation with a novel chest compression device in a porcine model of cardiac arrest: improved hemodynamics and mechanisms. *J Am Coll Cardiol* 2004; 44:2214–20.

42. Hallstrom A, Rea TD, Sayre MR, *et al.* Manual chest compression vs use of an automated chest compression device during resuscitation following out-of- hospital cardiac arrest: a randomized trial. *JAMA* 2006; 295:2620–8.

43. Wik L. Manual vs. integrated automatic load-distributing band CPR with equal survival after out of hospital cardiac arrest. The randomized CIRC trial. *Resuscitation* 2014; 85(6):741–48.

44. Rubertsson S. Mechanical chest compressions and simultaneous defibrillation vs conventional cardiopulmonary resuscitation in out-of-hospital cardiac arrest: The LINC randomized trial. *JAMA* 2014; 311(1):53–61.

45. Rubertsson S. A multicenter randomized trial comparing a mechanical CPR algorithm using LUCAS versus manual CPR in out-of-hospital cardiac arrest patients-per protocol analysis of the LINC study. *Circulation* 2013; 128(24).

46. Larsen AI, Hjornevik AS, Ellingsen CL, *et al.* Cardiac arrest with continuous mechanical chest compression during percutaneous coronary intervention. A report on the use of the LUCAS device. *Resuscitation* 2007; 75:454–9.

47. Wagner H, Terkelsen CJ, Friberg H, *et al.* Cardiac arrest in the catheterisation laboratory: a 5-year experience of using mechanical chest compressions to facilitate PCI during prolonged resuscitation efforts. *Resuscitation* 2010; 81:383–7.

48. Abella BS, Alvarado JP, Myklebust H, *et al.* Quality of cardiopulmonary resuscitation during in-hospital cardiac arrest. *JAMA* 2005; 293:305–10.

49. Abella BS, Sandbo N, Vassilatos P, *et al.* Chest compression rates during cardiopulmonary resuscitation are suboptimal: a prospective study during in-hospital cardiac arrest. *Circulation* 2005; 111:428–34.

50. Fletcher D, Galloway R, Chamberlain D, *et al.* Basics in advanced life support: a role for download audit and metronomes. *Resuscitation* 2008; 78:127–34.

51. Sugerman NT, Edelson DP, Leary M, *et al.* Rescuer fatigue during actual in-hospital cardiopulmonary resuscitation with audiovisual feedback: a prospective multicenter study. *Resuscitation* 2009; 80:981–4.

52. Eftestol T, Sunde K, Steen PA. Effects of interrupting precordial compressions on the calculated probability of defibrillation success during out-of-hospital cardiac arrest. *Circulation* 2002; 105:2270–3.

53. <http://www.feel-uk.com>

54. Edelson DP, Abella BS, Kramer-Johansen J, *et al.* Effects of compression depth and pre-shock pauses predict defibrillation failure during cardiac arrest. *Resuscitation* 2006; 71:137–45.

55. Gundersen K, Kvaloy JT, Kramer-Johansen J, *et al.* Development of the probability of return of spontaneous circulation in intervals without chest compressions during out-of-hospital cardiac arrest: an observational study. *BMC Med* 2009; 7:6.

56. Lloyd MS, Heeke B, Walter PF, *et al.* Hands-on defibrillation: an analysis of electrical current flow through rescuers in direct contact with patients during biphasic external defibrillation. *Circulation* 2008; 117:2510–4.

57. Sunde K, Eftestol T, Askenberg C, *et al.* Quality assessment of defibrillation and advanced life support using data from the medical control module of the defibrillator. *Resuscitation* 1999; 41:237–47.

58. Rea TD, Shah S, Kudenchuk PJ, *et al.* Automated external defibrillators: to what extent does the algorithm delay CPR? *Ann Emerg Med* 2005; 46:132–41.

59. Van Alem AP, Sanou BT, Koster RW. Interruption of cardiopulmonary resuscitation with the use of the automated external defibrillator in out-of-hospital cardiac arrest. *Ann Emerg Med* 2003; 42:449–57.

60. Eftestol T, Sunde K, Steen PA. Effects of interrupting precordial compressions on the calculated probability of defibrillation success during out-of-hospital cardiac arrest. *Circulation* 2002; 105:2270–3.

61. Bobrow BJ, Clark LL, Ewy GA, *et al.* Minimally interrupted cardiac resuscitation by emergency medical services for out-of-hospital cardiac arrest. *JAMA* 2008; 299:1158–65.

62. Rea TD, Helbock M, Perry S, *et al.* Increasing use of cardiopulmonary resuscita- tion during out-of-hospital ventricular fibrillation arrest: survival implications of guideline changes. *Circulation* 2006; 114:2760–5.

63. Steinmetz J, Barnung S, Nielsen SL, *et al.* Improved survival after an out-of-hospital car- diac arrest using new guidelines. *Acta Anaesthesiol Scand* 2008; 52:908–13.

64. Lin, S. Adrenaline for out-of-hospital cardiac arrest resuscitation: A systematic review and meta-analysis of randomized controlled trials. *Resuscitation* 2014; 85(6):732–40.

65. Hagihara A, Hasegawa M, Abe T, *et al.* Prehospital epinephrine use and survival among patients with out-of-hospital cardiac arrest. *JAMA* 2012; 307:1161–8.

66. Donnino MW, Salciccioli JD, Howell MD, *et al.* Time to administration of epinephrine and outcome after in hospital cardiac arrest with non-shockable rhythms: retrospective analysis of hospital episode statistics. *BMJ* 2014; 348:g3028.

67. Steiger HV, Rimbach K, Muller E, *et al.* Focused emergency echocardiography: lifesav- ing tool for a 14-year-old girl suffering out-of-hospital pulseless electrical activity arrest because of cardiac tamponade. *Eur J Emerg Med* 2009; 16:103–5.

68. Price S, Uddin S, Quinn T. Echocardiography in cardiac arrest. *Curr Opin Crit Care* 2010; 16:211–5.

69. Blaivas M, Fox JC. Outcome in cardiac arrest patients found to have cardiac standstill on the bedside emergency department echocardiogram. *Acad Emerg Med* 2001; 8:616–21.

70. Salen P, O'Connor R, Sierzenski P, *et al.* Can cardiac sonography and capnography be used independently and in combination to predict resuscitation outcomes? *Acad Emerg Med* 2001; 8:610–5.

71. Salen P, Melniker L, Chooljian C, *et al.* Does the presence or absence of sonographically identified cardiac activity predict resuscitation outcomes of cardiac arrest patients? *Am J Emerg Med* 2005; 23:459–62.

72. Takasu A, Saitoh D, Kaneko N, *et al.* Hyperthermia: is it an ominous sign after cardiac arrest? *Resuscitation* 2001; 49:273–7.

73. Zeiner A, Holzer M, Sterz F, *et al.* Hyperthermia after cardiac arrest is associated with an unfavorable neurologic outcome. *Arch Intern Med* 2001; 161:2007–12

74. Alzaga AG, Cerdan M, Varon J. Therapeutic hypothermia. *Resuscitation* 2006; 70:369–80.

75. The Hypothermia after Cardiac Arrest Study Group. Mild therapeutic hypothermia to improve neurological outcome after cardiac arrest. *New Engl J Med* 2002; 346:549–55.

76. Bernard S, Gray TW. Treatment of comatose survivors of out of hospital cardiac arrest with induced hypothermia. *NEJM* 2002; 346:557–63.

77. Hachimi-Idrissi S, Corne L, Ebinger G, *et al.* Mild hypothermia induced by a helmet device: a clinical feasibility study. *Resuscitation* 2001; 51(3):275–81.

78. Mori A. Multivariate analysis of prognostic factors in survivors of out-of-hospital cardiac arrest with brain hypothermia therapy. *Crit Care Med* 2000; 28:A168.

79. Holzer M, Bernard SA, Hachimi-Idissi S, *et al.* Hypothermia for neuroprotection after cardiac arrest: Systematic review and individual patient data meta-analysis. *Crit Care Med* 2005; 33:414–18.

80. Cheung KW, Green RS, Magee KD. Systematic review of randomized controlled trials of therapeutic hypothermia as a neuroprotectant in post cardiac arrest patients. *Canadian Journal of Emergency Medicine* 2006; 8(5):329–37.

81. Arrich J, Holzer M, Herkner H, *et al.* Hypothermia for neuroprotection in adults after cardiopulmonary resuscitation. *Cochrane Database of Systematic Reviews* 2009; Issue 4. Art. No.: CD004128. DOI:10.1002/14651858.CD004128.pub2

82. Bernard SA, Jones BM, Horne MK. Clinical trial of induced hypothermia in comatose survivors of out-of-hospital cardiac arrest. *Ann Emerg Med* 1997; 30:146–53.

83. Yanagawa Y, Ishihara S, Norio H, *et al.* Preliminary clinical outcome study of mild resuscitative hypothermia after out-of-hospital cardiopulmonary arrest. *Resuscitation* 1998; 39:61–6.

84. Busch M, Soreide E, Lossius HM, *et al.* Rapid implementation of therapeutic hypothermia in comatose out-of-hospital cardiac arrest survivors. *Acta Anaesthesiol Scand* 2006; 50(10):1277–83.

85. Castrejon S, Improved prognosis after using mild hypothermia to treat cardiorespiratory arrest due to a cardiac cause; comparison with a control group. *Rev Esp Cardiol* 2009; 62(7):733–41.

86. Sunde K, Pytte M, Jacobsen D, *et al.* Implementation of a standardised treatment protocol for post resuscitation care after out-of-hospital cardiac arrest. 82007; 73:29–39.

87. Belliard G, Catez E, Charron C, *et al.* Efficacy of therapeutic hypothermia after out-of-hospital cardiac arrest due to ventricular fibrillation. *Resuscitation* 2007; 75:252–9.

88. Oddo M, Schaller M-D., Feihl F, *et al.* From evidence to clinical practice: effective implementation of therapeutic hypothermia to improve patient outcome after cardiac arrest. *Crit Care Med* 2006; 34:1865–73.

89. Holzer M, Mullner M, Sterz F, *et al.* Efficacy and safety of endovascular cooling after cardiac arrest: Cohort study and Bayesian approach. *Stroke* 2006; 37:1792–7.

90. Storm C, Nee J, Krueger A, Schefold J, *et al.* 2-year survival of patients undergoing mild hypothermia treatment after ventricular fibrillation cardiac arrest is significantly improved compared to historical controls. *Scandinavian Journal of Trauma, Resuscitation and Emergency Medicine* 2010; 18:2.

91. Felberg RA, Krieger DW, Chuang R, *et al.* Hypothermia after cardiac arrest: feasibility and safety of an external cooling protocol. *Circulation* 2001; 104(15):1799–1804.

92. Zeiner A, Holzer M, Sterz F, *et al.* Mild resuscitative hypothermia to improve neurological outcome after cardiac arrest. A clinical feasibility trial. Hypothermia After Cardiac Arrest (HACA) Study Group. *Stroke* 2000; 31(1):86–94.

93. Scott BD, Hogue T, Fixley MS, et al. Induced hypothermia following out-of-hospital cardiac arrest; initial experience in a community hospital. *Clin Cardiol* 2006; 29:525–9.

94. Laish-Farkash A, Matetzky S, Kassem S, *et al.* Therapeutic hypothermia for comatose survivors after cardiac arrest. *Isr Med Assoc J* 2007; 9:252–6.

95. Kliegel A, Janata A, Wandaller C, *et al.* Cold infusions alone are effective for induction of therapeutic hypothermia but do not keep patients cool after cardiac arrest. *Resuscitation* 2007; 73(1):46–53.

96. Kliegel A, Losert H, Sterz F, *et al.* Cold simple intravenous infusions preceding special endovascular cooling for faster induction of mild hypothermia after cardiac arrest—a feasibility study. *Resuscitation* 2005; 64:347–51.

97. Al-Senani FM, Graffagnino C, Grotta JC, *et al.* A prospective, multicenter pilot study to evaluate the feasibility and safety of using the CoolGard System and Icy catheter following cardiac arrest. *Resuscitation* 2004; 62:143–50.

98. Sagalyn E, Band RA, Gaieski DF, *et al.* Therapeutic hypothermia after cardiac arrest in clinical practice: Review and compilation of recent experiences. *Crit Care Med* July 2009; 37 (Suppl. 7):S223–S226.

99. Nielsen N, *et al.* Outcome, timing and adverse events in therapeutic hypothermia after out-of-hospital cardiac arrest. *Acta Anaesthesiol Scand* 2009; 53(7):926–34.

100. Arrich J. The European Resuscitation Council Hypothermia After Cardiac Arrest Registry Study Group. Clinical application of mild therapeutic hypothermia after cardiac arrest. *Crit Care Med* 2007; 35:1041–7.

101. Oksanen T, Pettila V, Hynynen M, *et al.* Therapeutic hypothermia after cardiac arrest: implementation and outcome in Finnish intensive care units. *Acta Anaesthesiol Scand* 2007; 51:866–71.

102. Oddo M, Ribordy V, Feihl F, *et al.* Early predictors of outcome in comatose survivors of ventricular fibrillation and non-ventricular fibrillation cardiac arrest treated with hypothermia: a prospective study. *Crit Care Med* 2008; 36(8):2296–301.

103. Nielsen N, Wetterslev J, Cronberg T, *et al.* Targeted Temperature Management at 33ÅãC versus 36ÅãC after Cardiac Arrest. *N Engl J Med* 2013; 369:2197–206; doi: 10.1056/NEJMoa1310519

104. Wolff B, Machill K, Schumacher D, *et al.* Early achievement of mild therapeutic hypothermia and the neurologic outcome after cardiac arrest. *International J Cardiology* 2009; 133:223–8

105. Kim F, Nichol G. Effect of Prehospital Induction of Mild Hypothermiaon Survival and Neurological Status Among Adults With Cardiac Arrest. A Randomized Clinical Trial. *JAMA* 2014 1 Jan; 311(1):45–52; doi:10.1001/jama.2013.282173

106. Laver S, Padkin A, Atalla A, *et al.* Therapeutic hypothermia after cardiac arrest; a survey of practice in intensive care units in the United Kingdom. *Anaesthesia* 2006; 61, 873–7.

107. Sim M, Dean P, Booth M, *et al.* Uptake of therapeutic hypothermia following out of hospital cardiac arrest in Scottish intensive care Units. *Anaesthesia* 2008; 63:886–7.

108. Kilgannon JH, Jones AE, Shapiro NI, *et al.* Association between arterial hyperoxia following resuscitation from cardiac arrest and in-hospital mortality. *JAMA* 2010; 303:2165–71.

109. Sunde K, Pytte M, Jacobsen D, *et al.* Implementation of a standardised treatment protocol for post resuscitation care after out-of-hospital cardiac arrest. *Resuscitation* 2007; 73:29–39.

110. Hovdenes J, Laake JH, Aaberge L, *et al.* Therapeutic hypothermia after out-of-hospital cardiac arrest: experiences with patients treated with percutaneous coronary intervention and cardiogenic shock. *Acta Anaesthesiol Scand* 2007; 51:137–42.

111. Spaulding CM, Joly LM, Rosenberg A, *et al.* Immediate coronary angiography in survivors of out-of-hospital cardiac arrest. *N Engl J Med* 1997; 336:1629–33.

112. Bendz B, Eritsland J, Nakstad AR, *et al.* Long-term prognosis after out-of-hospital cardiac arrest and primary percutaneous coronary intervention. *Resuscitation* 2004; 63:49–53.

113. Keelan PC, Bunch TJ, White RD, *et al.* Early direct coronary angioplasty in survivors of out-of-hospital cardiac arrest. *Am J Cardiol* 2003; 91:1461–3. A6.

114. Quintero-Moran B, Moreno R, Villarreal S, *et al.* Percutaneous coronary intervention for cardiac arrest secondary to ST-elevation acute myocardial infarction. Influence of immediate paramedical/medical assistance on clinical outcome. *J Invasive Cardiol* 2006; 18:269–72.

115. Garot P, Lefevre T, Eltchaninoff H, *et al.* Six-month outcome of emergency percutaneous coronary intervention in resuscitated patients after cardiac arrest complicating ST-elevation myocardial infarction. *Circulation* 2007; 115:1354–62.

116. Nagao K, Hayashi N, Kanmatsuse K, *et al.* Cardiopulmonary cerebral resuscitation using emergency cardiopulmonary bypass, coronary reperfusion therapy and mild

hypothermia in patients with cardiac arrest outside the hospital. *J Am Coll Cardiol* 2000; 36:776–83.

117. Knafelj R, Radsel P, Ploj T, *et al*. Primary percutaneous coronary intervention and mild induced hypothermia in comatose survivors of ventricular fibrillation with ST-elevation acute myocardial infarction. *Resuscitation* 2007; 74:227–34.

118. Nielsen N, Hovdenes J, Nilsson F, *et al*. Outcome, timing and adverse events in therapeutic hypothermia after out-of-hospital cardiac arrest. *Acta Anaesthesiol Scand* 2009; 53:926–34.

119. Noc M, Fajadet J, Lassen JF, *et al*. Invasive coronary treatment strategies for out-of-hospital cardiac arrest: a consensus statement from the European Association for Percutaneous Cardiovascular Interventions (EAPCI)/Stent for Life (SFL) groups. *EuroIntervention* 2014; 10:31–7.

120. Galloway R, Sherren P. Therapeutic hypothermia following out of hospital cardiac arrest-does it start in the Emergency department? *Emergency Medicine Journal* 2010; 27:948–9.

121. Losert H, Sterz F, Roine RO, *et al*. Strict normoglycaemic blood glucose levels in the therapeutic management of patients within 12 h after cardiac arrest might not be necessary. *Resuscitation* 2008; 76(2):214–20.

122. Mullner M, Sterz F, Binder M, *et al*. Blood glucose concentration after cardiopulmonary resuscitation influences functional neurological recovery in human cardiac arrest survivors. *J Cereb Blood Flow Metab* 1997; 17:430–6.

123. Kramer-Johansen J, Myklebust H, Wik L, *et al*. Quality of out-of-hospital cardiopulmonary resuscitation with real time automated feedback: a prospective interventional study. *Resuscitation* 2006; 71:283–92.

124. <http://clinicaltrials.gov/ct2/show/NCT01400373>

3 Traumatic occult pneumothorax

Anthony Hudson

Expert commentary Sir Keith Porter

Case history

The trauma team is called to a 52-year-old woman who has fallen 8 metres from a balcony. She is complaining of severe pelvic pain with associated deformity of her lower limb and so consequently a pelvic binder has been applied in the pre-hospital phase. At the scene she is breathing spontaneously and there is no evidence of haemodynamic compromise.

On arrival to the ED she is in significant pain despite titrated doses of morphine; however, her airway and cervical spine, breathing, and circulation are all uncompromised. Intravenous analgesia is provided, blood investigations and electrocardiogram performed along with immediate supine radiographs in the resuscitation room of the chest and pelvis. The chest X-ray is unremarkable but there is an obvious pelvic fracture.

While awaiting CT imaging to further evaluate the patient, a FAST scan (focused abdominal sonography in trauma) is performed at the bedside by the ED registrar. An ED junior asks you as team leader if, aside from the classic role of detecting intra-abdominal free fluid and haemothorax, bedside ED ultrasound can have a role in the detection of pneumothorax that may not be picked up on a supine chest radiograph?

See Box 3.1 for a clinical summary of occult pneumothorax.

Box 3.1 Clinical summary of occult pneumothorax

Use of CT scanning in the assessment of trauma has led to the recognition of occult pneumothoraces. They are defined as a pneumothorax not suspected clinically or on plain radiography but present on subsequent CT images.[17]

In polytrauma cases this is a common problem, with occult pneumothoraces accounting for up to 76% of all traumatic pneumothoraces.[18-20]

The published incidence of traumatic occult pneumothorax in all trauma patients ranges from 2%[21] to as high as 64% (in a series of ventilated patients with an average injury severity score (ISS) greater than 30).[22]

Clearly the incidence is a reflection of the patient cohort studied and the use of CT in trauma which has increased dramatically over recent years, for example one series found a tenfold increase in the use of thoracic CT in blunt trauma from 1998 to 2004.[23]

> **Expert comment**
>
> A CT traumagram is the definitive triage tool and should be performed as early as possible, providing the patient's condition permits.
>
> In pre-hospital care ultrasound is increasingly used to detect pneumothoraces, which are notoriously difficult to recognize clinically, and also to confirm cardiac output in peri-arrest trauma patients.
>
> Similarly, in the critically unwell trauma patient in ED ultrasound in the hands of experienced practitioners can have the same application.

Clinical question: Does ultrasound have a role in the diagnosis of pneumothorax?

Early studies on the investigatation of the use of ultrasound in the diagnosis of pneumothorax used chest X-ray as reference standard. These papers indicated that ultrasound had potential but CT provides a far more robust gold standard.[1,2] The key papers to assess the use of ultrasound in pneumothorax are presented in Table 3.1.

Table 3.1 Assessment of the use of ultrasound in pneumothorax—key papers

Author, country, date	Patient group	Study type	Outcomes	Key results	Study weaknesses
Alrajhi et al., Canada, 2011[3]	Adult patients 6 papers relate to trauma 2 papers relate wto iatrogenic pneumothorax	Meta-analysis	Comparison of sensitivity and specificity	8 papers with a total of 1048 patients identified Ultrasound was found to be more sensitive than chest X-ray (90.9% vs 50.2%) Specificity was found to be similar (ultrasound 98.2% vs 99.4% for chest X-ray)	Some relevant papers not identified and included in analysis Paediatric population excluded

Relevant papers not included in the meta-analysis by Alrajhi et al.

Author, country, date	Patient group	Study type	Outcomes	Key results	Study weaknesses
Nagarsheth et al., USA, 2011[4]	All trauma patients	Prospective single blinded diagnostic study	Comparison of sensitivity and specificity of ultrasound and chest X-ray CT was used as gold standard	79 patients recruited Sensitivity 81.8% for ultrasound vs 31.8% for chest X-ray Both had a specificity of 100%	Convenience sampling Small sample size Incomplete blinding
Brook et al., Israel, 2009[5]	All trauma patients	Prospective diagnostic study	Comparison of ultrasound vs supine chest X-ray CT was used as gold standard	169 patients recruited Sensitivity 46.5% for ultrasound vs 16.3% for chest X-ray Specificity for ultrasound was 99% vs 100% for chest X-ray	Unclear if investigators were blinded Small sample size Low sensitivity of ultrasound compared to other studies thought to be due to use of low frequency convex ultrasound transducer
Dean et al., USA, 2006[6]	All trauma patients	Prospective diagnostic study	Assessment of diagnostic utility of ultrasound CT was used as gold standard	607 patient recruited but only 566 patients' data available for analysis Sensitivity for ultrasound was 57.1%, specificity was 99.4% Ultrasound reported to be superior to chest X-ray	Convenience sampling Significant number of patients excluded

Data from various sources (see references)

Answer

This body of evidence supports the use of ultrasound as a useful tool in the diagnosis of traumatic pneumothorax, highlighting that, importantly, it has consistently higher sensitivity than plain chest X-ray.

eFAST

Clinical detection of pneumothoraces is reported at a rate of 10–40 %[1] so clinicians have increasingly come to rely on imaging, traditionally chest X-ray, and increasingly, CT. However chest X-rays, particularly when patients are supine, have been shown to be poor at detecting pneumothorax.[7] It is vital to remember to perform an erect chest X-ray where possible. This is particularly important in penetrating trauma when the cervical spine has been cleared as it increases the sensitivity of chest X-ray for the detection of pneumothorax.

Detection of pneumothorax by ultrasound was first described in 1986 in a horse,[8] and then in humans in 1987.[9] The concept of eFAST (extendedFAST)[10] includes scanning the anterior thorax to assess for pneumothorax in trauma, the advantage being that it is immediately available at the patient's side, is non-invasive, and small handheld devices can be used in the pre-hospital setting.[11,12,13]

⑥ Expert comment

In clinical practice, the high sensitivity of ultrasound is useful to help eliminate a pneumothorax as a negative test can be used to rule out the condition. For example, a normal ultrasound will support the decision not to perform a thoracostomy in trauma patients who have been intubated in a pre-hospital setting, with the significant risk of contamination (a 'dirty finger' thoracostomy).

⊕ Clinical tip Signs used in the diagnosis of pneumothorax

Lung sliding

In normal patients the horizontal hyperechogenic line represents the pleural interface and the 'to and fro' sliding motion that is synchronized with respiration represents the movement of visceral over parietal pleura (see Figure 3.1). This is similar in appearance to an army of ants marching along this prominent white line, and absent in pneumothorax.[14]

Comet-tail sign

Comet tails are hyperechoic ray-like projections extending into the lung parenchyma caused by water-rich structures in the visceral pleura interfacing with the air-filled lung. Their presence therefore precludes the diagnosis of pneumothorax.[15] An example of this phenomenon can be seen in Figure 3.2. Note that they can be subtle or more pronounced, extending down into the lung parenchyma. This sign should be interpreted with caution as comet tails can be caused by subcutaneous emphysema and shotgun pellets.[1,2]

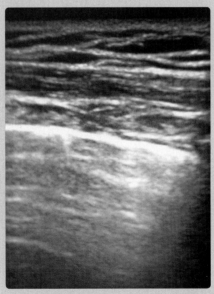

Figure 3.1 Ultrasound image demonstrating the sliding pleural line (a) and a comet tail (b).

➕ **Clinical tip** Seashore sign

This is a unique representation of lung sliding when captured in time motion-mode and depicts the motionless parietal pleura over movement artefact below.[16] This is illustrated in Figure 3.2 where you can imagine looking out across a beach to waves breaking in the distance. This is absent in pneumothorax and in Figure 3.3 where there is no differentiation between the beach and waves; i.e. this image demonstrates a pneumothorax.

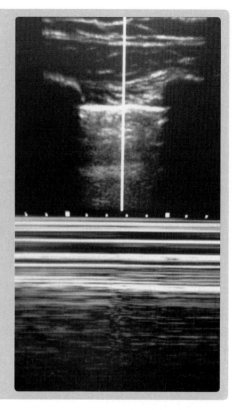

Figure 3.2 Ultrasound image of normal lung in motion mode demonstrating the seashore sign.

➕ **Clinical tip**

This is a unique representation of lung sliding when captured in time motion-mode and depicts the motionless parietal pleura over movement artefact below.[16] This is illustrated in Figure 3.2 where you can imagine looking out across a beach to waves breaking in the distance. This is absent in pneumothorax and in Figure 3.3 where there is no differentiation between the beach and waves; i.e. this image demonstrates a pneumothorax.

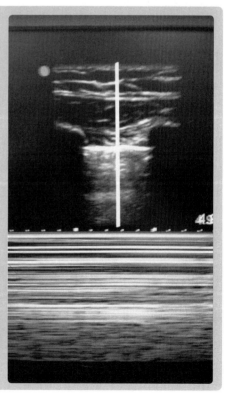

Figure 3.3 Ultrasound image demonstrating loss of the seashore appearance.

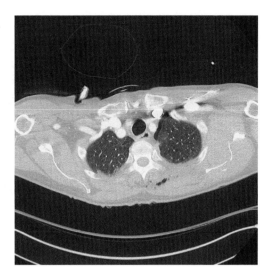

Figure 3.4 CT of occult apical pneumothorax.

Case progression

The patient remains haemodynamically stable both in the ED and during transfer to and whilst undergoing CT. This imaging confirms the presence of a complex pelvic fracture and an anterior pneumothorax despite the normal chest X-ray (see Figure 3.4).

Clinical question: Can occult pneumothoraces in spontaneously breathing patients be managed by observation alone?

ATLS guidelines[25] state that any pneumothorax is best managed by insertion of an intercostal drain due to the risk of progression and possible tension pneumothorax. The guidelines acknowledge that observation of an asymptomatic pneumothorax may be appropriate but the choice should be made by a qualified doctor. ATLS guidelines go on to state that those patients with a pneumothorax who are mechanically ventilated should have an intercostal drain inserted.[25]

It is important to follow the guidelines surrounding any topic, however, the insertion of an intercostal drain should not be considered a benign procedure. It is reasonable to question whether tube thoracostomy is necessary in cases where, prior to the commonplace use of CT scanning, clinicians were unaware of the underlying pneumothorax. This is particularly important when taking into consideration that complication rates associated with tube thoracostomy are reported as high as 21 %.[18]

> **Clinical tip** Chest tube complications
>
> Incorrect tube position
>
> Pain
>
> Infective sequelae (empyema and pneumonia)
>
> Vascular and solid organ injury
>
> Intercostal nerve injury with resulting neuralgia
>
> Persistent or recurrent pneumothorax
>
> Subcutaneous emphysema
>
> Anaphylaxis associated with surgical preparation or local anaesthetic[25,26]

> **Expert comment**
>
> The dilemma as to placing the chest tube is a difficult one. Traditional practice was a plain chest X-ray invariably taken in the supine position in polytrauma patients. In 15 years of consultant practice in a hospital without CT access, I can recall only 2 patients who deteriorated acutely during positive pressure ventilation and required needle decompression followed by tube thoracostomy.
>
> The morbidity and mortality associated with chest tube placement is significant. Providing there is clinical awareness of the risk of progression and the patient is cared for in an appropriate place, I would always choose to avoid chest drains in these circumstances.

Case progression

The trauma team are not keen to place bilateral chest drains at this juncture because the incidental pneumothoraces are both less than 2 cm in size on each side. The patient is reviewed and deemed to require emergency operative management to stabilize her pelvis. Obviously she will thus be exposed to positive pressure ventilation during general anaesthesia.

Clinical question: Can occult pneumothorax be managed conservatively even if under positive pressure ventilation?

A clinical dilemma exists in how to manage these previously undiagnosed pneumothoraces. Does the potential for progression of the pneumothorax outweigh the risk of complications associated with immediate tube thoracostomy? The evidence is presented in Table 3.2.

Key evidence to support a definitive management strategy in each clinical scenario is limited. Three randomized controlled trials have been published, all are small, under-powered, and they appear to produce contradictory results. A total of 106 patients have been included across the three trials. Each trial randomized patients to either immediate tube thoracostomy or observation alone, regardless of whether they were exposed to positive pressure ventilation or not (a total of 67 were mechanically ventilated).

The papers by Ouellet et al.[20] and Brasel et al.[28] concluded observation alone is safe for all patients even those who are mechanically ventilated. The trial by Enderson et al.[27] was small but the most methodologically robust; they reported that observation was not safe in patients under positive pressure ventilation with significantly more complications (including progression of pneumothorax or tension pneumothorax) in the ventilation group ($p=0.02$). Enderson et al.[27] did not rule out observation in spontaneously breathing patients. A potential cause for this disparity could be differing ventilation strategies.

A review of the topic by Yadav et al.[31] identified the papers by Brasel et al.,[28] Enderson et al.,[27] and Ouellet et al.[20] discussed in the previous paragraph and drew similar conclusions. The authors concluded that observation was reasonable but urged caution in the observation of those patients under positive pressure in view of the limited evidence and potential risk.[31] They also reiterated the opinion that the clinician must also consider the risk of complications associated with tube thoracostomy.

The trial by Moore et al.[29] has the largest sample size, recruiting 569 patients across 16 trauma centres. They reported 6 % of all patients failed observation and required tube thoracostomy (for pneumothorax progression, respiratory distress, or haemothorax). In those under positive pressure ventilation 14 % failed observation. However, no patients suffered any adverse event, in particular tension pneumothorax[29] due to delayed tube thoracostomy.

These figures should be considered in the context of the high complication rate associated with tube thoracostomy (reported as up to 21 %).[18]

Table 3.2 Evidence for management of occult pneumothoraces

Author, country, date	Patient group	Study type	Outcomes	Key results	Study weaknesses
Enderson et al., USA, 1993[27]	40 adult trauma patients 21 randomized to observation alone (with 12 being exposed to positive pressure ventilation) 19 treated with immediate tube thoracostomy (15 exposed to positive pressure ventilation)	Prospective RCT	Primary outcomes: Complications of observation Secondary outcome 1: Length of stay in ITU (days) Secondary outcome 2: Length of hospital stay (days)	Observation group had significantly more complications (p=0.02) 8 occult pneumothoraces progressed including 3 tension pneumothorax No significant difference Observation 3.2 +/– 1.3 Tube thoracostomy 2.8 +/– 0.8 No significant difference Observation 17.6 +/– 4.3 Tube thoracostomy 12.9 +/– 1.8	No blinding Small study No power calculation Unclear if treatment was otherwise identical, e.g. ventilation strategies No long-term follow-up of patients
Brasel et al., USA, 1999[28]	39 adult trauma patients with 44 occult pneumothoraces 24 randomized to observation alone (with 9 being exposed to positive pressure ventilation) 20 randomised to immediate tube thoracostomy (with 9 exposed to positive pressure ventilation)	Prospective RCT	Primary outcomes: Need for late tube thoracostomy Incidence of respiratory distress Key secondary outcomes: Length of stay in ITU and hospital Ventilator days	3 occult pneumothoraces progressed (2 whilst under positive pressure ventilation) requiring late tube thoracostomy No emergency tube thoracostomies required No statistical difference	No blinding Small study No power calculation Only enrolled 45.3% of eligible patients Unclear randomization No long-term follow-up of patients
Ouellet et al., Cananda, 2009[20]	22 adult trauma patients 13 randomized to observation only 9 randomised to immediate tube thoracostomy All exposed to positive pressure ventilation	Prospective RCT (Pilot study)	Primary outcomes: Pneumothorax progression or need for late tube thoracostomy Key secondary outcomes: Respiratory distress (defined as increased oxygen requirements) Days on mechanical ventilation Median ITU length of stay Median hospital length of stay	4 pneumothoraces in the observation group required late tube thoracostomy (none urgent) 1 for progression, 2 for effusion, 1 for haemodynamic instability No statistical difference	No blinding Small study This study excluded 'large' occult pneumothoraces Only recruited stable patients Unclear if 2 groups were similar, e.g. ISS No long-term follow-up Convenience sampling

(continued)

Author, country, date	Patient group	Study type	Outcomes	Key results	Study weaknesses
Moore et al., USA, 2011[29]	569 patients (all ages) across 16 trauma centres 121 received immediate tube thoracostomy 448 managed by observation alone (73 of which required positive pressure ventilation)	Prospective observational study	Primary outcome: Need for late tube thoracostomy (failure of observation due to pneumothorax progression) Key secondary outcomes: Days on mechanical ventilation Length of ITU stay Length of hospital stay	6% patients in observation group required delayed tube thoracostomy for pneumothorax progression, respiratory distress or haemothorax 14% of mechanically ventilated patients required delayed tube thoracostomy No patients who failed observation developed tension pneumothorax or adverse events due to delayed tube thoracostomy Those patients who failed observation had more days on ventilation and longer ITU and hospital stays	No randomization No blinding No long-term follow-up No standardized management across centres, e.g. ventilation strategies
Paediatric studies					
Holmes et al., USA, 2001[30]	12 occult pneumothoraces in 11 blunt trauma patients under 16 11 treated by observation alone (2 exposed to positive pressure ventilation)	Prospective observational study	Primary outcome: Need for late tube thoracostomy Secondary outcome: Respiratory or haemodynamic compromise	None required No complications reported	Small sample size No randomization No blinding Limited control group (1 patient)

Data from various sources (see references)

Answer

The published evidence supports observation of patients with occult pneumothorax over immediate tube thoracostomy even if under positive pressure ventilation. This is the safest management strategy and avoids the risks associated with insertion of an intercostal drain. It is important to consider that the presence of respiratory or haemodynamic compromise should lower the threshold for tube thoracostomy.

It is worth noting that none of these trials demonstrated that size of an occult pneumothorax had a significant effect on outcome. Likewise, there is no evidence that managing a patient by observation alone reduces ITU or hospital stay.

> **⑥ Expert comment**
>
> Avoidance of chest drain is controversial but in my clinical experience, no patient has suffered long-term by adopting an 'observation' policy. It is essential the patient is observed vigilantly in an appropriate environment so in the event of deterioration appropriate action by trained staff can occur.

Safe observation of occult pneumothorax

When considering this management strategy, it appears that there are two distinct clinical scenarios. The patients at highest risk who are managed in the safest environment (i.e. those under positive pressure ventilation) are monitored closely in theatres or ITU where clinicians capable of intervention are immediately available. In contrast, patients who continue to self-ventilate and thus are at lower risk of pneumothorax progression may be managed in an environment with less intensive monitoring. In short, if patients are to be managed by observation alone it is the quality of observation that ensures patient safety, as clinicians we must strive to ensure this. The following will help achieve this:

1. Any case should be discussed with the admitting team, especially the anaesthetist or intensivist responsible for the patient under positive pressure ventilation.
2. Remember to administer 100 % oxygen to all patients during the initial phase of their admission as this is thought to increase re-absorption of the pneumothorax up to fourfold.[18]
3. All patients should be regularly reviewed and repeat chest X-ray performed at 24 hours (sooner if the patient becomes symptomatic).
4. Handover of care: careful handover is essential (medical and nursing); key information includes the need for regular review (including documentation of vital signs) and which side is affected. This can be facilitated by use of a coloured wristband to identify clearly the affected side.
5. Remember to inform the patient about possible symptoms and educate them about the risks associated with flying and diving.

Indications for tube thoracostomy include respiratory or haemodynamic compromise, progression of the pneumothorax (i.e. increasing size on subsequent chest X-ray), and clinical concern. It is worth noting careful consideration should be given before undertaking inter-hospital transfer without an intercostal drain in-situ.

> **✪ Learning point** An approach to pelvic trauma
>
> Although this chapter focuses on occult pneumothorax, this patient's significant injury was a pelvis fracture. This has significant morbidity and mortality associated with it including the potential for catastrophic haemorrhage, and urethral and bladder injuries.
>
> Consider the pelvis in the same way as the cervical spine in trauma. Immobilize immediately if there is the potential for pelvic injury. This should ideally be done with an appropriate splinting device.
>
> (continued)

Having immobilized the pelvis, limit any further movements to reduce the risk of clot disruption and further injury to the pelvic contents. Gently palpate the pelvis to examine it; do not 'spring' it.

Do not log-roll the patient until pelvic fracture has been excluded, and use split scoop stretchers to move the patient rather than extrication boards whenever possible.

Plain X-ray images of the pelvis during the primary survey maybe a useful adjunct in the early assessment of trauma patients, however, it is important not to consider the pelvis clear if there is strong clinical suspicion of pelvic injury, a highly suggestive mechanism of injury, or the patient has altered mental state, is sedated, or has distracting injuries.

Rapid access to CT with immediate reporting is transforming trauma management with the concept rightly considered as a FACT scan (Focused Assessment by CT in Trauma) looking at key areas for life-threatening injuries prior to reviewing and reporting the scan in great detail.

Case progression

This patient was managed without insertion of any intercostal drains prior to and during theatre. Thankfully she made a good recovery after pelvic surgery and had no adverse clinical sequelae as a result of her pneumothoraces.

A Final Word from the Expert

Occult pneumothoraces in the trauma patient should always be considered and early detection by bedside ultrasound is recommended.

The use of ultrasound techniques is gaining increasing popularity in both the pre-hospital and in-hospital assessment of the trauma patient and these techniques now have an established role in central line placement.

Their use routinely to exclude pneumothoraces is a transferable skill that could be taught to advanced paramedics. The use of ultrasound to detect cardiac function in peri-arrest patients will have increasing application.

References

1. Dulchavsky SA, Schwartz KL, Kirkpatrick AW, *et al*. Prospective evaluation of thoracic ultrasound in the detection of pneumothorax. *J Trauma* 2001; 50:201–5.
2. Knudtson JL, Dort JM, Helmer SD, *et al*. Surgeon-performed ultrasound for pneumothorax in the trauma suite. *J Trauma* 2004; 56:527–30.
3. Alrajhi K, Woo MY, Vaillancourt C. Test Characteristics of Ultrasonography for the Detection of Pneumothorax: A Systematic Review and Meta-analysis. *Chest* Published online before print, August 25, 2011, doi:10.1378/chest.11-0131.
4. Nagarsheth K, Kurek S. Ultrasound detection of pneumothorax compared with chest x-ray and computed tomography scan. *Am Surg* 2011; 77:480–3.
5. Brook OR, Beck-Razi N, Abadi S, *et al*. Sonographic detection of pneumothorax by radiology residents as part of Extended Focused Assessment with Sonography for Trauma. *J Ultrasound Med* 2009; 28:749–55.

6. Dean AJ, Carr BC, Gracias VH, *et al*. Ultrasound evaluation of the thorax as component of the Focused Assessment by Sonography in Trauma. *Ann Emerg Med* 2006; 48:87.

7. Tam MM. Occult pneumothorax in trauma patients: should this be sought in focused assessment with sonography for trauma examination. *Emerg Med Australas* 2005; 17: 488–93.

8. Ratanen NW. Diagnostic ultrasound: diseases of the thorax. *Vet Clin North Am* 1986; 2: 49–66.

9. Wernecke K, Galanski M, Peters PE, *et al*. Pneumothorax: evaluation by ultrasound – preliminary results. *J Thorac Imaging* 1987; 2:76–8.

10. Kirkpatrick AW, Sirois M, Laupland KB, *et al*. Hand-held thoracic sonography for detecting post-traumatic pneumothoraces: the extended Focused Assessment with Sonography for Trauma (EFAST). *J Trauma* 2004; 57:288–95.

11. Blaivas M, Lyon M, Duggal S. A prospective comparison of supine chest radiography and bedside ultrasound for the diagnosis of traumatic pneumothorax. *Acad Emerg Med* 2005; 12:844–9.

12. Zhang M, Liu ZH, Yang JX, *et al*. Rapid detection of pneumothorax by ultrasonography in patients with multiple trauma. *Crit Care* 2006; 10:R112–R118.

13. Soldati G, Testa A, Sher S, *et al*. Occult traumatic pneumothorax: Diagnostic accuracy of lung ultrasonography in the emergency department. *Chest* 2008; 133:204–11.

14. Lichtenstein DA, Menu Y. A bedside ultrasound sign for ruling out pneumothorax in the critically ill. *Chest* 1995; 108:1345–8.

15. Lichtenstein DA, Meziere G, Biderman P, *et al*. The comet tail artefact: an ultrasound sign ruling out pneumothorax. *Intensive Care Med* 1999; 25:383–8.

16. Lichtenstein DA, Meziere G, Lascols N, *et al*. Ultrasound diagnosis of occult pneumothorax. *Crit Care Med* 2005; 33:1231–8.

17. Lee KL, Graham CA, Yeung JHH, *et al*. Occult pneumothorax in Chinese patients with significant blunt chest trauma: Incidence and management. *J Injury* 2010; 41:492–4.

18. Ball CG, Hameed SM, Evans D, *et al*. Occult pneumothorax in the mechanically ventilated trauma patient. *Can J Surg* 2003; 46:373–9.

19. de Moya MA, Seaver C, Spaniolas K, *et al*. Occult pneumothorax in trauma patients: Development of an objective scoring system. *J Trauma* 2007; 63:13–7.

20. Ouellet JF, Trottier V, Kmet L, *et al*. The OPTICC trial; a multi-institutional study of occult pneumothoraces in critical care. *Am J Surg* 2009; 197:581–6.

21. Wall SD, Federle MP, Jeffrey RB, *et al*. CT diagnosis of unsuspected pneumothorax after blunt abdominal trauma. *Am J Radiol* 1983; 141:919–21.

22. Guerrero-Lopez F, Vazquez-Mata G, Alcazar-Romero PP, *et al*. Evaluation of the utility of computed tomography in the initial assessment of the critical care patient with chest trauma. *Crit Care Med* 2000; 28:1370–5.

23. Plurad D, Green D, Demetriades D, *et al*. The increasing use of chest computer tomography for trauma: Is it being overused? *J Trauma* 2007; 62:631–5.

24. Laws D, Neville E, Duffy J. BTS guidelines of the insertion of a chest drain. *Thorax* 2003; 58(suppl):53–9.

25. American College of Surgeons Committee on Trauma. Advanced Trauma Life Support for Doctors: ATLS Student Course Manual. 8th Edition. Chicago: American College of Surgeons; Chapter 4; Thoracic Trauma, pp. 85–101.

26. Ball CG, Kirkpatrick AW, Feliciano DV. The occult pneumothorax: What have we learned? *Can J Surg* 2009; 52:174–9.

27. Enderson BL, Abdalla R, Frame SB, *et al*. Tube thoracostomy for occult pneumothorax: A prospective randomised study of its use. *J Trauma* 1993; 35:726–30.

28. Brasel KJ, Stafford RE, Weigelt JA, *et al*. Treatment of occult pneumothoraces from blunt trauma. *J Trauma* 1999; 46:987–91.

29. Moore FO, Goslar PW, Coimbra R, *et al*. Blunt traumatic occult pneumothorax: is observation safe?-results of a prospective, AAST multicenter study. *J Trauma* 2011; 70:1019–25.

30. Holmes JF, Brant WE, Bogren HG, *et al*. Prevalence and importance of pneumothoraces visualized on abdominal computed tomographic scan in children with blunt trauma. *J Trauma* 2001; 50:516–20.

31. Yadav K, Jalili M, Zehtabchi S. Management of traumatic occult pneumothorax. *Resuscitation* 2010; 81:1063–8.

4 Facial burns and inhalation injury

Duncan Bootland

☞ Expert Commentary Baljit Dheansa

Case history

A 66-year-old lady is brought to the emergency department from a house fire. The paramedic crew report the fire appears to have started in the bedroom where the patient was found lying unconscious in bed next to her husband. Her husband has been declared dead at the scene.

An accompanying relative is able to give a past medical history of congestive cardiac failure, type 2 diabetes mellitus with peripheral neuropathy, and ischaemic heart disease.

On arrival in the ED it is noted that the paramedic has already sited a naso-pharyngeal airway. Her observations are: respiratory rate 24 min^{-1}, oxygen saturations 99 % on high flow oxygen via a reservoir mask, blood pressure 115/55, pulse 90 min^{-1}, and temperature 33 °C.

See Box 4.1 for a clinical summary of burns.

Box 4.1 Clinical summary of burns

- Approximately 175 000 people attend UK emergency departments with burns every year,[1] accounting for between 0.5–1.5 % of total attendances[1,2]

- Around 13 000 burns patients per year are admitted to hospital (40 % to non-specialist units) with 300 going on to die from their injury[3]

- Observational studies of large series of burns patients have shown an incidence of inhalational injury of between 4 % and 19.6 %[4,5,6]

- Inhalation injury is strongly associated with mortality; death rates of burns patients admitted to burns units without inhalation injury are around 4 %, but those with the injury comprise up to 30 %[4,5,6]

- The proportion of patients intubated for suspected inhalation injury has risen dramatically in the last 15 years but in over half of these an inhalation burn cannot subsequently be demonstrated[7]

- Inhalation injury can be divided into a) injury to the upper airway including the glottis, b) injury to the lower airways, and c) systemic injury due to inhalation of toxic substances such as carbon monoxide or cyanide[8]

☞ Expert comment

It is important to get a history of level of consciousness (Glasgow coma scale) at the scene and any changes that occur. This may help inform decisions regarding airway management as well as raise the possibility of any other causes of altered consciousness such as drugs, alcohol, or cardiovascular incident.

In addition, finding out what was burning within the house may be able to offer clues as to risk of cyanide poisoning as this may occur in concert with carbon-monoxide poisoning.

Clinical question: In patients with suspected inhalation injury, who should we intubate?

Inhalation injury carries a high mortality and as such early, intubation of appropriate patients is crucial. However, the process of intubation can be difficult and mechanical ventilation of burns patients, particularly those with an inhalation injury, not only carries a substantial risk of ventilator associated pneumonia but has also been associated with higher rates of fluid administration and poorer outcomes[7,9,10,11].

The Advanced Trauma Life Support (ATLS) course[12] teaches that there are clinical indicators of inhalation injury and hence these should be actively looked for in patients with burns. These include face and/or neck burns, singeing of the eyebrows and nasal vibrissae, carbon deposits and acute inflammatory change in the oropharynx, carbonaceous sputum, hoarseness, a history of impaired mentation and/or confinement in a burning environment, explosion with burns to head and torso, or carboxyhaemoglobin level greater than 10 %. It has been suggested that the widespread adoption of the ATLS course as a standard for trauma care may well explain the increased rates of intubation of burns patients over the last 15 years[7].

⊘ Evidence base Intubation in suspected inhalational injury

Madnani et al. (2006):[13] conducted a retrospective review of 41 patients presenting to the ED of a regional US burn centre where fibre-optic laryngoscopy is a routine part of the assessment of all patients in whom an inhalation burn is suspected. Eight patients subsequently needed intubation: 4 for worsening hoarseness, 2 for a change in mental status due to hypoxia, 1 after developing stridor, and 1 for airway protection after becoming agitated. No symptoms (hoarseness, drooling, stidor, dysphagia) were significantly associated with the need for intubation. On physical examination, soot in the oral cavity ($p < 0.001$), facial burns ($p = 0.025$), and body burns ($p = 0.025$) were all significantly associated with the need for intubation. At laryngoscopic examination, oedema of the true vocal cords ($p < 0.001$) or false vocal cords ($p < 0.01$) were associated with the need for intubation.

Muehlberger et al. (1998):[14] prospectively studied 62 consecutive patients with suspected inhalation injuries admitted to a regional US burn centre. Eleven patients were subsequently enrolled; 6 had clinical findings and symptoms that traditionally would have suggested they be intubated. All patients went on to have fibre-optic laryngoscopy and although 4 patients had 'moderate to severe supraglottic and/or glottis oedema', the airway diameter was deemed sufficient in all patients to allow observation rather than endotracheal intubation.

Answer

The decision to intubate patients with suspected inhalation injuries should not be based on symptoms alone and is likely to be facilitated by the use of fibre-optic laryngoscopy, particularly in those with soot in the oral cavity or facial or body burns.

Although the decision to intubate or not is relatively easy in the most extreme cases, those who appear well but have facial burns or soot in the oral cavity present more of a dilemma. The current evidence highlights this difficulty and suggests that whilst symptoms of stridor, hoarseness, drooling, or dysphagia do not predict the need for intubation, those with soot in the mouth or facial or body burns should be further assessed with fibre-optic laryngoscopy to assess the need for intubation.

❝ Expert comment

The decision to intubate is difficult and should be made by someone who is experienced in airway management. Soot on the face can sometimes be misleading and should not be taken as an indication for intubation. However significant facial burns with swelling will require assessment. As with many situations, this is a dynamic process and so constant re-assessment is essential. During the assessment and observation phase it is essential to keep the patient as upright as possible to reduce oedema and aid breathing. A further concern is the patient's temperature as she is at risk of

(continued)

hypothermia, and it is essential to keep the patient warm to help reduce the negative impact of this low temperature on the patient's physiology.

In addition to the airway, one must also take into consideration the extent of any acidosis on blood gas analysis. A low pH with a raised lactate may indicate a metabolic as well as a respiratory acidosis which may require intubation and ventilation. This is especially likely in cases of cyanide poisoning or when associated with large burns.

Case progression

The examining doctor reports bilateral wheeze in the chest, singed eyebrows, a superficial dermal burn to the right cheek, right arm, torso, and leg estimated at 15 % total body surface area. Soot is noted around and in the mouth. The Glasgow Coma Score is 10/15 (Eyes 2, Verbal 3, Motor 5) but there is no evidence of head or other injury.

Due to her reduced conscious level and the clinical impression of a high likelihood of inhalation injury, the patient is intubated by rapid sequence induction. At laryngoscopy she is found to have soot visible down to the larynx with swollen vocal cords. An initial arterial blood gas (ABG) on high flow oxygen immediately post-intubation shows: pH 7.16, pCO_2 4.1 kPa, pO_2 60 kPa, base excess–9.1 mmol/l, lactate 8.9 mmol/l, and a carboxyhaemoglobin (COHb) level of 33 %.

The history of having been found confined and unconscious in a house fire along with the clinical findings of soot in the mouth and COHb level of 33 % point to a diagnosis of inhalation injury. In a neurologically normal patient it might have been appropriate to further assess the airway with fibre-optic laryngoscopy but in this case the findings, in association with her significantly reduced conscious level, make it clear that the patient needs to be intubated.

The arterial blood gas result highlights the presence of tissue hypoxia. The COHb of 33 % directs us to a diagnosis of carbon-monoxide poisoning but given the markedly high lactate, a diagnosis of cyanide poisoning must be considered.

⊗ **Learning point** Cyanide poisoning

Hydrogen cyanide gas is produced during incomplete combustion of nitrogen containing components including plastic, polyurethane, silk, or wool. Cyanide is a small lipid soluble molecule and is easily absorbed, and rapidly distributed, via ingestion, inhalation, or dermal or eye exposure[15,16]. Cyanide is highly toxic and death may occur within seconds or minutes of a large dose.

Cyanide's primary toxic effect is caused by blockage of the intracellular respiration chain responsible for the formation of intracellular adenosine triphosphate. Cyanide binds to the ferric ion of the cytochrome (a–a_3) complex, an essential intra-mitochondrial enzyme used in the electron transport chain. Cells and organs that are particularly dependent on high oxygen usage such as the central nervous system and myocardium are particularly affected[15]. High levels of cyanide have been seen to result in pulmonary oedema and it is hypothesized that this is due to a direct pulmonary arteriolar and/or coronary artery vasoconstriction[17].

Clinical question: In suspected cyanide poisoning, what is the best antidote?

The College of Emergency Medicine recommends that dicobalt edetate or hydroxocobalamin or sodium nitrite and sodium thiosulphate be available in EDs for use in cyanide poisoning[18]. The ideal antidote would 'have rapid onset of action, neutralize cyanide without interfering with cellular oxygen use, tolerability and safety profiles conducive to prehospital use, safe for use with smoke-inhalation victims, not [be] harmful when administered to non-poisoned patients, [and] easy to administer'.[19] Important considerations in the decision on which antidote to use include; the failure of sodium thiosulphate to act quickly in reactivating cellular respiration, the contraindication to the use of sodium nitrite and other methaemoglobin-inducing antidotes in the presence of carbon-monoxide poisoning, and the toxic side-effects of dicobalt edetate, particularly in the absence of cyanide poisoning—a real possibility if a presumptive diagnosis is being made. Although there is no consensus on the best antidote of these options, increasingly hydroxocobalamin is being recognized as fulfilling many of the ideal requirements.

> ### ✅ Evidence base Hydroxocobalamin in cyanide poisoning
>
> **Bebarta et al. (2010):**[20] performed a comparison of hydroxocobalamin and sodium thiosulphate vs sodium nitrite and sodium thiosulphate in treatment of intravenous cyanide poisoning of a swine model. Twenty-four pigs were anaesthetized and ventilated and an intravenous protocol of cyanide was given to induce a reduction in mean arterial pressure of 50%, a degree of poisoning the group had previously shown to be lethal in 100% of cases. Subjects were then randomized to one of the two antidotes. The pigs were monitored until 40 mins after the start of the antidote infusion. The hydroxocobalamin group had a significantly quicker return to baseline mean arterial pressure and reduction in serum cyanide levels compared to the sodium nitrite group, although there was no difference in mortality over the time period studied.
>
> **Boron et al. (2007):**[21] conducted a prospective observational study of 69 adult smoke-inhalation patients suspected of cyanide poisoning as judged by soot in the face, mouth, or nose, or expectorations and neurologic impairment. All the patients were given an intravenous infusion of 5 g of hydroxocobalamin either at the scene or on admission to a toxicology ICU. Cyanide poisoning, as defined as a blood level of ≥ 39 µmol/L and measured in a pre-antidote sample, was found *a posteriori* to have been present in 42 patients. Fifty of the 69 patients survived after admission to the ICU and hydroxocobalamin was not associated with any serious adverse events. Although given the lack of a control group the study was unable to comment on the effectiveness of hydroxocobalamin, it did suggest that it was a safe intervention in critically ill patients suspected of cyanide poisoning.

Answer

Although the data are limited, in suspected cyanide poisoning, hydroxocobalamin appears to be safe and as equally effective as other cyanide antidotes and it does not have many of their limitations.

> ### ➕ Clinical tip When to use a cyanide antidote
>
> As already discussed, there are problems with most of the potential antidotes for cyanide, and in the current economic climate the relatively high cost of hydroxocobalamin should not be underestimated. Making the diagnosis of cyanide poisoning can be challenging given that in inhalation injury it will often co-exist with the easier to diagnose and also toxic carbon-monoxide poisoning. Equally, in a setting where only dicobalt edetate is available, the knowledge that using it in someone who is not cyanide toxic may cause significant side effects makes the decision to treat even more difficult.
>
> As cyanide measurement is not available in routine practice, the following may guide the clinician in making the diagnosis of cyanide poisoning:[15,16]
>
> * Altered mental status, unconsciousness and convulsions
> * Soot in the mouth or expectoration
> * Blood lactate > 7 mmol/L

(continued)

- Elevated anion gap acidosis
- Reduced arterio-venous oxygen gradient

As with any critically ill patient, the response to treatment will be more valuable than any one-off finding, and in patients who do not improve and whose blood lactate does not fall despite adequate resuscitative efforts, cyanide poisoning should be considered.

> **❝ Expert comment**
>
> The diagnosis of cyanide poisoning is very difficult and in cases of concern it is best to liaise with the local burns service who will be able to guide the decision-making process. Many burns services now tend to use hydroxocobalamin as their treatment for cyanide poisoning.

Case progression

In view of the clinical history and the blood gas results it is decided to administer hydroxycobalamin and the patient is then intubated. Post-intubation, you turn your attention to your patient's carbon-monoxide level and wonder if there is a role for hyperbaric oxygen therapy.

Clinical question: In patients with carbon monoxide poisoning, should we refer for hyperbaric oxygen therapy?

> **✪ Learning point** Carbon monoxide poisoning
>
> Carbon monoxide, a colourless, tasteless, and odourless gas, is generated during the incomplete combustion of carbon-containing substances. Carbon monoxide combines with haemoglobin with an affinity of more than 200 times that of oxygen, shifting the oxygen dissociation curve to the left and hence impairing oxygen delivery to the tissues. Other mechanisms of toxicity include increasing cytosolic heme levels, resulting in oxidative stress, and by interrupting cellular respiration by binding to platelet heme protein and cytochrome c oxidase.[22] The resulting hypoxia is responsible for the many symptoms and signs seen in acute poisoning: headache, nausea, irritability, and weakness leading to dizziness, agitation, impaired consciousness, and respiratory failure.
>
> Markers of severity are considered to be one or more of:[23]
>
> - Any new objective acute neurological signs
> - Need for ventilation
> - ECG indication of infarction or ischaemia
> - Clinically significant acidosis
> - Initial carboxyhaemoglobin > 30% (although it is to be noted that the correlation between carboxyhaemoglobin level and clinical outcome is weak)
>
> Although the majority of patients can be expected to recover uneventfully, some are noted to develop neuropsychological sequelae with one trial reporting cognitive sequelae in 46% and affective sequelae in 45% of poisoned patients treated with normobaric oxygen therapy. The half-life of carbon monoxide in air is 4 hours, when breathing 100% oxygen at sea level it is 40 mins, and at 2.5 atmospheres it will drop to approximately 20 mins. Despite the relatively unimpressive drop in half-life by providing hyperbaric oxygen, and the inherent risks and cost in transferring a carbon monoxide poisoned patient to one of the few centres that provide it, some authors have suggested that the hyperbaric oxygen is effective in reducing the neurological sequelae seen in carbon monoxide poisoning and hence should be adopted.

> **✔ Evidence base** Hyperbaric oxygen therapy in carbon monoxide poisoning
>
> Weaver *et al.* (2002):[24] conducted a double-blind randomized controlled trial to look at normobaric versus hyperbaric oxygen therapy in patients with all degrees of carbon-monoxide poisoning including intubated patients. Patients with symptomatic acute carbon-monoxide poisoning were randomized to three chamber sessions within 24 hours of either three hyperbaric oxygen treatments or one normobaric oxygen treatment plus two sessions of exposure to normobaric room air.

(continued)

The trial enrolled 152 patients but was stopped early after the third of 4 planned interim analyses showed a significant reduction in cognitive sequelae in the hyperbaric group at 6 weeks (25 % vs 46.1 %, $p = 0.007$ and 12 months ($p = 0.04$) according to the intention to treat analysis.

Scheinkestel *et al.* (1999):[25] conducted a randomized double-blind trial of 230 patients with all degrees of carbon-monoxide poisoning. They were randomized to daily, 100 minute treatments with 100 % oxygen in a hyperbaric chamber over three days, with the intervention group receiving 60 minutes at 2.8 atmospheres and the control group being at 1.0 atmosphere throughout. Hyperbaric oxygen patients had a worse outcome in learning test at completion of treatment ($p = 0.01$), a greater number of abnormal test results at completion of treatment ($p = 0.02$), and delayed neurological sequelae were restricted to the hyperbaric group ($p = 0.03$). They concluded hyperbaric oxygen did not benefit and may have worsened outcomes.

Buckley *et al.* (2011):[26] in a cochrane review which analysed 6 trials, including the 2 trials just mentioned, concluded that there was insufficient evidence to support the use of hyperbaric oxygen for the treatment of patients with carbon monoxide poisoning.

Answer

The available evidence is not sufficient to recommend the use of hyperbaric oxygen therapy in acute carbon-monoxide poisoning.

> **☆ Learning point**   Advances in the ED management of inhalation injury
>
> Whilst it is self-evident that patients with a significant inhalation injury should be discussed with a burns unit and managed in a critical care setting at the very minimum, they will often spend a considerable time in the ED awaiting transfer. There is an increasing evidence base for the use of nebulized therapy in these patients. Nebulized heparin and N-acetylcysteine has been shown in children with massive burns and smoke inhalation to reduce mortality and re-intubation rates, albeit with historical controls.[27]
>
> The commencement of nebulized therapy in the ED is feasible and as with other interventions early in the course of the critically unwell patient, it has the potential to have positive impact on outcomes. Further good quality multi-centre trials would be needed to drive a change in the current practice of providing only supportive care.

Case progression

In view of the extensiveness of the patient's burns together with the likely inhalation injury, it is decided to transfer the patient to the local burns unit. She is ventilated with 100 % oxygen and fluid resuscitation is commenced according to the Parkland formula[28] prior to transfer.

> **✚ Clinical tip**   The Parkland formula
>
> The profound inflammatory response seen after a burn results in high fluid requirements. The most commonly employed resuscitation formula to calculate the fluid requirement in a burns patient is the Parkland formula.[28]
>
> - 4 mls (Ringers Lactate) × % total body surface area of burn × weight (kg)
> - The first half being given in the first 8 hours and the remainder in the following 18 hours
> - Fluid should be titrated to maintain a urine output 0.5–1.0 mL/Kg/hr
>
> Research is ongoing in this area and debate continues into optimum volumes, the use of colloids, resuscitation protocols, and hypertonic fluids.

❝ Expert comment

In addition to the lack of clear evidence for the benefit of hyperbaric oxygen one also has to note that in the UK such facilities are not close to any burns service and therefore the management of any concomitant burn will be compromised.

❝ Expert comment

Fluid requirements often exceed those predicted by the Parkland formula because of the lung injury. Usually such injuries deteriorate at about 48–72 hours because of inflammation generated by the soot in the lungs and therefore they require increased ventilatory support. They may also require further therapeutic bronchoscopies to reduce the amount of soot in the lungs.

A Final Word from the Expert

Inhalation injury is a life threatening complication in the patient with burns. Early recognition and treatment can reduce morbidity and mortality in this group of patients. Early liaison with the burns team will help guide management regarding intubation, treatment for cyanide poisoning, and early inhalation therapy.

References

1. Chipp E, Walton J, Gorman DF, *et al.* A 1 year study of burn injuries in a British Emergency Department. *Burns* 2008; 34(4):516–20.
2. Khan AA, Rawlins J, Shenton AF, *et al.* The Bradford Burn Study: the epidemiology of burns presenting to an inner city emergency department. *Emerg Med J* 2007; 24(8):564–6.
3. NBC, National Burn Care Review; 2000. <http://www.ibidb.org/downloads/doc_download/1-2001-national-burn-care-review>
4. Muller MJ, Pegg SP, Rule MR. Determinants of death following burn injury. *Br J Surg.* 2001; 88(4):583–7.
5. Saffle JR, Davis B, Williams P. Recent outcomes in the treatment of burn injuries in the United States: a report from the American Burn Association Patient registry. *J Burn Care Rehabil* 1995; 16:219–32.
6. Smith DL, Cairns BA, Ramadan F, *et al.* Effect of inhalational injury, burn size, and age on mortality: a study of 1447 consecutive burn patients. *J Trauma* 1994; 37(4):655–9.
7. Mackie DP, van Dehn F, Knape P, *et al.* Increase in Early Mechanical Ventilation of Burn Patients: An Effect of Current Emergency Trauma Management? *J Trauma* 2011; 70(3):611–15.
8. Cancio LC. Current concepts in the pathophysiology and treatment of inhalation injury. *Trauma* 2005; 7:19–35.
9. Cook D, Walter S, Cook R, *et al.* Incidence of and risk factors for ventilator-associated pneumonia in critically ill patients. *Ann Intern Med* 1998; 129(6):433–40.
10. Soni N, Williams P. Positive pressure ventilation: what is the real cost? *Br J Anaesth.* 2008; 101(4):446–457.
11. Shirani KZ, Pruitt BA, Jr, Mason AD, Jr. The influence of inhalation injury and pneumonia on burn mortality. *Ann Surg* 205(1): 82–87.
12. American College of Surgeons Committee on Trauma. *Advanced Trauma Life Support, Student Course Manual*, 8th Edition. Chicago: American College of Surgeons, 2008.
13. Madnani DD, Steele NP, de Vries E. Factors that predict the need for intubation in patients with smoke inhalation injury. *ENT J* 2006; 85(4):278–80.
14. Muehlberger T, Kunar D, Munster A, *et al.* Efficacy of Fiberoptic Laryngoscopy in the Diagnosis of Inhalation Injuries. *Arch Otolaryngol Head Neck Surg.* 1998; 124(9):1003–7.
15. Lawson-Smith P, Jansen EC, Hyldegaard O. Cyanide intoxication as part of smoke inhalation-a review on diagnosis and treatment from the emergency perspective. *Scand J Trauma Resusc Emerg Med.* 2011; 19:14.
16. National Poisons Information Service Toxbase Guidance. <http://www.toxbase.org/Poisons-Index-A-Z/C-Products/Cyanide-----------/>
17. Beasley DM, Glass WI. Cyanide poisoning: pathophysiology and treatment recommendations. *Occup Med (Lond)* 1998; 48(7):427–31.
18. College of Emergency Medicine Guideline on Antidote Availability for Emergency Departments May 2008. <http://www.collemergencymed.ac.uk/Shop-Floor/Clinical%20Guidelines/College%20Guidelines>

19. Hall AH, Saiers J, Baud F. Which cyanide antidote? *Crit Rev Toxicol*. 2009; 39(7):541–52.

20. Bebarta VS, Tanen DA, Lairet J, *et al*. Hydroxocobalamin and Sodium Thiosulfate Versus Sodium Nitrite and Sodium Thiosulfate in the Treatment of Acute Cyanide Toxicity in a Swine (Sus scrofa) Model. *Ann Emerg Med* 2010; 55(4):345–51.

21. Boron SW, Baud FJ, Barriot P, *et al*. Prospective Study of Hydroxocobalamin for Acute Cyanide Poisoning in Smoke Inhalation. *Ann Emerg Med* 2007; 49(6):794–801.

22. Weaver LK. Carbon monoxide poisoning. *N Engl J Med* 2009; 360(12):1217–25.

23. National Poisons Information Service Toxbase Guidance, <http://www.toxbase.org/ Poisons-Index-A-Z/C-Products/Carbon-monoxide-A/>

24. Weaver LK, Hopkins RO, Chan KJ, *et al*. Hyperbaric oxygen for acute carbon monoxide poisoning. *N Engl J Med* 2002;347(14):1057–67.

25. Scheinkestel CD, Bailey M, Myles PS, *et al*. Hyperbaric or normobaric oxygen for acute carbon monoxide poisoning: a randomised controlled trial. *Med J Aust* 1999; 170(5):203–10

26. Buckley NA, Juurlink DN, Isbister G, *et al*. Hyperbaric oxygen for carbon monoxide poisoning. *Cochrane Database of Systematic Reviews* 2011, Issue 4. Art. No.: CD002041. doi: 10.1002/14651858.CD002041.pub3.

27. Desai MH, Micak R, Richardson J, *et al*. Reduction in Mortality in Pediatric Patients with Inhalation Injury with Aerosolized Heparin/Acetylcystine Therapy. *J Burn Care Rehabil* 1998; 19(3):210–12.

28. Baxter CR, Shires GT. Physiological response to crystalloid resuscitation of severe burns. *Ann NY Acad Sci* 1968; 150(3):874–94.

5 Paediatric head injury

Fleur Cantle

Expert Commentary Emer Sutherland

Case history

A 6-year-old boy is brought to the ED after falling 2 meters from a tree. The children with him report that he fell backwards from the tree and landed on his head and upper back, and confirmed that he was lying on the ground not moving until the ambulance crew arrived. The paramedics found he had a Glasgow Coma Scale (GCS) of 14 (E=4, V=4, M=6) with evidence of a 6 cm bleeding wound on the occiput. They were able to move him on a scoop but he became distressed when they tried to put a cervical collar on and his neck is therefore not immobilized.

See Box 5.1 for a clinical summary of paediatric trauma.

Box 5.1 Clinical summary of paediatric trauma

- Injury is the main cause of death and disability in children worldwide.[1]
- Head injury in children is a common presentation to the ED, the majority of attendances pertain to minor head injuries which require no further intervention.
- The incidence of head injuries requiring admission to paediatric intensive care unit (PICU) has been estimated at 5.6 per 100 000 population per year.[2] The mechanism of injury shows significant variation with age. In this study the most common mechanism was a pedestrian accident (36%) followed by falls (24%). In infants, 'suspected assault' accounted for 52% of injuries.

> **Learning point** Important considerations in paediatric head injury
>
> - The relative size of head to body particularly in young children leads to a higher centre of gravity and a predisposition to head trauma.
> - The cranial bones are thinner in children and therefore do not protect the contents of the skull as well as thicker adult bones.
> - The anterior fontanelle, which can be palpated in children up to around 18 months of age, may be tense in the setting of trauma due to raised intracranial pressure, or sunken due to volume loss.
> - Until the cranial sutures fuse there is room for limited expansion in the presence of raised intracranial pressure.

Case progression

On arrival at the hospital the child's primary survey revealed no evidence of airway compromise. The cervical spine was not immobilized but the child was lying still and not distressed. The chest examination was normal with no evidence of chest injury, oxygen saturations of 100%, and a respiratory rate of 16. The abdomen was soft and non-tender with no evidence of external injuries. The pelvis and long bones were stable and the pulse was 90 and BP 100/60. The GCS was still 14 E=3, V=5, M=6, and pupils were equal size 3 and reactive. A CT was requested, however the radiologist was reluctant to perform this advising instead close observation and a CT scan if any deterioration in the GCS occurred.

> **⊕ Expert comment**
>
> The immobilization of the cervical spine in the young child is a source of debate for the paediatric trauma team. The objective, to minimize movement, will not be achieved by restraining a resistant child. In these situations paediatric specialist nurses, play therapists, and the supported presence of a reassuring parent can achieve a position of safety. Cervical spine injuries in children are rare and associated with high-energy injuries. In such a situation general anaesthesia would be indicated to maintain safety and allow prompt and comprehensive imaging.
>
> If a young child is immobilized due consideration must be given to the anatomical variance of the occiput. Without additional support under the thorax the large occiput will push the neck into flexion, potentially exacerbating neurological injury. Forty per cent of the paediatric population also manifest a pseudosubluxation at the C2/C3 joint that can mimic true pathology due to ligament laxity, posing yet another challenge to the ED physician.

Clinical question: Which children require a CT of their head?

A CT scan of the head is the most frequently requested CT examination in young people and the number of CT scans being performed is increasing.[3] This reflects the increased diagnostic accuracy of CT scanners and their increased availability in recent years. It is too early to measure the lifetime risks of cancer following paediatric CT directly as the latency period may be over 40 years.[4] A recent large cohort study from Australia[5] concluded that for people exposed to at least one CT scan before the age of 20, cancer incidence was increased by 24% and that the proportional increase in cancer risk was greater after scans at young ages.

The balance of risk and benefit in this population has lead to the development of decision rules which use clinical data from original research to provide 3 or more predictor variables from history and examination[6] to reduce the uncertainty in medical decision-making by standardizing the collection and interpretation of clinical data.[7] A recent comparison[8] identified 3 high-quality clinical decision rules for the use of CT head in children with head injury (summarized in Table 5.1).

Table 5.1 Comparison of the CATCH, CHALICE, and PECARN decision rules for CT head requests

Paper	CATCH 2010 (Canada)[9] Aimed to derive a tool to identify children who require a CT scan	CHALICE 2006 (UK)[10] Aimed to derive a tool to identify children who require a CT scan	PECARN (USA)[11] Aimed to derive a tool to identify children who DID NOT require a CT scan
Population	3866 children (under 17) 10 tertiary paediatric teaching institutions emergency departments Blunt head trauma (GCS 13–15)	22772 children (under16) 10 emergency departments in north-west England Any history of signs of injury to the head	42412 children (under 18) Head trauma within 24 hrs GCS 14–15
Primary outcome	Need for neurological intervention	Clinically significant intracranial injury	Clinically important traumatic brain injury

(continued)

Comparison of predictor variables[8]

	CATCH	CHALICE	PECARN	
Mechanism of injury	Dangerous mechanism of injury	High-speed RTA as paedestrian, cyclist occupant (>40 miles/h) Fall >3 m in height High-speed injury from projectile or object	PECARN <2 years old Severe mechanism of injury	PECARN ≥2 years old Severe mechanism of injury
History	History of worsening headache*	Witnessed LOC >5 mins ≥3 discrete vomits Amnesia (retrograde/ anterograde >5 mins Suspicion on NAI Seizure in patient with no history of epilepsy	LOC ≥5 seconds Not acting normally per parent	LOC Severe headache Vomiting
Examination	GCS <15, 2h after injury* Irritability on examination* Any signs of a basal skull fracture Suspected open* or depressed skull fracture Large boggy scalp haematoma *high-risk factors	GCS <14 or <15 if less than 1 year old. Abnormal drowsiness Positive focal neurology Signs of a basal skull fracture Suspicion of penetrating or depressed skull injury or tense fontanelle Presence of bruise/ swelling/laceration >5 cm if <1 year old	GCS <15 Other signs of altered mental status Palpable or unclear skull fracture Occipital, parietal or temporal scalp haematoma	GCS <15 Other signs of altered mental status Clinical signs of basilar skull fracture
Accuracy of clinical decision rule	Need for neurological intervention (4 high-risk factors) Sensitivity 24/24 100% Specificity 2698/3842 70.2%	Clinically significant intracranial injury Sensitivity 277/281 98.6% Specificity 19558/22491 86.9%	Clinically important brain injury Sensitivity 72/73 98.6% Specificity 4528/8429 53.7%	Clinically important brain injury Sensitivity 208/215 96.7% Specificity 14656/25068 58.5%

CATCH: Data from Osmond MH, Klassen TP, Wells GA, et al., 'CATCH: a clinical decision rule for the use of computed tomography in children with minor head injury', Canadian Medical Association Journal, 2010, 182, 4, pp. 341–348. CHALICE: Adapted from Archives of Disease in Childhood, Dunning J, Daly JP, Lomas JP et al., 'Derivation of the children's head injury algorithm for the prediction of important clinical events decision rule for head injury in children', 91, 11, pp. 885–891, copyright 2006, with permission from BMJ Publishing Group Ltd. PECARN: Reprinted from The Lancet, 274, Kuppermann N, Holmes JF, Dayan PS, et al., 'Identification of children at low risk of clinically-important brain injuries after head trauma: a prospective cohort study', pp. 1160–1170, Copyright 2009, with permission from Elsevier.

Dunning J, Daly JP, Lomas JP et al. Derivation of the children's head injury algorithm for the prediction of important clinical events decision rule for head injury in children. Arch Dis Child 2006;91:885-891.

Kuppermann N, Holmes JF, Dayan PS, et al. Identification of children at low risk of clinically-important brain injuries after head trauma: a prospective cohort study. Lancet 2009 vol 274. 1160-1170.

The paper highlighted the comparable accuracy of the clinical decision rules (CDRs) despite heterogeneity of the studies in outcomes, age limits, inclusion and exclusion criteria, and differing severity of head injuries. This leads to uncertainty as to which would be most appropriate to implement. The CHALICE clinical decision rules have been incorporated into the 2007 NICE guidance for the management of head injuries and hence are likely to be used widely across the UK. It is recognized that implementation of the CHALICE rule leads to more CT scans;[12,13,14] however, there is no conclusive evidence that this increase is detrimental.

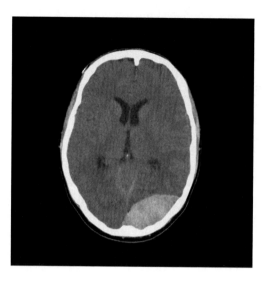

Figure 5.1 Extradural haemorrhage.

Answer

Validated decision rules aid decision making on the shop floor. It is important to be aware of which rules are being used locally (usually NICE), but to also appreciate that occasionally deviation from such guidelines may be necessary.

Case progression

It was decided to observe the child in the clinical decision unit. Twenty minutes later the GCS falls to 12 (E=4, V=3, M=5) and the patient is taken for an urgent CT scan (see Figure 5.1). The child continues to deteriorate and is taken to resuscitation area where the GCS is now 8 and the pulse is 45. The left arm and face are twitching abnormally and the anaesthetist decides to intubate the child. There are no neurosurgeons on site and the anaesthetist suggests using hypertonic saline to reduce intracranial pressure.

Clinical question: In paediatric head injury does hypertonic saline (HS) reduce intracranial pressure?

> ⭐ **Learning point** Osmotherapy for raised ICP
>
> Primary brain injury occurs at the time of impact and hence medical intervention is not able to influence its severity. Medical therapies are directed at strategies to reduce secondary brain damage which is mediated by multiple mechanisms but hypoxia and ischaemia pose the greatest threat.[15] Cerebral oedema (an increase in brain water resulting in an increase in total brain mass)[16] from the inflammatory response to trauma leads to increased intracranial pressure (ICP) leading to hypoxia and ischaemia.[15] In a damaged brain the normal mechanisms of ICP homeostasis are impaired or simply exceeded.[17]
>
> Osmotherapy uses substances to increase the osmotic pressure of plasma and hence encourage movement of water from the interstitial space to the vascular space to reduce ICP.

HS differs from isotonic saline (normal/0.9 %) in the number of osmoles of sodium and chloride contained in the solution. The mechanisms of action leading to a reduction in oedema and ICP are likely to be complex and multiple.[18] The primary mechanism is thought to be through dehydration of brain tissue by creating an osmotic gradient and drawing water into the intravascular space through an intact blood–brain barrier.

HS is available in commercially available 2.7 % solutions or can be made up to a 3 % solution from 30 % saline.[19] HS is recommended in the Advanced Paediatric Life Support Course[20] for clinical signs of raised intracranial pressure.

There are no randomized controlled trials on paediatric subjects in this area. Overall the studies are heterogeneous in terms of the regimes and concentrations of hypertonic saline used. The studies have mostly taken place in the Paediatric Intensive care unit where the population differ greatly from the ED population in terms of time from injury and other concurrent interventions. See Table 5.2.

Clinical tip Hypertonic saline in head injury

The London Air ambulance in its pre-hospital care head injury standard operating procedure[21] recommends 6 mls of 5 % (to a maximum of 350 mls) by a well-secured, large bore (>18G) cannula to patients with signs of actual or impending herniation secondary to head injury:

- Unilateral or bilateral pupil dilation and GCS of <8 (usually 3)
- Progressive hypertension (SBP > 160 mmHg) and bradycardia (pulse < 60) and GCS < 8 (usually 3)

Table 5.2 Summary of evidence of the use of hypertonic saline in paediatric head injury

Study	Design, subjects, and Intervention	Main results
Fisher et al. (1992)[22]	Double-blind randomized crossover study 18 Children traumatic brain injury PICU Bolus (10 ml/kg) of 0.9 % and 3 % saline the first 2 times the patient met the entry criteria Followed up for 2 hrs post each bolus	No significant change in ICP in 0.9 % saline group ($p=0.32$) 4 % increase in ICP Significant change in ICP in 3 % group ($p=0.003$) 21 % reduction in ICP in 3 % saline group No evidence of morbidity of mortality associated with saline infusion
Simma et al. (1998)[23]	Open randomized prospective study 35 consecutive children Head injury GCS <8 Entered trial at time of first ICP measurement Paediatric intensive care Ringers lactate (Group 1) or Hypertonic saline (Group 2) as maintenance 1200 mL/m² for 72 hrs Standard scheme of interventions if ICP >15 mmHg increased in the study period	Inverse relationship between serum sodium concentrations and ICP 1) r=−13 ($p<0.03$) 2) r=−29 ($p<0.001$) Survival 94 % The 2 patients who died were in group 1 Group 1 patients significantly longer in ICU ($p<0.04$) Significantly more interventions in group 1 ($p<0.01$)
Khanna et al. (2000)[24]	Prospective descriptive study 10 children Severe head injury GCS <8 Paediatric Intensive care. Failure of conventional treatment. A continuous infusion of 3 % saline on 'sliding scale' to achieve a target serum sodium level that would maintain ICP <20 mmHg. (rescue therapy)	Significant decrease in ICP spike frequency vs time zero ($p<0.01$) Significant increase in CPP vs time zero ($p<0.01$) Mean GOS 4 (moderate disability) 1 patient died of uncontrollable ICP 2 patients developed renal failure (associated with sepsis)
Peterson et al. (2000)[25]	Retrospective observational study Closed traumatic head injury Intracranial pressure >20 mmHg 68 Children PICU Continuous infusion of 3 % saline to raise serum sodium to the level required to reduce ICP to <20 mmHg and <15 mmHg in those with an open fontanelle	41 predicted survivors and 58 actual survivors (Z=6, W=17) Mean Glasgow outcome score for all patients 3.9 (+/- 1.4) Correlation with highest Na and outcome: Na160-169 14/19 (72 %) had a good to moderate outcome Na 170-179 4/7 (57 %) had good to moderate outcome Na 180+ did poorly; 3 died and 1 severe No renal failure

Data from various sources (see references)

Answer

Currently there is insufficient evidence to mandate changes in standards of care in
the ED, but these studies suggest the use of HS as rescue therapy is safe.

Case progression

You are waiting for the retrieval team and a discussion starts between the anaesthetist and the ED FY2 about cooling and cerebral protection. You wonder whether
there would be any benefit to cooling this child.

Clinical question: Does cooling a child after traumatic brain injury improve long-term outcome?

Therapeutic hypothermia is thought to reduce cerebral metabolism and attenu-
ates multiple cellular injury cascades,[30] hence may reduce secondary brain injury.
Induced hypothermia has been found to lead to improved neurological outcome
in neonates with hypoxic ischaemic encephalopathy,[31,32] and in adults after cardiac arrest due to ventricular fibrillation.[33] The possibility of a beneficial effect of
hypothermia after head injury was raised in the 1950s in a retrospective trial of 18
children.[34] This study concluded that systemic cooling after head injury was a 'useful adjunct' and could improve outcome. Since then there have been a number of
randomized trials which have considered this intervention. See Table 5.3.

Table 5.3 Summary of evidence of the use of hypothermia after paediatric head injury

Study	Design and intervention	Main results
Adelson et al. (2005)[35]	Multicentre randomized controlled trial 48 children <13 years with severe traumatic brain injury (GCS</=8) Additional parallel single institution trial of 27 excluded patients (delay in transfer, unknown time of injury and adolescence) Moderate hypothermia (32–33 °C) for 48 hrs or normothermia (36.5–37.5 °C)	No difference in mortality between the groups No difference in complications between the 2 groups No significant difference between groups on neurocognitive measures at 3 and 6 months
Hutchinson et al. (2008)[36]	Multicenter (17), international (3 countries) randomized controlled trial Children with severe traumatic brain injury GCS <8 (225 children randomized) Block-stratified randomization to hypothermia therapy (32.5 °C for 24 hrs—within 8 hrs after injury) or normothermia (37 °C)	At 6 months 31 % in the hypothermia group compared to 22 % of patients in the normothermia group had an unfavourable outcome RR (1.41 (95 %CI 0.89–2.22 p=0.14) 23 deaths (21 %) in the hypothermia group, and 14 (12 %) in the normothermia group RR 1.40 (95 %CI 0.9–2.27 p =0.06)
Li et al. (2009)[37]	Single-centre randomized controlled trial. 22 children with severe traumatic brain injury Moderate hypothermia (intracranial temperature of 34.5 +/- 0.2 °C for 72 hrs or normothermia (intracranial temperature of 38.0+/-0.5 °C)	ICP level in the moderate hypothermia group was lower than the control group at every time point) p<0.01) At 24, 48, and 72 hrs the NSE, S-100, and CK-BB levels in the moderate group were lower than the levels in the normothermia group (p<0.01).

Data from various sources (see references)

The largest multicentre randomised controlled trial found no difference in outcome in cooled patients. Another large multicentre RCT was commenced in February 2007[38] (the Cool Kids trial) but terminated in February 2011 on the grounds of futility. At present there is one unpublished but completed study registered with <http://www.clinicaltrials.gov>.[39]

Answer

Routine therapeutic hypothermia cannot be recommended after severe traumatic brain injury in children, but the topic should be the subject of ongoing investigation.

> **❻ Expert comment**
>
> Hypothermia in trauma is controversial having previously been regarded as part of the 'triad of death'[40]—hypothermia, coagulopathy, and acidosis. Head-injured patients require strict medical/critical care management as well as neurosurgical intervention.
>
> It was recognized in the work of Hutchinson[36] that one limitation of this work is that it might be more effective if initiated earlier as has been seen in animal models.[41] One of the difficulties facing research in emergency medicine which is particularly evident in the paediatric population is the ethical challenges associated with consent at the front door.

Case progression

The child is safely transferred to the local neurosurgical centre where the child has a decompressive craniectomy and a bolt inserted.

See Box 5.2 for future advances in the management of head injury.

Box 5.2 Future advances

S100b is a protein released by astrocytes that can be used as peripheral biomarker of brain injury if the blood–brain barrier is damaged.[42] In a review of predominantly adult patients,[43] it was found that high levels of S100b is a marker of poor long-term outcome following minor and major head injury, however it is also being considered as a marker to be used at the front door in order to omit unnecessary CT scans. Whilst there have been some promising results,[44] a recent literature review of the use of S100b in children with mild traumatic brain injury[45] concluded that whilst a normal value could rule out injury associated abnormalities on CT scan in the majority of cases the variability in normal level due to age, sex, blood sampling time, and extra-cranial S100b release may make interpretation difficult. Work continues in this area.

A Final Word from the Expert

Whilst accident prevention policies and public education both attempt to reduce the incidence of serious trauma at source, we continue to see large numbers of injured children within the ED. Robust studies on a paediatric population are difficult to achieve, particularly at the front door, but the anatomical and physiological differences between children and adults make extrapolation from adult studies problematic. This, together with differing injury patterns should encourage us to strive to find answers from exclusive paediatric studies when available.

References

1. Segul-Gomez, M. Mackenzie EJ. Measuring the public health impact of injury. *Epidemiol. Rev* 2003; 25:3–19.
2. Parslow RC, Morris KP, Tasker RC, *et al*. UK Paediatric Traumatic Brain Injury Study Steering Group; Paediatric Intensive Care Society Study Group. Epidemiology of traumatic brain injury in children receiving intensive care in the UK. *Arch Dis Child*. 2005 Nov; 90(11):1182–7.
3. Pearce MS, Salotti JA, Howe NL, *et al*. CT Scans in Young People in Great Britain: Temporal and Descriptive Patterns, 1993–2002 *Radiology Research and Practice* 2012; Article ID 594278, 8 pages. doi:10.1155/2012/594278.
4. Brenner DJ, Elliston CD, Hall EJ, *et al*. Estimates of the cancer risks from pediatric CT radiation are not merely theoretical: Comment on 'Point/Counterpoint: In x-ray computed tomography, technique factors should be selected appropriate to patient size. Against the Proposition'. *Medical Physics* November 2001; 28(11):2387–8.
5. Mathews JD, Forsythe AV, Brady Z, *et al*. Cancer risk in 680 000 people exposed to computed tomography scans in childhood or adolescence: data linkage study of 11 million Australians. *BMJ* 21 May 2013; 346:f2360. doi:10.1136/bmj.f2360.
6. Laupacis A, Sekar N, Stiell IG. Clinical prediction rules: a review and suggested modifications of methodological standards. *JAMA* 1997; 277:488–94.
7. Steil IG. Clinical decision rules in the emergency department. *CMAJ* 2000; 163:1465–6.
8. Lyttle M, Crowe L, Oakley E, *et al*. Comparing CATCH, CHALICE and PECARN clinical decision rules for paediatric head injuries. *Emerg Med J* 2012; 29(10):785–94.
9. Osmond MH, Klassen TP, Wells GA, *et al*. CATCH: a clinical decision rule fro the use of computed tomography in children with minor head injury. *CMAJ* March 9 2010; 182(4): 341–8.
10. Dunning J, Daly JP, Lomas JP, *et al*. Derivation of the children's head injury algorithm for the prediction of important clinical events decision rule for head injury in children. *Arch Dis Child* 2006; 91:885–91.
11. Kuppermann N, Holmes JF, Dayan PS, *et al*. Identification of children at low risk of clinically-important brain injuries after head trauma: a prospective cohort study. *Lancet* 2009; 274:1160–70.
12. Harty E, Bellis F. CHALICE head injury rule: an implementation study. *Emerg Med J* 2010; 27:750–2.
13. Bowler T, Te Water Naude J, Tuthill D. How does the CHALICE rule affect CT scanning in children with head injuries. *Arch Dis Child* 2011; 96(8):782.
14. Crowe L, Anderson V, Babl FE. Application of the CHALICE clinical prediction rule for intracranial injury in children outside the UK: impact on head CT rate. *Arch Dis Child* 2010; 95(12):1017–22.
15. Parto A, Nohanty S. Pathophysiology and treatment of traumatic brain edema. *Indian J Neurotr* 2009; 6(1):11–16.
16. Fishman RA. Brain edema. *New Eng J Med* 1975; 293:706–11.
17. Enevoldsen EM, Jensen FT. Autoregulation and CO_2 responses of cerebral blood flow in patients with acute severe head injury. *J Neurosurg* 1978; 48:689–703.
18. Suarez JI. Hypertonic saline for cerebral edema and elevated intracranial pressure. *Clev Clin J Med* January 2004; 71(Sup1):S9–S11.
19. South Thames retrieval service guideline. *Hypertonic saline*. Available at <http://www.strs.nhs.uk/resources/pdf/guidelines/hypertonicNa.pdf>
20. Advanced Life Support Group. *Advanced Paediatric Life Support: The Practical Approach*. 5th Edition. Oxford: Wiley-Blackwell, 2011.
21. London Air ambulance pre-hospital standard operating procedure. *Head Injury*. <http://www.ukhems.co.uk/ukhemssops.html>

22. Fisher B, Thomas D, Peterson B. Hypertonic saline lowers raised intracranial pressure in children after head trauma. *J of Neurosurg Anesth* 1992; 4(1):4–10.

23. Simma B, Burger R, Falk M, *et al.* A prospective, randomized and controlled study of fluid management in children with severe head injury: Lactated Ringers solution versus hypertonic saline. *Crit Care Med.* 1998; 26(7):1265–70.

24. Khanna S, Davis D, Peterson B, *et al.* The Use of hypertonic saline in the treatment of severe refractory post traumatic intracranial hypertension in paediatric traumatic Brain injury. *Crit Care Med* April 2000; 28(4):1144–51.

25. Peterson B, Khanna S, Fisher B, *et al.* Prolonged Hyponatremia controls elevated intracranial pressure in head injured pedaitric Patients. *Crit Care Med* April 2000; 28(4):1136–43.

26. Wakai A, Roberts IG, Schierhout G. Mannitol for acute traumatic brain injury. *Cochrane Database of Systematic Reviews.* 2007; 1: Art. No.: CD001049. doi:10.1002/14651858. CD001049.pub4.

27. Rickard A. Best evidence topic reports. Hypertonic sodium solutions versus mannitol in reducing ICP in traumatic brain injury. *Emerg Med J* 2011; 28:75–6.

28. Dorman HR, Sondheimer JH, Cadnapaphornchai P. Mannitol-induced acute renal failure. *Medicine (Baltimore)* 1990; 69(3):153.

29. Davis M, Lucatorto M. Mannitol revisited. *J of Neurosci Nurs* 1994; 26(3):170–4.

30. Hutchinson JS, Doherty DR, Orlowski JP, *et al.* Hypothermia therapy after cardiac arrest in paediatric patients. *Pediatr Clin North Am* 2008; 55:529–44.

31. Azzopardi DV, Strohm B, Edwards AD, *et al.* Moderate hypothermia to treat perinatal asphyxial encephalopathy. *N Engl J Med* 2009; 361:1349–58.

32. Gluckman PD, Wyatt JS, Azzopardi D, *et al.* Selective head cooling with mild systemic hypothermia after neonatal encephalopathy: multicentre randomised trial. *Lancet* 2005; 365:663–70.

33. Bernard SA, Gray TW, Buist MD, *et al.* Treatment of comatose survivors of out of hospital cardiac arrest with induced hypothermia. *N Engl J Med* 2002; 346:557–63.

34. Hendrick EB, Harwood-Nash DC, Hudson AR. Head Injuries in children: A survey of 4454 consecutive cases at the Hospital for Sick children, Toronto, Canada. *Clin Neurosurg* 1963; 11:46–65.

35. Adelson PD, Ragheb J, Kanev P, *et al.* Phase II clinical trial of moderate hypothermia after severe traumatic brain injury in children. *Neurosurgery* April 2005; 56(4):740–54.

36. Hutchinson JS, Ward RE, Lacroix J, *et al.* Hypothermia after traumatic brain injury in children. *N Engl J Med* 2008; 358(23):2447–56.

37. Li H, Lu G, Shi W, Zheng S. Protective effect of moderate hypothermia on severe traumatic brain injury in children. *Journal of Neurotrauma* 2009; 26(11):1905–9.

38. <http://clinicaltrials.gov/ct2/show/record/NCT00222742>

39. <http://clinicaltrials.gov/ct2/show/NCT00282269?term=hypothermia+AND+Head+injury &rank=9>

40. Mitra B, Tullio F, Cameron PA, *et al.* Trauma patients with the 'triad of death'. *Emerg Med J* 2012 Aug; 29(8):622–5.

41. Markgraf CG, Clifton GL, Moody MR. Treatment window for hypothermia in brain injury. *J Neurosurg* 2001; 95:979–83.

42. Homlkova H, Prchlik M, Tomek P. The relationship between S100B protein serum levels, injury severity and Glasgow Outcome Scale in children with CNS injuries. *Neuroendocrinology Letters* 2012; 33(2):207–11.

43. Lomas JP, Dunning J. S-100b protein levels as a predictor for long term disability after head injury. *Emerg Med J* 2005; 22:885–91.

44. Cervellin G, Benatti M, Carbucicchio A, *et al.* Serum levels of protein S100B predict intracranial lesions in mild head injury. *Clinical Biochemistry* 2012; 45(6):408–11.

45. Lo TY, Jones PA, Minns RA. Combining coma scores and serum biomarker levels to predict unfavourable outcome following childhood brain trauma. *Journal of Neurotrauma* 2010; 27(12):2139–45.

6 Vaginal bleeding in early pregnancy

Rita Das

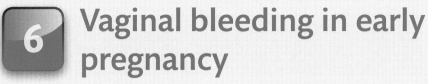

❝ **Expert Commentary** Lindsey Stevens

Case history

A 38-year-old Caucasian woman presents to the ED with mild abdominal pain and vaginal bleeding.

The pain started gradually 3 hours before presentation. It is in her left lower abdomen, of mild severity, and does not radiate. She has no bowel or bladder disturbance and no fever.

Her vaginal bleeding started 2 hours earlier. It is dark brown with no clots and she has only used one pad. She is not short of breath or dizzy.

Her last menstrual period was 9 weeks ago. She has been undergoing fertility treatment and has had a positive pregnancy test at home. She has had 2 spontaneous abortions in the last 2 years. Her periods have been irregular, but not painful or very heavy. She denies a history of fibroids, sexually transmitted diseases, or previous ectopic pregnancies. She has been with a regular male partner for 4 years. Her last cervical smear was normal 2 years ago.

See Box 6.1 for a clinical summary of the likelihood of pregnancy.

Box 6.1 In the Emergency Department population

- Pregnancy must be considered in all women of childbearing age.
- A recent observational study demonstrated that patient assessment of the likelihood of pregnancy has been shown to be reliable,[1] however another study suggested that there was a 10% chance of a patient being pregnant despite a patient stating that this was unlikely.[2]
- A pregnancy test should therefore be done in all female patients of childbearing age presenting with abdominal pain or vaginal bleeding.
- Women attending with gastrointestinal or urinary tract symptoms should also have a pregnancy test as these symptoms may indicate an ectopic pregnancy.[3]
- Urinary qualitative pregnancy tests measure the β-subunit of human chorionic gonadotrophin which is produced by the trophoblast once implantation of the fertilized ovum has occurred at about 7 days post-fertilisation. Serum quantitative ß-hCG tests reflect the volume of living trophoblast tissue (and so can be positive when the fetus itself has died).
- The sensitivity of urinary tests for diagnosing pregnancy is 99.4% approximately 3 weeks from the last menstrual period. This correlates to a serum ß-hCG level of >25 mmIU/ml. False negatives occur if the test is done too early or if the urine is dilute (specific gravity <1.015).

❝ **Expert comment**

Always take a detailed menstrual history. It is not unusual for a patient in early pregnancy to deny amenorrhoea but to admit to a change in quantity or timing of menstrual bleeding over the previous 2–3 months.

(continued)

➕ **Clinical tip Consider the diagnosis**

If a female patient of childbearing age has collapsed or is shocked always consider a ruptured ectopic pregnancy as a possible cause. In order to confirm or exclude pregnancy, the patient should be catheterized and the urine tested immediately for ß-hCG. The gynaecology team should be involved immediately as resuscitation may require surgical haemorrhage control.

Although rare, patients with ectopic pregnancy may have a negative urine ß-hCG test. Ectopic pregnancies can rupture even at serum ß-hCG levels below the discriminatory range for normal pregnancy.[4] Transvaginal ultrasound should, therefore, always be performed where an ectopic is suspected, even in the presence of negative urine and serum ß-hCG tests.

Case progression

The patient's urinary ß-hCG is positive and urinalysis is normal.

On examination she is haemodynamically normal with a pulse of 88 bpm and blood pressure of 125/60 mmHg.

Her abdomen is soft with tenderness suprapubically and guarding over the left iliac fossa.

She has a normal perineum. Speculum examination shows a normal vagina, with a small amount of dark red blood. Her cervical os is closed. On bimanual examination she does not have any cervical motion tenderness. Her uterus feels bulky but is not tender. There is some adnexal tenderness on the left side but no palpable mass.

The gynaecology team are contacted and they state they are unable to scan the patient in ED and as the patient is haemodynamically stable the patient should attend the Early Pregnancy Assessment Unit the next day. The gynaecologists state that they are unavailable to scan the patient in the ED.

🕪 Expert comment

The most common differential diagnosis in the emergency physician's mind is between a threatened miscarriage and a possible ectopic. Abdominal pain, abdominal tenderness (which is often generalized or bilateral), shoulder tip pain, rebound, dysuria, and rectal pressure or pain on defecation all point to an ectopic but the evidence suggests that neither history nor examination findings can reliably rule ectopic pregnancy in or out though an assessment of cervical motion tenderness can be helpful. A transvaginal ultrasound is the most reliable diagnostic tool.

🕪 Expert comment

The guidance of the RCOG[7] (RCOG guideline 21) on the management of ectopic pregnancy is based on a combination of serum ß-hCG and ultrasound findings. Given the difficulty of diagnosing ectopic pregnancy and the lack of correlation between clinical findings and the risk of rupture, patients with suspected ectopics should be kept in hospital until serum ß-hCG and transvaginal ultrasound results are available.

⭐ Learning point Ectopic pregnancies

Ectopic pregnancies have a prevalence of 1–2% of all pregnancies. The prevalence is as high as 7.5% in pregnant women presenting to EDs with suspicious clinical features.[5] It remains the leading cause of early pregnancy related deaths in the United Kingdom.

The clinical features of ectopic pregnancy are notoriously variable. Abdominal pain tends to occur in tubal miscarriage with consequent bleeding through the fibrial end of the tube into the peritoneal cavity. Pain secondary to tubal rupture is more severe and sudden in onset.

The likelihood of an ectopic pregnancy in the presence of abdominal pain and vaginal blood loss in the first trimester with no other risk factors is may be as high as 39%.[6] However, 10–20% of women with ectopic pregnancies report an absence of vaginal bleeding, and 10% deny the presence of abdominal pain.

Four of the 6 women who died from ectopic pregnancies reported in the Confidential Enquiry into Maternal Deaths published in 2011, complained of vomiting or diarrhoea. Clinicians failed to consider an ectopic pregnancy in their differential diagnosis of these patients, despite these atypical presentations being highlighted in previous reports.[3]

Clinical question: Is there are role for ED physicians to perform early pregnancy scanning in the ED?

Most emergency departments have an ultrasound machine although few have a transvaginal probe. A transvaginal scan has the advantage of being able to detect an intrauterine pregnancy earlier at around 5.5 weeks and also visualizes the adnexal region better than a trans-abdominal scan.

Emergency physicians have varying degrees of competency in ultrasound scanning leading to variability within departments as to the quality of ultrasound scanning available.

✔ **Evidence base** Early pregnancy scanning in the ED

Stein *et al.* (2010) conducted a meta-analysis of 10 studies (3 retrospective and 7 prospective) evaluating the use of bedside pelvic ultrasound by emergency physicians in the diagnosis of ectopic pregnancy.[5]

The pooled population was 2057 patients at risk of ectopic pregnancy, of which 152 (7.5%) had an ectopic confirmed from radiology ultrasound, gynaecology ultrasound, and/or clinical notes follow-up.

The scans were done at the bedside by emergency physicians. In 3 of the studies there was exclusive use of transabdominal scans.

The pooled sensitivity estimate was 99.3% (95% confidence interval [CI] 96.6–100%), negative predictive value was 99.96% (95% CI 99.6–100%), and negative likelihood ratio was 0.08 (95% CI 0.025–0.25), all without significant heterogeneity.

The studies did not have a consistent reference standard. Furthermore, those scans which did not identify an intrauterine pregnancy were more likely to have a more expedient reference test performed leading to verification bias.

🄶 **Expert comment**

With emergency ultrasound becoming a core skill for emergency physicians it is likely that as practice evolves, emergency physicians in the UK will increasingly be able to perform transvaginal ultrasound in the ED as a screening test for ectopic pregnancies. There is evidence to suggest that pelvic scanning in the ED by emergency physicians reduces length of stay in ED, unnecessary referrals to gynaecology,[8] as well as a decrease in the incidence of complications from ruptured ectopics.[9]

Answer

Authors concluded that the use of ultrasound to diagnose an ectopic pregnancy by emergency physicians provides excellent sensitivity and negative predictive value. The visualization of an intrauterine pregnancy is useful in the exclusion of an ectopic pregnancy but it does not rule out a heterotopic pregnancy.

Case progression

One of the ED consultants is qualified in gynaecological scanning and performs a transvaginal scan which does not reveal an intrauterine pregnancy but shows an adnexal mass and free fluid suggestive of haemoperitoneum.

🄶 **Expert comment**

Serum ß-hCG measurement should not be used as a determinant of the site of a pregnancy. A 'pregnancy of unknown location' (one where no intrauterine or ectopic pregnancy is seen on ultrasound but the pregnancy test is positive) should be treated as an ectopic until proved otherwise. A level above 5000 IU/l mandates surgical treatment.

Clinical question: Does a normal intrauterine pregnancy on ultrasound exclude an ectopic pregnancy?

✔ **Evidence base** Heterotopic pregnancy

There are several case reports[10-14] documenting the coexistence of an intrauterine pregnancy with an ectopic pregnancy, the majority of which result in a live term baby. If the concurrent ectopic is live, it should be removed preferably laparoscopically. If the ectopic is small and not growing, it may be managed conservatively.

✪ **Learning point** Heterotopic pregnancy

A heterotopic pregnancy is one in which implantation occurs at two or more sites, at least one of these sites being extra uterine. The uterus will show an intrauterine yolk or gestational sac yet there is a concurrent ectopic pregnancy (see Figure 6.1). Heterotopic pregnancies occur in 1 in 30 000 spontaneous pregnancies. With the increased incidence of pelvic inflammatory disease and assisted reproductive therapies, they are increasing in frequency.

In pregnancies conceived by assisted reproductive therapies, the incidence of a heterotopic pregnancy is as high as 1 in 100. In women receiving in vitro fertilization, embryo placement

(continued)

near the tubal ostia, excessive force during embryo transfer, and the transfer of multiple embryos increase the risk.

The visualization of free fluid or an adnexal mass in conjunction with a viable intrauterine pregnancy should arouse the suspicion of a heterotopic pregnancy, especially in a woman who has had assisted conception.

In early pregnancy an ultrasound which fails to identify an intrauterine sac should stimulate active exclusion of an ectopic pregnancy.

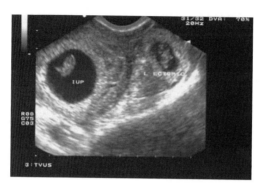

Figure 6.1 Ultrasound image of heterotopic pregnancy.

Reprinted from Best Practice & Research Clinical Obstetrics and Gynaecology, 18, 1, Condous G, 'The management of early pregnancy complications', pp. 37–57, Copyright 2004, with permission from Elsevier.

Answer

Visualisation of an intrauterine pregnancy does not necessarily rule out an ectopic pregnancy, especially in patients who have received embryo transfer.

Case progression

You call the gynaecology doctor back. He is pleased that the scan has been performed and a diagnosis of ectopic pregnancy has been made but advises no further action today.

Clinical question: Can patients presenting to the ED with ectopic pregnancies be treated conservatively?

Management of a tubal pregnancy in a haemodynamically shocked patient should be by resuscitation and the most expedient surgical method to control haemorrhage.

Ectopic pregnancies that have not ruptured in a haemodynamically normal patient can be managed surgically, medically, or expectantly.

⭐ Learning point Medical treatment for ectopic pregnancies

This approach is a treatment option in women with unruptured ectopic pregnancies, who are haemodynamically normal and have minimal symptoms. Selection criteria include the size of the

(continued)

tubal ectopic pregnancy, maximum serum hCG concentrations, and the absence of fetal cardiac activity on ultrasound. Patient preference and access to expert follow up also play a key role.

Intramuscular methotrexate is the most successful and most widely used medical treatment. Methotrexate is a folic acid antagonist which inhibits de novo synthesis of purines and pyrimidines, thereby interfering with DNA synthesis and cell division. The drug targets the proliferation of cytotrophoblast cells halting hormonal support for the ectopic pregnancy.

In practice only 25% of ectopic pregnancies meet the selection criteria for medical management.[16]

The new NICE guidance[17] recommends that systemic methotrexate be offered as first-line treatment to women with an ectopic pregnancy who have all of the following:

- No significant pain
- An unruptured ectopic pregnancy with an adnexal mass <35 mm with no visible heartbeat
- Serum βHCG <1500 IU/L
- No intrauterine pregnancy

Expectant management is based on the knowledge that the natural course of many early ectopic pregnancies is a self-limiting process ultimately resulting in tubal abortion or reabsorption.[18]

✔ Evidence base Management of ectopic pregnancies

A systematic review[19] of 35 randomized controlled trials comparing different treatment strategies for tubal ectopic pregnancies was published in 2009. A total of 25 different treatment comparisons were made including different surgical methods, systemic and local medical treatment, and expectant management. The primary outcome measure was complete elimination of trophoblast tissue with an uneventful decline of serum ß-hCG to undetectable levels after the index treatment.

Conclusions

- Systemic methotrexate is less invasive, easier to administer, and less dependent on clinical skill than locally administered (transvaginal ultrasound guided or laparoscopic guided) methotrexate.
- The short- and long-term outcomes of variable dose regimen systemic methotrexate are comparable to laparoscopic salpingostomy, although patients had more significant side-effects from methotrexate.
- An evaluation of expectant management of tubal pregnancy cannot adequately be made yet.

Answer

Some patients with ectopic pregnancies can be treated conservatively, however this group of patients require a gynaecology review and clear management plan if they are to be discharged from the ED.

Case progression

You become concerned that the ectopic pregnancy has ruptured as her abdominal tenderness has suddenly increased with rebound. Her blood results are as follows:

- Hb 11.1g/dl
- Blood group O negative
- Serum ß-hCG 7000 IU/l

You call the gynaecology team back and explain that, due to her level of tenderness, possible free fluid on the scan, and the high serum ß-hCG level, you would like them to come immediately to ED to review the patient. The gynaecology team decide to

❝ Expert comment

Expectant or medical treatment must lie with the gynaecology team as follow-up and easy access to skilled review will be needed; at least 15% of women will require more than 1 dose of methotrexate, 7% will have a tubal rupture, 75% will have abdominal pain and conjunctivitis, stomatitis and gastrointestinal upset also occur.[7]

admit her for a laparoscopic salpingostomy. You consider if this patient requires anti D given her rhesus status.

Clinical question: What is the role of the ED in using Anti D in rhesus-negative women with ectopic pregnancies?

> ✪ **Learning point** Anti D immunoglobulin
>
> Approximately 16% of women in the UK are RhD-negative, and in about 10% of all pregnancies the mother is RhD-negative and the fetus RhD positive.[20] During these pregnancies, the mother is at risk of becoming sensitized by transplacental haemorrhage, with the development of anti-D antibodies in the RhD negative mother. Sensitization depends on the volume of fetal blood entering the mother's circulation and the magnitude of the mother's immune response.
>
> If in a subsequent pregnancy the fetus is again RhD positive, the anti-D antibodies of the RhD negative mother attack the red cell fetal RhD-positive antigens causing haemolytic disease of the newborn. This is a spectrum of disease ranging from jaundice of the newborn which is responsive to phototherapy, to severe haemolytic anaemia causing cardiac failure, hydrops, and intrauterine death, or severe physical disability and mental retardation in the neonate.
>
> The anti-D immunoglobulin administered neutralizes this fetal antigen preventing the production of maternal anti-D antibodies.
>
> For successful immunoprophylaxis the anti-D immunoglobulin should be given as soon as possible after the potentially sensitizing event, and always within 72 hours. There is evidence that some protection may still be conferred if given within 10 days. The immunoglobulin is given ideally into the deltoid as gluteal injections often lead to delayed absorption. If a woman is coagulopathic the anti-D immunoglobulin can be given subcutaneously or intravenously.

> ✅ **Evidence base** Anti-D in rhesus-negative patients with ectopic pregnancies
>
> There has been no randomized controlled trial on pregnant RhD-negative women to evaluate whether anti-D immunoglobulin prevents seroconversion. One study used RhD-negative males who were injected with either 0.1 ml of RhD-positive blood[21] - or with Rh-positive cells which had been coated with Rh antibody in vitro. Fifty per cent of the first group became immunized to RhD-positive blood cells whereas none of the second group developed antibodies.
>
> Alloimmunisation has been reported in 25% of ruptured ectopic pregnancies.[22]
>
> The Royal College of Obstetricians and Gynaecologists national guidelines recommend the administration of 250 IU of anti-D immunoglobulin to be given to all non-sensitized women who are rhesus negative and who have a confirmed or suspected ectopic pregnancy.[7,22]
>
> The NICE guidelines on this matter reserve anti-D for ectopics undergoing surgical treatment.[22]

> ➕ **Clinical tip** Indications for Anti-D Immunoprophylaxis in non-sensitized RhD-negative women in early pregnancy
>
> - **NICE** [17] **recommends 250 IU anti-D rhesus prophylaxis to all RhD-negative women who have a surgical procedure to manage an ectopic or miscarriage in the first trimester.**
> - **It advises that anti D is NOT given to women who:**
>
>   ○ Receive solely medical management for an ectopic pregnancy or miscarriage
>   ○ Have a threatened miscarriage
>
> (continued)

- Have a complete miscarriage
- Have a pregnancy of unknown location

- **The Royal College of Obstetricians and Gynaecologists Green-top Guideline on Anti-D Prophylaxis**[22] refers to later gestations and recommends anti-D prophylaxis in the following circumstances:
  - **Spontaneous complete or incomplete miscarriage** after 12 weeks
  - **Threatened miscarriage** after 12 weeks
  - **Termination of pregnancy—all patients** regardless of gestation and whether medical or surgical method
  - **Invasive prenatal diagnosis** (amniocentesis, chorion villus sampling)
  - **Any abdominal trauma**

For all events at or after 20 weeks of gestation, a minimum dose of 500 IU anti-D Ig IM should be given.

A Final Word from the Expert

Vaginal bleeding in early pregnancy may culminate in the loss of a pregnancy and causes significant anxiety for patients and their partners. The emergency physician should approach this vulnerable group with expediency and sensitivity. Ectopic pregnancy is a potentially life-threatening diagnosis and should be considered in any woman of childbearing age, remembering that the problem may present atypically. If an ectopic is suspected, ideally a transvaginal ultrasound scan should be performed by a qualified practitioner at first presentation to enable a risk assessment to be performed and a clear follow-up plan devised involving the gynaecology team. Ongoing management decisions related to a diagnosed ectopic pregnancy should rest with the gynaecology team, but for those patients who are discharged home clear safety netting is required.

Lastly, PV bleeding is a *haemorrhage* and should be approached in the same way as any other haemorrhage with the performance of full blood counts for all patients, group and saves for prolonged or heavy bleeding, and clotting studies where indicated; missed and septic miscarriages are particularly associated with disseminated intravascular coagulopathy.

References

1. Minnerop MH, Garra G, Chohan JK, *et al*. Patient history and physician suspicion accurately exclude pregnancy. *Am J of Emerg Med* 2011 Feb; 29(2):212–5.
2. Ramoska EA. Sacchetti AD, Nepp M. Reliability of patient history in determining the possibility of pregnancy. *Ann of Emerg Med* 1989 Jan; 18(1):48–50.
3. Centre for Maternal and Child Enquiries (CMACE). Saving Mothers' Lives: reviewing maternal deaths to make motherhood safer: 2006–08. The Eighth Report on Confidential Enquiries into Maternal Deaths in the United Kingdom. *BJOG* 2011 Mar; 118(Suppl.1):1–203.
4. Lee Y-A A, Farina G, Lhamon H. Ruptured ectopic pregnancy with a negative urine pregnancy test. *JUCM* 2007 Nov; 2(2):26–8.
5. Stein JC, Wang R, Adler N, *et al*. Emergency physician ultrasonography for evaluating patients at risk for ectopic pregnancy: a meta-analysis. *Ann Emerg Med* 2010 Dec; 56(6):674–83.

6. Mol BW, Van der Veen F, Bossuyt PM. Implementation of probabilistic decision rules improves the predictive values of algorithms in the diagnostic management of ectopic pregnancy. *Hum Reprod* 1999 Nov; 14(11):2855–62.

7. RCOG Guideline No. 21. Management of Tubal Pregnancy 2004, Reviewed 2010.

8. Burgher SW, Tandy TK, Dawdy MR. Transvaginal Ultrasonography by Emergency Physicians Decreases Patient Time in the Emergency Department. *Acad Emerg Med* 1998 Aug; 5(8) 802–7.

9. Mateer JR, Valley VT, Aiman EJ, *et al.* Outcome analysis of a protocol including bedside endovaginal sonography in patients at risk for ectopic pregnancy. *Ann Emerg Med* 1996 Mar; 27(3):283–9.

10. Qiong Z, Yanping L, Deep JP, *et al.* Treatment of cornual heterotopic pregnancy via selective reduction without feticide drug. *J Minim Invasive Gynecol* 2011 Nov–Dec; 18(6):766–8.

11. Kumbak B. Ozkan ZS. Simsek M. Heterotopic pregnancy following bilateral tubal ligation: case report. *Eur J Contracep Reprod Health Care* 2011 Aug 16(4):319–21.

12. Sijanovic S, Vidosavljevic D, Sijanovic I. Methotrexate in local treatment of cervical heterotopic pregnancy with successful perinatal outcome: Case report. *J Obstet Gynaecol Res* 2011 Sept. 37(9):1241–5.

13. Majumdar A, Gupta SM, Chawla D. Successful management of post-in-vitro fertilization cervical heterotopic pregnancy. *J Hum Reprod Sci* 2009 Jan; 2(1): 45–6.

14. Eigbefoh, JO. Mabayoje, PS. Aliyu, JA. Heterotropic pregnancy: a report of two cases. *Niger J Clin Pract* 2008 Mar; 11(1):85–7.

15. Hassanik IM, El Bouazzaoui A, Khatouf M, *et al.* Heterotopic pregnancy, a diagnosis we should suspect more often. *J Emerg Trauma Shock* 2010 Jul; 3(3):304.

16. Sowter MC, Farquhar CM, Petrie KJ, *et al.* A randomised trial comparing single dose systemic methotrexate and laparoscopic surgery for the treatment of unruptured tubal pregnancy. *BJOG* 2001 Feb; 108(2):192–203.

17. National Institute for Health and Care Excellence. Ectopic Pregnancy and Miscarriage: Diagnosis and Initial Management in Early Pregnancy of Ectopic Pregnancy and Miscarriage NICE Clinical Guideline 154. London: National Institute for Health and Care Excellence, 2012.

18. Sivalingam VN, Duncan WC, Kirk E, *et al.* Diagnosis and management of ectopic pregnancy. *J Fam Plann & Reprod Health Care* 2011 Oct; 37(4):231–40.

19. Hajenius PJ, Mol F, Mol BWJ, *et al.* Interventions for tubal ectopic pregnancy. *Cochrane Database of Systematic Reviews* 2007, Issue 1. Art. No.: CD000324.

20. Chilcott J, Lloyd Jones M, Wight J, *et al.* A review of the clinical effectiveness and cost-effectiveness of routine anti-D prophylaxis for pregnant women who are rhesus-negative. *Health Technol Assess* 2003; 7(4) iiii–62.

21. Stern K, Goodman HS, Berger M. Experimental iso-immunization to hemo antigens in man. *J Immunol* 1961; 87:189–98.

22. RCOG Green-top Guideline No. 22. The Use of Anti-D Immunoglobulin for Rhesus D Prophylaxis. March 2011.

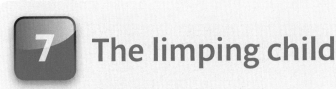

7 The limping child

Lalarukh Khan

ⓘ **Expert commentary** Tina Sajjanhar

Case history

An 18-month-old boy is brought to the paediatric ED by his parents who have noticed that he is limping on the right side since the previous day. They are unable to recall any history of trauma and report that other than a mild coryzal illness he has been well. He has been walking normally prior to this.

He has no past history of note, is not on any regular medications and his immunizations are up-to-date. He is an only child. His father had Perthes' disease as a child, and is naturally concerned that this may be similar.

See Box 7.1 for a clinical summary of limp presentations.

Box 7.1 Clinical summary of limp presentations

Children may be brought to the ED with a spectrum of disorders which might be classified as a 'limp'. These range from a change in gait which is difficult for the assessing clinician to see, to a child who is totally non-weight-bearing.

A change in gait can cause significant anxiety to parents particularly as it often occurs in the absence of a history of trauma.

The annual incidence of non-traumatic limping in children was identified as 1.5 cases in 1000 in a recent study from the Netherlands.[1]

The number appears to vary geographically and in Scotland was higher at 3.6 cases per 1000 children aged 0–14 years.[2]

Limp is a common presentation within the ED, from both traumatic and atraumatic causes; atraumatic limp should prompt a careful search for children who are at high risk of serious disease or pathology (see Table 7.1 and Table 7.2).

> ✪ **Learning point** Causes of limp in children
>
> **Table 7.1 Causes of limp in children**
>
> | Common causes | Incidence (I) or Prevalence (P) | Key features |
> |---|---|---|
> | Trauma (fracture or soft tissue injury, including NAI) | I: leading cause of limp[3] | Relevant history, point of injury tenderness (often difficult to localize in young children) |
> | Infection (all ages)-septic arthritis or osteomyelitis | I: 5–37 per 100 000[4,5] | Fever, painful limp, restricted range of movement (RROM) |
> | Transient synovitis (irritable hip) | I: 5–20 per 10 000[6-7] | Recent viral illness, self-limiting |
>
> (continued)

Common causes	Incidence (I) or Prevalence (P)	Key features
Perthes' disease	I: 5.7 in 100 000[8]	Predominant in boys aged 4–8 years, painful limp, RROM, leg length discrepancy, and muscular atrophy present later
Slipped upper femoral epiphysis (SUFE)	I: 10.8 per 100 000[9]	Predominantly age 8–14, pain on internal rotation of hip, male, and obesity predominance
Primary anatomical abnormality, e.g. limb length inequality	High	Postural problems (scoliosis)
Metabolic disease e.g. rickets, vitamin D deficiency	Rickets incidence: <1:200 000[10]	At-risk group for rickets (dark-skinned, breastfed, poor diet), bowing of legs or widened wrists
Developmental dysplasia	P: up to 28 per 1000[11]	Delayed walking, asymmetrical skin crease Incidence does not pertain to ED presentation as often picked up shortly after birth.
Neurological disease, e.g. cerebral palsy, cerebral tumours, spinal tumours	Cerebral palsy prevalence: >2 per 1000[12]	Stormy perinatal course or prematurity, cerebellar signs, developmental regression, unsteady gait
Malignancy, e.g. leukaemia, primary or secondary bone tumours	I: 14 per 100 000[13-14]	Persistent unexplained bone pain, pallor, fatigue, unexplained fever. Nocturnal pain.
Haematological disease, e.g. sickle cell disease (SCD)	I: 0.25 per 1000 SCD and 0.03 per 1000 thalassemia major or intermedia[15]	Usually known diagnosis or family history of anaemia
Rheumatological disease, e.g. juvenile idiopathic arthritis	P: 1 per 1000[16]	Joint involvement (pain, warmth, stiffness and swelling), eye involvement (inflammation, pain, redness), fevers, rash, myalgia, lymphadenopathy, weight loss, growth disturbance, plus multi-organ manifestations
Referred pain, e.g. testicular torsion, appendicitis	Torsion incidence: 1 per 4000[17]	Testicular torsion: testicular pain, testicular or scrotal oedema, abdominal pain, and nausea or vomiting.
	Appendicitis incidence: 1.17 per 1000[18]	Appendicitis: abdominal pain, nausea and vomiting, loss of appetite, low-grade fever, diarrhoea, dysuria or frequency

✚ **Clinical tip** Primary differential diagnosis for limp by age

Table 7.2 Memory aid for primary differential diagnosis for limp by age: ChIPS 4 T

Age	Aid memoire	Cause	4 T
Less than 24 months	Ch	Congenital hip (developmental dysplasia) and infection	Trauma
24 months to <4 years	I	Infection/Inflammation	Trauma
>4 to <10 years	P	Perthes' disease and infection	Trauma
>10–16 years	S	SUFE (slipped upper femoral epiphysis)	Trauma

Reproduced from MS Kocher et al., 'Differentiating between septic arthritis and transient synovitis of the hip in children: an evidence-based clinical prediction algorithm', *Journal of Bone and Joint Surgery American*, 81, 12, pp. 1662-1670, Copyright 1999, with permission from *Journal of Bone and Joint Surgery* Inc. http://jbjs.org/

🔒 **Expert comment**

Children presenting with a limp, or where a parent reports a limp, must have a careful evaluation with a full history and examination bearing in mind the long list of possible causes. The differential diagnosis will vary with the age of the child. Remember the cause may be in the bone (hip, knee, shaft), the brain (neurological), or the blood (leukaemia, vitamin D deficiency).

Case progression

On examination he is apyrexial with all observations within normal limits. He is reluctant to bear any weight on the right side and is noted to have a mild limp on walking. On undressing him, the legs appear normal, there are no signs of trauma, there is no joint swelling, and he has a full range of movements of his joints, although there is slight discomfort on rotating his right hip. There is no sign of any focal tenderness over the spine or legs, and he is neurologically intact. You suspect the child has transient synovitis but want to rule out septic arthritis.

Clinical question: What investigations may assist in differentiating transient synovitis from septic arthritis and when should they be performed as part of the initial assessment of a limping child?

In this age group, patients may present within a few hours of the onset of limp or a few days later. With a very short history, unless there are symptoms that raise concerns of serious pathology or the presence of a high temperature, it is reasonable to delay investigations as it is unlikely that they will yield any positive findings in the early stages of disease, and the vast majority will have transient synovitis (TS).[15,19] This is usually a well-looking, non-toxic child with a mild limp. A longer history over 2 days OR the presence of symptoms of concern should prompt urgent investigations as correct identification and prompt treatment of infections, especially septic arthritis (SA), is essential to avoid later complications.[20,24] The 1999 work of Kocher et al (see Table 7.3 and Table 7.4) highlighted 4 independent variables which could help distinguish septic arthritis from transient synovitis. In the older child, diagnosing and treating SUFE early is essential for a good prognosis, and it is vital to consider conditions such as Perthes' or malignancies, including both bony tumours and leukaemia, although these may not be evident on initial investigations.

Since Kocher's work from 1999 there have been additional studies which have looked to replicate and validate his findings (see Table 7.5).

Table 7.3 Differentiating between septic arthritis and transient synovitis in children

Author and date	Patient group Study type Outcome	Key results
Kocher et al. (1999)[25]	Retrospective study of 168 children presenting with an acutely irritable hip and diagnosed with septic arthritis (true or presumed if WCC >50×10⁹/L in joint fluid) or transient synovitis Analysis of the diagnostic value of presenting variables for differentiating between SA and TS of the hip in children and to develop an evidence-based clinical prediction algorithm for this differentiation	4 independent multivariate clinical predictors were identified to differentiate between SA and TS: History of fever Non-weight-bearing Erythrocyte sedimentation rate of at least 40 mm/hr Serum white blood-cell count of >12.0×109 cells/l 99.6% predicted probability for all 4 variables. The area under the receiver operating characteristic curve was 0.96 for the 4 multivariate predictors in identifying SA

Data from Kocher M, Zurakowski D, Kasser JR. Differentiating between septic arthritis and transient synovitis of the hip in children: an evidence-based clinical prediction algorithm. *J Bone Joint Surg Am* 1999; 81(12):1662-70.

Table 7.4 Kocher's prediction rules

No. of predictors	Transient synovitis ($n = 86$) (no. of patients)	Septic arthritis ($n = 82$) (no. of patients)	Predicted probability of septic arthritis (per cent)
0	19 (22.1%)	0 (0%)	<0.2
1	47 (54.7%)	1 (1.2%)	3.0
2	16 (18.6%)	12 (14.6%)	40.0
3	4 (4.7%)	44 (53.7%)	93.1
4	0 (0%)	25 (30.5%)	99.6

Data from Kocher M, Zurakowski D, Kasser JR. Differentiating between septic arthritis and transient synovitis of the hip in children: an evidence-based clinical prediction algorithm. *J Bone Joint Surg Am* 1999; 81(12):1662-70.

Table 7.5 Evidence base from Investigations in the limping child

Author and date	Patient group Study type Outcome	Key results
Luhmann et al. (2004)[26]	Retrospective study of 163 children with 165 involved hips who underwent hip arthrocentesis for the evaluation of irritable hip	Found the predicted probability of SA using Kocher's algorithm was 59%, whereas it was 71% using a combination of: history of fever, serum total white blood-cell count of >12.0×10^9 cells/l, and a previous healthcare visit
	Application of Kocher's clinical prediction algorithm to diagnose SA correctly	
Kocher et al. (2004)[27]	Prospective study of 154 children presenting with an acutely irritable hip and diagnosed with SA or TS (according to previous study[20] criteria)	Found a 93.0% predicted probability for all 4 variables, compared with 99.6% previously, and the area under the receiver operating characteristic curve was 0.86 for the 4 multivariate predictors in identifying SA, compared with 0.96
	Validation of their previous clinical prediction rule in a new patient population	
Reed et al. (2009)[28]	Retrospective study of 350 children aged <12 years presenting with an acute limp	Fever, non-weight-bearing, raised WCC, raised ESR and raised CRP were all associated with increased risk of infection. Having >3 of these variables gave 71.4% sensitivity and 97.3% specificity. The optimum inflammatory marker was CRP, with a count of >12 having a sensitivity of 87% and specificity of 91%
	Examined the utility of clinical findings, laboratory markers and X-ray radiographs in the assessment of children presenting with an acute non-traumatic limp	

Data from various sources (see references)

Answer

If the limp lasts more than 48 hrs with or without fever then the first step is to do simple blood tests to risk-stratify the patient. In this case, as the limp was of short onset with no other adverse features, it was reasonable to wait and review the child.

> **❝ Expert comment**
>
> Most children have a minor limp and few cannot completely weight bear. A child who is unable to weight bear at all must not be discharged without a further assessment, investigation, and a careful follow-up plan. A child with a persistent limp, a fever, or evidence of being systemically unwell also requires further investigation.
>
> Useful investigations for evaluating the child with a limp are blood tests, X-rays, and ultrasound, although more high-level investigations may be necessary if symptoms are persistent and there is no diagnosis (bone scan, MRI scan)
>
> (continued)

Blood tests should at minimum include a full blood count, CRP, and ESR. Blood culture should be performed in the febrile child, blood film in persistent limp with no other cause, and a metabolic work up may be indicated by the history.

If X-rays are being considered, then a frog-leg view is essential if SUFE is suspected as the findings may be subtle on an AP view.

An ultrasound will help to exclude a hip effusion, although it may be useful in other conditions, depending on the operator, e.g. osteomyelitis.

Case progression

As the examination is unremarkable the parents are reassured and agree to observe at home and return for review in 2 days' time, with an earlier attendance if further concerns arise. The doctor suggests giving regular ibuprofen until the review as if this seems to resolve the problem then a simple inflammatory process may be the cause.

The child attends the review clinic after 2 days. His mother says he was unsettled overnight and appears lethargic this morning but there were no specific symptoms that she could describe. When assessed he is noted to have spiked a temperature of 39.4 °C with a tachycardia of 130 bpm. The rest of his observations are normal. His limp has become more marked and he will not put his leg on the floor. Examination of his limbs reveals a right hip that is warm and tender to touch with restricted movement. Neurovascular examination is unremarkable. In view of his fever and hip examination he undergoes blood testing for FBC, CRP, and ESR, and is sent urgently for an ultrasound scan.

Clinical question: Is there a role for plain radiographic imaging in addition to ultrasound when assessing the limping child?

Plain radiographs alone have a place evaluating the cause of limp in children where specific bony changes are being sought, including Perthes Disease, SUFE, or bony tumours (see Table 7.6). Suspected toddler's fracture may be difficult to pick up on X-ray due to the subtle nature of the fracture. Children can be managed expectantly if the clinical picture fits with this diagnosis, but repeat X-ray may be required to confirm the diagnosis.

While radiography is of use if the pain appears to be in the lower limb, in the hip radiographic abnormalities are less likely. If there is hip involvement an ultrasound will identify an effusion, which may then prompt aspiration for Gram stain and culture. The echogenicity of the fluid may indicate the cause of the effusion as haemorrhages and exudates are usually echogenic, transudates less so.[29,21]

❝ Expert comment

It is clear that ultrasound is superior to plain X-ray in assessing joint effusion, and urgent orthopaedic intervention is required in a child with an effusion secondary to a probable septic arthritis. However, if hip ultrasound is not available out of hours, assessment of the clinical picture with blood laboratory investigations will aid the clinician in suspecting the diagnosis.

Answer

Ultrasound is the best modality for detecting a hip effusion and may help in the management of suspected SA.

Table 7.6 Evidence base for imaging in the limping child

Author and date	Patient group Study type Outcome	Key results
Wright (BestBets) 2003[31]	6 papers, 5 of which looked at children only, comparing ultrasound with plain radiographs Detection of effusion with 2 papers also analysing change in clinical care	Ultrasound is better than X-ray at detecting hip effusions in the limping child
Martin 2005[32]	Retrospective study of children between the ages of 1 and 6 years who had radiological investigations for an acute atraumatic limp Relationship between pain and radiological findings and value of plain radiographs and ultrasound in the investigation of limping children	Highly significant association between pain and radiological findings ($p<0.05$). Where there was hip joint pain, an ultrasound scan had sensitivity of 100% compared with 26.6% for plain radiographs
Zamzam 2006[33]	Retrospective study of 154 children with differential diagnosis of SA or TS based upon clinical, laboratory, and plain radiographic findings who were admitted Identification of role of US in diagnosing SA	The sensitivity, specificity and positive predictive value for US diagnosing SA were 86.4%, 89.7%, and 87.9% respectively. Out of 127 patients 4 had false-negative results; all these were done within the first 24 hrs from symptom onset, which was statistically significant ($p \leq 0.0084$). The ability of US to detect SA over the chosen clinical, laboratory, and radiographic parameters was also significant ($p \leq 0.005$)
Baskett *et al.* 2009[34]	Retrospective study of 310 children between 2 and 11 years presenting with hip pain Diagnostic accuracy of radiographs in urgent and non-urgent pathology	Radiographs had 18% sensitivity, 99% specificity, and a positive predictive value of 63% for detecting 'urgent pathology' (sepsis, SUFE). The sensitivity was a little higher (36%) in those above 9 yrs old

Data from various sources (see references)

Case progression

The blood tests reveal white cell count 11.79×10^3 cells/L, CRP 10.9 mg/dL, and ESR 68.8 mm/hr.[6] The ultrasound examination shows a marked effusion on the right side. He is referred urgently to the orthopaedic team who take him to theatre for aspiration. The resultant synovial fluid was Gram-stain positive and cultured *S. aureus*. He is started on intravenous antibiotics and the question of concomitant steroids is raised.

The organism responsible for septic arthritis in children varies according to the child's age.

★ **Learning point** Organisms that cause septic arthritis in children

First 2 months of life	*Group B streptococcus* *S. aureus* *Gram negative enteric bacilli* *Candida* spp. *N. gonorrhoea*

(continued)

2 months to adolescence	S. aureus
	H. influenzae type b
	Group A streptococci
	S. pneumoniae
Adolescents	N gonorrhoea
	S. aureus

Clinical question: Is there a role for steroids in addition to antibiotics in the treatment of septic arthritis?

The traditional treatment of SA is arthrocentesis (both for diagnostic and therapeutic purposes) followed by a course of antibiotics, initially intravenously (IV) and then orally, together with analgesia (see Table 7.7). The duration of intravenous antibiotics is guided by clinical improvement and normalizing inflammatory markers. In children with an acute hematogenous septic arthritis, a short total course of 10 days of antimicrobials is sufficient in uncomplicated cases.[35]

Following experimental studies in rabbits[36,22] which suggested that there was less joint destruction with the addition of steroids to traditional antibiotic treatment, 2 more recent studies have investigated this in the paediatric population.

Table 7.7 Evidence base for the role of steroids in septic arthritis

Author and date	Patient group Study type Outcome	Key results
Odio et al. 2003[38]	Prospective randomized controlled trial of 123 children between 3 months and 13 yrs old were randomly administered IV dexamethasone or IV saline as adjuvant therapy to antibiotics in haematogenous septic arthritis	In the dexamethasone group, the complication rate was far lower than in the control group at all time points ($p<0.005$), notably at 12 months only 2% of dexamethasone patients had residual dysfunction compared with 26% in the control group
	Complications at the end of therapy and at 6 and 12 months of follow-up	Secondary outcome analyses showed the steroid group had quicker resolution of symptoms (2.34 ± 5.06 days) compared with the saline group (7.81 ± 2.04), $p=0.001$, and the CRP normalized
	Fall of serum C-reactive protein and speed of clinical recovery in the cute phase	quicker (2.04 ± 1.25 days vs 4.68 ± 6.23), $p=0.01$
Harel et al. 2011[39]	Prospective randomized controlled trial of 49 children with septic arthritis treated with antibiotics and randomized to receive dexamethasone 0.15 mg/kg 6 hourly for 4 days or placebo	Statistically significant differences were noted for duration of fever ($p=0.021$), local inflammatory signs ($p=0.021$), levels of acute phase reactants ($p=0.003$), and duration of IV treatment ($p=0.007$)
	Time to clinical and laboratory normalisation	The duration of hospital stay decreased in steroid group
	Duration of hospitalization	

Data from various sources (see references)

Answer

Intravenous dexamethasone appears to be of benefit as an adjuvant therapy in septic arthritis, but more robust study needs to be conducted in order for its routine use to be recommended.

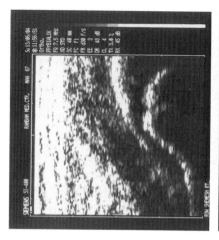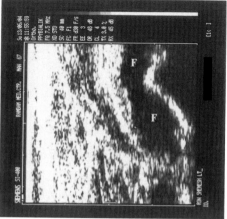

Figure 7.1 Ultrasound image of normal hip and fluid within the hip joint. Fluid within the hip joint denoted by 'F'.
Images courtesy of Dr Itai Shavit, MD, Director of Pediatric Emergency Department, Rambam Health Care Campus, Haifa, Israel.

Future advances

Although hip ultrasonography is sensitive for the detection of joint effusion, it is not as good at picking up other causes of hip problems such as pelvic musculoskeletal problems. One study has looked at the use of MRI in evaluation of the child with non-traumatic limp and suggested that in conjunction with inflammatory markers this modality may discriminate between those children who can be treated expectantly or those who require aggressive management.[41] The limited access to this form of investigation in the acute phase for most centres makes this impractical for many children, as a potential diagnosis of SA needs to be treated immediately. However, where it is readily available and the child is cooperative, it is an option.

With the increasing expertise of ED physicians in the use of ultrasound to aid diagnosis, such as focused abdominal sonography in trauma, one study looked at its use for the evaluation of children presenting with a limp.[23] This described a new modality called Sonography of the Hip joint by the Emergency Physician (SHEP), a bedside test to rapidly detect fluid in the hip joint (see Figure 7.1).

Three more recent studies have also promoted the training of ED physicians in bedside ultrasonography for detecting hip effusions.[40-42] Following more rigorous prospective study, together with the history and examination this may prove to be a useful triage tool to guide the management of the limping child.

A Final Word from the Expert

Children presenting with limp is a common complaint. Careful history and examination are required to ascertain the site of the pathology, remembering that the cause may not always be in the lower limbs, but may involve other systems.

Assessment of the gait is an essential part of this; non-weight-bearing children require careful further consideration.

Investigation should be tailored to the possible pathology; it is vital not to miss a diagnosis of septic arthritis or SUFE.

Ultrasound is a useful modality, even if it is to rule out a hip effusion so that other causes can be considered.

References

1. Krul M, van der Wouden JC, Schellevis FG, *et al*. Acute non-traumatic hip pathology in children: incidence and presentation in family practice. *Fam Pract* 2010; 27:166–70.
2. Fischer S, Beattie TF. The limping child: epidemiology, assessment and outcome. *J Bone Joint Surg Br* 1999; 81(6):1029–34.
3. Laine J, Kaiser SP, Diab M. High-risk pediatric orthopedic pitfalls. *Emerg Med Clin North Am* 2010; 28(1):85–102.
4. Riise ØR, Handeland KS, Cvancarova M, *et al*. Incidence and characteristics of arthritis in Norwegian children: a population-based study. *Pediatrics* 2008; 121(2):e299–306.
5. Yagupsky P, Bar-Ziv Y, Howard CB, *et al*. Epidemiology, etiology, and clinical features of septic arthritis in children younger than 2 months. *Arch Pediatr Adolesc Med* 1995; 149(5):537–40.
6. Kunnamo I, Kalilio P, Pelkonen P. Incidence of arthritis in urban Finnish children. A prospective study. *Arthritis Rheum* 1986; 29(10):1232–8.
7. Von Koskull S, Truckenbrodt H, Holle R *et al*. Incidence and prevalence of juvenile arthritis in an urban population of southern Germany: a prospective study. *Ann Rheum Dis* 2001; 60(10):940–5.
8. Landin LA, Danielsson LG, Wattsgard C. Transient synovitis of the hip. Its incidence, epidemiology and relation to Perthes' disease. *J Bone Joint S* 1987; 69(2):238–42.
9. Perry D, Bruce CE, Pope D, *et al*. Legg-Calvé-Perthes disease in the UK: geographic and temporal trends in incidence reflecting differences in degree of deprivation in childhood. *Arthritis Rheum*. 2012 May; 64(5):1673–9.
10. Lehmann C, Arons RR, Loder RT, *et al*. The epidemiology of slipped capital femoral epiphysis: an update. *J Pediatr Orthop*. 2006; 26(3):286–90.
11. <http://www.nhs.uk/conditions/Rickets/Pages/Introduction.aspx>
12. Leck I. Congenital dislocation of the hip 2000. In Wald N, Leck I (eds) Antenatal and neonatal screening. 2nd edition. New York. Oxford University Press.
13. Odding E, Roebroeck ME, Stam HJ. The epidemiology of cerebral palsy: Incidence, impairments and risk factors. *Disabil Rehabil* 2006; 28(4):183–91.
14. Office for National Statistics, Cancer Statistics registrations: Registrations of cancer diagnosed in 2008, England. (Series MB1) 2010, National Statistics: London.
15. Welsh Cancer Intelligence and Surveillance Unit. Cancer Incidence in Wales, 2004–2008. 2010.
16. ISD Online. Information and Statistics Division, NHS Scotland, 2010.
17. Northern Ireland Cancer Registry 2010. Cancer Incidence and Mortality.
18. Davies S, Cronin E, Gill M, *et al*. Screening for sickle cell disease and thalassaemia: a systematic review with supplementary research. *Health Technol Assess* 2000; 4(3):i–v, 1–99.
19. Paediatric Rheumatology Report. National Steering Group for Specialist Children's Services. <http://www.specialchildrensservices.scot.nhs.uk/Documents/org00003.pdf>
20. Somani BK, Watson G, Townell N. Testicular torsion. *BMJ* 2010; 341:c3213.
21. Williams NM, Jackson D, Everson NW *et al*. Is the incidence of acute appendicitis really falling? *Ann R Coll Surg Engl* 1998; 80(2):122–124.

22. Mattick A, Turner A, Ferguson J *et al.* Seven year follow up of children presenting to the accident and emergency department with irritable hip. *J Accid Emerg Med* 1999; 16:345–7.
23. Fabry G, Meire E. Septic arthritis of the hip in children: poor results after late and inadequate treatment. *J Pediatr Orthop* 1983; 3(4):461–5.
24. Belthur MV, Palazzi DL, Miller JA *et al.* A clinical analysis of shoulder and hip joint infections in children. *J Pediatr Orthop* 2009 (7); 29:828–33.
25. Kocher M, Zurakowski D, Kasser JR. Differentiating between septic arthritis and transient synovitis of the hip in children: an evidence-based clinical prediction algorithm. *J Bone Joint Surg Am* 1999; 81(12):1662–70.
26. Luhmann SJ, Jones A, Schootman M *et al.* Differentiation between septic arthritis and transient synovitis of the hip in children with clinical prediction algorithms. *J Bone Joint Surg Am* 2004; 86-A (5):956–62.
27. Kocher MS, Mandiga R, Zurakowski D *et al.* Validation of a clinical prediction rule for the differentiation between septic arthritis and transient synovitis of the hip in children. *J Bone Joint Surg Am* 2004; 86-A(8):1629–35.
28. Reed L, Baskett A, Watkins N. Managing children with acute non-traumatic limp: the utility of clinical findings, laboratory inflammatory markers and X-rays. *Emerg Med Australas* 2009; 21(2):136–42.
29. Marchal GJ, Van Holsbeeck MT, Raes M *et al.* Transient synovitis of the hip on children: role of US. *Radiol* 1987; 162(3):825–8.
30. Miralles M, Gonzalez G, Pulpeiro JR *et al.* Sonography of the painful hip in children: 500 consecutive cases. *Am J Roentgenol* 1989; 152(3) 579–82.
31. Wright N. Ultrasound is better than X-ray at detecting hip effusions in the limping child. BestBets. <http://www.bestbets.org/bets/bet.php?id=108>
32. Martin A. Investigating the limping child: The role of plain radiographs and ultrasound. *Radiol* 2005; 11(2):99–107.
33. Zamzam M. The role of ultrasound in differentiating septic arthritis from transient synovitis of the hip in children. *J Pediatr Orthop* 2006; 15(6): 418–22.
34. Baskett A, Hosking J, Aickin R. Hip radiography for the investigation of nontraumatic, short duration hip pain presenting to a children's emergency department. *Pediatr Emer Care* 2009; 25(2):76–82.
35. Peltola H, Paakkonen M, Kallio P *et al.* Prospective, randomized trial of 10 days versus 30 days of antimicrobial treatment, including a short-term course of parenteral therapy, for childhood septic arthritis. *Clin Infect Dis* 2009; 48(9):1201–10.
36. Stricker SJ, Lozman PR, Makowski AL *et al.* Chondroprotective effect of betamethasone in lapine pyogenic arthritis. *J Pediatr Orthop* 1996; 16(2):231–6.
37. Wysenbeek AJ, Leirman M, Amit M *et al.* Experimental septic arthritis in rabbits treated by a combination of antibiotic and steroid drugs. *Clinical and Experimental Rheumatology* 1996; 14(5):507–12.
38. Odio CM, Ramirez T, Araia G *et al.* Double-blind, randomized, placebo-controlled study of dexamethasone therapy for hematogenous septic arthritis in children. *Pediatr Infect Dis* 2003; 22:883–8.
39. Harel L, Prais D, Bar-on E, *et al.* Dexamethasone therapy for septic arthritis in children. *J Pediatr Orthop* 2011; 31(2):211–5.
40. Shavit I, Eidelman M, Galbraith R. Sonography of the hip joint by the emergency physician. *Ped Emerg Care* 2006; 22(8):570–3.
41. Vieira RL, Levy JA. Bedside Ultrasonography to Identify Hip Effusions in Pediatric Patients. *Ann Emerg Med* 2010; 55(3):284–9.
42. McLaughlin R, Collum N, McGovern S, *et al.* Emergency department ultrasound (EDU): clinical adjunct or plaything? *Emerg Med J* 2005; 22(5):333–5.
43. White PM, Boyd J, Beattie TF, *et al.* Magnetic resonance imaging as the primary imaging modality in children presenting with acute non-traumatic hip pain. *Emerg Med J* 2001; 18(1):25–9.

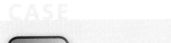

8 Corneal injury

Shweta Gidwani

Expert Commentary Mike Beckett

Case history

A 25-year-old construction worker presents to the ED with a painful red eye. He was hammering some metal rods at work about 3 hrs earlier and thinks that something may have gone into his right eye. His eye has been painful and watering profusely since the injury. He is finding it difficult to open the eye and the lids look red and swollen. He is otherwise well and has no significant medical history or any allergies and is fully immunized against tetanus.

On examination his right eye is swollen, slightly red and inflamed, and is watering profusely. He is unable to open his eye for you to evaluate his visual acuity. The other eye is normal in appearance and the triage nurse has documented a visual acuity of 6/6 in his left eye. He has been given oral NSAIDs for pain relief.

He is seen by the emergency nurse practitioner (ENP) who checks his visual acuity (VA) using a Snellen's chart. His VA is 6/12 in the affected eye. The ENP asks you to review the patient, as she is concerned about an embedded corneal foreign body.

See Box 8.1 for a clinical summary of corneal injuries.

Box 8.1 Clinical summary of corneal injuries

- The cornea is a transparent refractive layer of the eye anterior to the iris and accounts for nearly two-thirds of the optical power of the eye. Therefore, in any injury involving the cornea a formal visual acuity must be performed (see Figure 8.1)

- The cornea has no direct blood supply and gets its oxygen from the external environment. It is extremely well innervated from the ophthalmic division of the trigeminal nerve and thus very sensitive to pain.

- Corneal injuries cause severe pain and blepharospasm making it difficult to open and examine the eye adequately initially. Often a drop of topical anaesthesia is needed before the eye can be opened for examination.

- Corneal inflammation usually produces a characteristic circumcorneal injection sparing the palpebral conjunctiva, rather than diffused injections see in conjunctival inflammation.

Expert comment

Any injury to the eye involving glass or metal should raise the question of a penetrating foreign body. Patients hammering or drilling often assume they have dust in their eye when it may be a penetrating fragment of metal from the hammer, etc. The only way to be completely sure there is not a penetrating foreign body is to directly visualize it and remove it from the surface of the cornea. The back of the eye has no pain sensation so the pain of penetrating injury may be similar to that of a corneal foreign body and the pain will be abolished by local anaesthetic applied to the cornea.

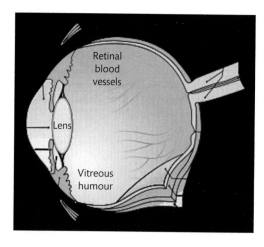

Figure 8.1 Cross-sectional view of eye.

With kind permission from Dr Reza Jarral, SHO, Emergency Medicine.

Case progression

Initially, the patient is in a lot of discomfort and is unable to keep his eye open for long enough to be examined properly. You decide to instil a single drop of a local anaesthetic 1 % tetracaine into the right eye to relieve the pain and allow a thorough examination.

A detailed examination of the eye reveals circumcorneal injection of the sclera, a symmetric pupil that reacts to light normally, and a normal anterior chamber.

The eye is then examined with a slit lamp after instilling a drop of fluoroscein dye using a blue filter. A corneal abrasion, which stains green, is seen along with an embedded metallic corneal foreign body. You also evert the eyelids to inspect the eye for any other foreign bodies.

You perform a Seidel's test which is negative (see Figure 8.2).

The ENP asks you about the indications for further imaging in patients with a possible ocular foreign body.

> **⊕ Clinical tip** Seidel's Test
>
> Seidel's test is used to test for a full thickness corneal injury. This can be performed with either a concentrated fluoroscein strip or 2 % fluoroscein drops placed in the region of the corneal injury. When there is a full thickness laceration, the aqueous flows out and dilutes the fluoroscein strip or concentrated dye to reveal a 'tear drop' when the eye is examined with a blue filter.

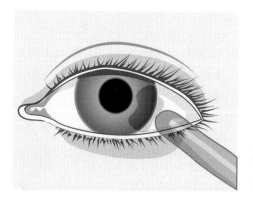

Figure 8.2 Siedels test to test for full thickness corneal injury.

With kind permission from Dr Reza Jarral, SHO, Emergency Medicine.

Clinical question: What is the best imaging modality in the presence of a suspected intraocular foreign body?

There have been no prospective diagnostic studies directly comparing the accuracy of plain films, ultrasound, and CT in detecting orbital foreign bodies (see Table 8.1). In a study[1] comparing helical CT, axial CT, and MR imaging using 42 fresh porcine eyes in which different sizes of glass were implanted on the corneal surface and the anterior and posterior chambers, it was found that detection rates were 57.1 % for helical CT, 41.3 % for axial CT, and 11.1 % for T1-weighted MR imaging ($n = 63$ fragments p<0.0001). It was concluded that helical CT was the most sensitive. The sensitivity of detection was unaffected by hyphema but was determined by the type of glass, size, and location.

Table 8.1 Evidence base: routine imaging for metallic corneal foreign body

Author	Design, subjects, and intervention	Results
Saeed A et al. (2008)[2]	A retrospective review of 177 patients with eye injuries from suspected high-velocity metallic projectiles in the absence of any clinically evident ocular penetration, and 27 patients with clinically evident foreign bodies who had plain X-ray films to rule out foreign bodies	None of the patients who had no clinical evidence of foreign body had intraocular foreign bodies (IOFB) visible on X-rays However, in patients with clinical evidence of ocular penetration as demonstrated by the Seidel's test, IOFB was visible in 19 of 27 patients who had plain X-ray and all 12 patients who had a CT scan

Data from Saeed A, Cassidy L, Malone DE et al. Plain X-ray and computed tomography of the orbit in cases and suspected cases of intraocular foreign body. *Eye* (Lond). 2008 Nov 22(11):1373-7.

Answer

The authors concluded that in the absence of clinically evident ocular penetration plain X-ray and CT were non-contributory, while in the presence of high clinical suspicion, CT was the imaging of choice.

> **❻ Expert comment**
>
> The most appropriate imaging modality for a suspected intraorbital foreign body will depend on the skills and resources within a given facility. The Royal College of Radiologists[3] states that a single lateral X-ray is the only projection required to exclude a metallic foreign body, and that a CT is only required if a plain film has failed to show a highly suspected foreign body, if the foreign body is not metallic, or if there are suspected multiple foreign bodies. The use of ultrasound within the ED by ED physicians has increased greatly in recent years and has been shown to facilitate early diagnosis of orbital trauma[4] and raised intraocular pressure,[5] and hence it could be of some value in the diagnosis of an orbital foreign body. The small size of such foreign bodies together with poor patient cooperation make the procedure challenging and hence the use of ultrasound is currently limited to specialists using an ultrasound biomicroscope at present.[6]

Case progression

Since a metallic foreign body is visible on direct examination, you decide that this patient does not need further imaging. However, the embedded corneal foreign body needs to be removed. A drop of local anaesthetic is instilled in each eye and the metallic foreign body is carefully removed under direct visualization using the slit lamp for magnification and a 25-gauge needle.

> **❻ Expert comment**
>
> On the day of injury, corneal foreign bodies are usually fairly easy to remove. After a day or so they may become embedded due to corneal overgrowth and rubbing the eye. Removing them may then be more difficult. Common methods for removal in the ED include the use of a sterile needle or wet cotton bud using a slit lamp.
>
> (continued)

> **✪ Learning point** Foreign bodies of different materials
>
> Inert, non-toxic, sterile materials such as plastic and glass are well tolerated within the eye, but most intra-ocular foreign bodies occur from metal striking metal. The majority of these are magnetic, and particles containing iron oxidize to set up an inflammatory reaction within the eye (siderosis). Vegetable matter may also induce a severe response with endophthalmitis. Therefore, it is vital that these foreign bodies are removed without delay.

Most EDs do not have a co-located eye unit and most medical students get minimal exposure to ophthalmology in their training. An ED needs a good working relationship with its local eye unit and ED doctors need to be clear how much they can safely diagnose and treat and when to refer with the appropriate degree of urgency.

Case progression

Having removed the metallic foreign body, you re-examine the eye and notice that there is a residual rust ring that you have only been able to remove partially.

> ✪ **Learning point** Rust rings
>
> Metallic foreign bodies often leave a rust ring behind and this usually starts to form within the first 2–4 hrs. This is toxic to the cornea and must also be removed carefully and thoroughly. When it has not been possible to remove all the rust in the ED, it is appropriate to bring the patient back the next day as the rust ring will soften overnight, making it easier to remove. It may be necessary to refer to ophthalmology to remove the ring using a low-speed rotatory sterile burr.

On re-staining the eye you also note a small abrasion in the area where a foreign body was embedded. The ENP asks you about the use of antibiotics and appropriate analgesia to treat this corneal abrasion.

Clinical question: Are routine antibiotics indicated in the acute management of corneal abrasions?

See Table 8.2.

Table 8.2 Evidence base: prophylactic antibiotics in corneal trauma

Author	Design, subjects, and intervention	Results
Kruger et al. (1990)[7]	In a prospective randomized controlled trial which recruited 94 patients with corneal foreign-body induced abrasion randomized to receive antibiotic or placebo	No difference seen between the groups in healing (symptoms, visual acuity/corneal appearance)
King and Brison (1993)[8]	In a prospective non-comparative cohort study, 351 patients with corneal trauma were recruited during a 4 month period. None of the patients were given topical or systematic antibiotics. Patients were followed up 16–36 hrs after presentation	290 patients followed up. 2/290 patients developed infection (0.7 % 95 % CI 0.09 %–1–8 %)
Upadhyay et al. (2001)[9]	In a cohort study which recruited 551 patients who presented with corneal abrasion within 48 hrs of injury without sign of infection were given 1 % chloramphenicol for 3 days. Patients were followed up for 2 yrs	442 patients followed up 424/442 (96 %) healed with no complication None of the 284 who commenced treatment within 18 hrs developed an ulcer 4/109 (3.7 %) who commenced treatment in 18–24 hrs developed an ulcer and 14/49 (28.6 %) who commenced treatment between 24–48 hrs developed an ulcer

Data from various sources (see references)

Answer

Topical antibiotics are prescribed routinely as prophylaxis[10] following a corneal abrasion although the evidence is weak and contradictory and infection rates are low. Despite evidence to the contrary, routine practice in many departments would be to prescribe antibiotics and such embedded behavior is difficult to change. It may be that some corneal ulcers are a higher risk for infection and maybe selective use of antibiotics in these groups may warrant further investigation.

When topical antibiotics are considered, traditionally ointments, due to the additional lubricant effect are preferred; however, in a prospective study[11] of 144 patients which compared Fucithalmic eye drops and chloramphenicol eye ointment, no difference was found between the groups in healing time or level of discomfort.

> ⊕ **Clinical tip** Patients who wear contact lenses
>
> Contact-lens wearers are at high risk of developing a rapidly progressing bacterial keratitis from corneal abrasions.[12] This may progress to corneal scarring and perforation which may limit sight. They should also be advised to avoid wearing lenses till the abrasion if fully healed and be routinely followed up in an ophthalmology clinic. Abrasions in contact-lens wearers should always be treated with prophylactic antibiotics as such patients are at high risk of developing infections with pseudomonas and proteus which may be resistant to Chloramphenicol. For this reason, guidance from an ophthalmologist regarding the choice of antibiotic and the follow-up arrangements should always be sought in these patients.

Clinical question: What is the most appropriate form of analgesia in the ED for corneal abrasions?

Corneal abrasions are notoriously painful but there are inconsistencies in what emergency physicians prescribe and advise for pain (see Table 8.3).[10] The relief that patients describe on application of topical anesthetics required to facilitate examination often leads to a request for an ongoing supply of anesthetic but these should be avoided after the initial examination as they can retard healing and any further corneal damage may go unnoticed due to the insensate cornea.

Table 8.3 Evidence base: topical NSAIDs for corneal abrasions

Author	Design, subjects, and intervention	Results
Brahma AK *et al.* 1996[13]	In a prospective randomized controlled trial, 401 patients with corneal abrasions presenting to the ED were treated with either (i) lubricant alone vs (ii) 2% homatropine (single dose) vs (iii) flubiprofen 0.03% vs (iv) flubiprofen 0.03% QDS and homatropine (single dose) Treatments given for 4 hrs	Usable responses obtained from 224/401 participants (55.8%) At 6 hrs the group who received 0.03% flubriprofen had significantly less pain
Jayamanne DG *et al.* (1997)[14]	In a prospective randomized double-blind placebo controlled trial 40 patients with traumatic corneal abrasions presenting to the ED had chloramphenical oitment + either diclofenac sodium 0.1% or normal saline	On day 1 ($p<0.001$) and day 2 ($p<0.02$) pain in the diclofenac group was significantly less. Using VAS of 0–100 mm and categorical pain scale

(continued)

Author	Design, subjects, and intervention	Results
Kaiser PK and Pineda R 1997[15]	In a prospective single-center randomized double-blind placebo controlled trial, 100 patients with corneal abrasions were randomized to receive ketoroloac tromethamine 0.5% or control vesicle drops. All patients also received a topical cycloplegic and topical antibiotics	In the ketorolac group the mean pain intensity reduction at 24 hrs was 2.7 vs 1.4 in the control group ($p=0.002$) using scale 1–10. Further, foreign body sensation ($p<0.003$), photophobia ($p<0.009$), and ocular pain ($p<0.002$) was significantly lower
Szucs et al. 2000[19]	In a prospective randomized double-blind placebo controlled trial, 49 patients with corneal abrasions were given either diclofenac 0.1% ophthalmic NSAID solution or artificial tears. Both groups had ED treatment with topical anaesthetic (proparacaine hydrochloride 0.5% + 2 drops gentamicin 0.3% +/–1 drop cyclopentolate at physicians' discretion	Patients receiving diclofenac had a mean pain-intensity reduction at 2 hrs of 3.1 compared with 1.0 in control group (difference 2.1+/–1.3 95% CI 0.8–3.4). 20% of diclofenac group took rescue medication compared with 42% of control subjects. (difference 42% 95% CI –4% to 47%)
Alberti MM et al. 2001[17]	In a multicenter randomized double blinded parallel study, 123 patients with traumatic corneal abrasions were given a fixed combination of 0.1% indomethacin and gentamicin or gentamicin alone 4 times daily for 5–6 days	The global difference in pain relief from day 0 today 4/5 was significantly better in the Indomethacin group ($p=0.015$) but no difference was seen in use of supplemental analgesia or time to healing
Goyal et al. 2001[18]	In a prospective single-center randomized placebo controlled double-blind trial, 85 patients presenting to an ophthalmology practice with abrasion or foreign body removal of <48 hrs duration were given Ketrorolac 0.5% 4 times daily or artificial tears together with cyclopentolate and topical chloramphenicol ointment	There was no significant difference in the two group at 24-hr follow-up in 5 subjective symptoms including pain. 16% of ketorolac group took rescue medication compared with 50% of control subjects (95% CI 15–53% $p=0.001$)
Calder LA et al. 2005[16]	In a meta-analysis of randomized trials 11 trials were included involving a total of 459 patients with corneal abrasions. Patients were given routine treatment+/–topical NSAIDs	The overall weighted mean difference in pain score at 24 hrs in the topical NSAIDs score was 1.3 (95% CI –1.56 to –1.03) which was statistically significant

Data from various sources (see references)

Answer

It can be seen that topical non-steroidal anti-inflammatory drugs such as 0.1% diclofenac and 0.05% ketorolac do reduce pain and decrease the use of oral analgesics and opiates in patients with corneal abrasions, however not all departments stock these and hence oral medication is often given in preference. There have been no studies to compare these drugs with oral preparations.

Mydriatics such as cyclopentolate or tropicamide have traditionally been prescribed in corneal abrasions to ease spasm of the ciliary muscle and improve pain but the evidence is not strong (see Table 8.4).

Table 8.4 Evidence base: topical mydriatics for corneal abrasions

Author	Design, participants, and intervention	Results
Brahma *et al.* 1996, UK.[20]	In a prospective randomized controlled trial, 401 patients with corneal abrasions presenting to the ED 401 patients with corneal abrasions were treated with either (i) lubricant alone vs (ii) 2% homatropine (single dose) vs (iii) flubiprofen 0.03% vs. (iv) flubiprofen 0.03% QDS and homatropine (single dose) Treatments given for 4 hrs	No difference between the lubricant alone and homatropine group or either of the 2 groups receiving flubiprofen
Meek *et al.* (2010)[21] Australia	In a triple-blind randomized controlled trial of a convenience sample of 40 patients with corneal abrasions randomized to 6 hrly Homatropine drops or placebo. Visual analogue scale (VAS) pain ratings at 0, 6, 12, 18, 24 hrs.	No significant difference in pain score reduction found. Percentage of patients reporting >20 mm VAS at 12 hrs 50% in Homatropine group (95% CI −27.2–72.8) and 60% in the placebo group (95% CI −36.1–80.9)

Data from various sources (see references)

Answer

The evidence is limited but the experimental work which has been done suggests limited benefit of using such medications.

> **⊗ Learning point** Eye patches
>
> Eye patches are no longer recommended for corneal abrasions.[22–24] A meta-analysis of 5 RCTs failed to reveal an increase in healing rate or improvement in pain scale.[24] Two subsequent RCTs (1 in children, 1 in adults) reported similar results.[22,23] Furthermore, patching can result in decreased oxygen delivery, increased moisture, and a higher chance of infection. Thus, patching may actually retard the healing process.[25,26] A Cochrane review[27] of 7 trials reporting complete healing rates on the first day of follow-up showed that more participants in the no-patch group had complete healing (risk ratio = 0.89; 95% confidence interval, 0.79–0.99).

Case progression

You discharge your patient with topical antibiotic ointment, analgesia and a follow-up appointment the next day in the eye clinic to remove the rest of the rust ring.

A Final Word from the Expert

Most corneal abrasions will heal within 48–72 hrs. Despite the lack of strong evidence, antibiotics and mydriatics are still often prescribed. The patient will be most distressed by the pain these injuries cause and hence the provision of some analgesia, preferably topical NSAIDS if available, should be given. All corneal abrasions should be re-evaluated within 48 hrs. In those that involve the visual axis or are greater than one-quarter, the corneal surface should have urgent ophthalmology follow-up and be seen the next day.

References

1. Gor DM, Kirsch CF, Leen J, *et al.* Radiologic Differentiation of Intraocular Glass: evaluation of imaging techniques, glass types, size and effect of intraocular hemorrhage. *Am J Roentgenol* 2001 Nov; 177(5):1199–203.
2. Saeed A, Cassidy L, Malone DE, *et al.* Plain X-ray and computed tomography of the orbit in cases and suspected cases of intraocular foreign body. *Eye* (Lond). 2008 Nov; 22(11):1373–7.
3. Royal College of Radiologists. Making the best use of a Clinical Department of Radiology. Guidelines for Doctors, Fifth Edition. London: Royal College of Radiologists, 2003.
4. Nunn K, Thompson PK. Towards evidence based emergency medicine: best BETs from the Manchester Royal Infirmary. Can the nature and extent of orbital trauma be optimally assessed with ultrasound imaging in the Emergency Department? *Emerg Med J* 2011 (Sept); 28(9):809–10.
5. Tayal VS, Neulander M, Norton HJ, *et al.* Emergency department sonographic measurement of optic nerve sheath diameter to detect findings of increased intracranial pressure in adult head injury patients. *Ann Emerg Med* 2007 Apr; 49(4):508–14.
6. Deramo VA, Shah GK, Baumal CR, *et al.* Ultrasound biomicroscopy as a tool for detecting and localizing occult foreign bodies after ocular trauma. *Ophthalmology* 1999 Feb; 106(2):301–5.
7. Kruger RA, Higgins J, Rashford S, *et al.* Emergency eye injuries. *Aust Fam Physician* 1990; 19(6):934–8.
8. King, JW, Brison RJ. Do topical antibiotics help corneal epithelial trauma? *Can Fam Physician* 1993 Nov; 39:2349–52.
9. Upadhyay MP, Karmacharya PC, Koirala S, *et al.* The Bhaktapur eye study: ocular trauma and antibiotic prophylaxis for the prevention of corneal ulceration in Nepal. *Br J Ophthalmol* 2001 Apr; 85(4):388–92.
10. Calder L, Balasubramanian S, Stiell I. Lack of consensus on corneal abrasion management: results of a national survey. *CJEM* 2004 Nov; 6(6):402–7.
11. Boberg-Ans, G, Nissen KR. Comparison of Fucithalmic viscous eye drops and Chloramphenicol eye ointment as a single treatment in corneal abrasion. *Acta Ophthalmol Scand* 1998 Feb; 76(1):108–11.
12. Quinn SM, Kwartz J. Emergency management of contact lens associated corneal abrasions. *Emerg Med J* 2004 Nov; 21(6):755.
13. Brahma AK, Shah S, Hillier VF, *et al.* Topical analgesia for superficial corneal injuries. *J Accid Emerg Med* 1996 May; 13(3):186–8.
14. Jayamanne DG, Fitt AW, Dayan M, *et al.* The effectiveness of topical diclofenac in relieving discomfort following traumatic corneal abrasions. *Eye* (Lond) 1997; 11(Pt 1):79–83.
15. Kaiser PK, Pineda R 2nd. A study of topical nonsteroidal anti-inflammatory drops and no pressure patching in the treatment of corneal abrasions. *Ophthalmology* 1997 Aug; 104(8):1353–9.
16. Calder LA, Balasubramanian S, Fergusson D. Topical nonsteroidal anti-inflammatory drugs for corneal abrasions: meta-analysis of randomized trials. *Acad Emerg Med* 2005 May; 12(5):467–73.
17. Alberti MM, Bouat CG, Allaire CM, *et al.* Combined indomethacin/gentamicin eye-drops to reduce pain after traumatic corneal abrasion. *Eur J Ophthalmol* 2001 Jul–Sept; 11(3):233–9.
18. Goyal R, Shankar J, Fone DL, *et al.* Randomised controlled trial of ketorolac in the management of corneal abrasions. *Acta Ophthalmol Scand* 2001 Apr; 79(2):177–9.
19. Szucs PA, Nashed AH, Allegra JR, *et al.* Safety and efficacy of diclofenac oph- thalmic solution in the treatment of corneal abrasions. *Ann Emerg Med* 2000 Feb; 35(2):131–7.
20. Brahma AK, Shah S, Hillier VF, *et al.* Topical analgesia for superficial corneal injuries. *J Accid Emerg Med* 1996 May; 13(3):186–8.

21. Meek R, Sullivan A, Favilla M, *et al*. Is homatropine 5% effective in reducing pain associated with corneal abrasion when compared with placebo? A randomized controlled trial. *Emerg Med Australas* 2010 Dec; 22(6):507–13.

22. Le Sage N, Verreault R, Rochette L. Efficacy of eye patching for traumatic corneal abrasions: a controlled clinical trial. *Ann Emerg Med* 2001 Aug; 38(2):129–34.

23. Michael JG, Hug D, Dowd MD. Management of corneal abrasion in children: a randomized clinical trial. *Ann Emerg Med* 2002 Jul; 40(1):67–72.

24. Flynn CA, D'Amico F, Smith G. Should we patch corneal abrasions? A meta-analysis. *J Fam Pract* 1998 Oct; 47(4):264–70.

25. Campanile TM, St Clair DA, Benaim M. The evaluation of eye patching in the treatment of traumatic corneal epithelial defects. *J Emerg Med* 1997 Nov–Dec; 15(6):769–74.

26. Kaiser PK. A comparison of pressure patching versus no patching for corneal abrasions due to trauma or foreign body removal. Corneal Abrasion Patching Study Group. *Ophthalmology* 1995 Dec; 102(12):1936–42.

27. Turner A, Rabiu M.Patching for corneal abrasion. *Cochrane Database Syst Rev* 2006 Apr 19;(2):CD004764.

9 Procedural sedation in the emergency department

Sophie Parker

Expert commentary Tim Harris

Case history

A 30-year-old man presents to the ED at 11 p.m. having sustained a right-sided shoulder injury after tripping on a wet step whilst out with his friends. He has drunk 3 pints of beer but denies taking any illicit drugs and he has not eaten since the morning. The triage nurse that saw him has ordered an X-ray and has given the patient 1 g paracetamol and 400 mg ibuprofen. You are asked to see him as the radiographer has called to say that she thinks the shoulder could be dislocated.

You go and see the patient in the minors area of the ED and note that he is relatively comfortable while sitting still with his right arm supported, but in significant pain whenever he moves. He denies any other injuries and has no past medical history of note. On examination his right shoulder is deformed and there is loss of pinprick sensation over the lateral aspect of his upper arm. The radial and ulna pulses were felt equally in both arms, with capillary refill times of less than 2 seconds in each. His observations are HR 100 bpm BP 110/80mmHg RR 18 breaths per minute O2 saturations 95 % on room air.

The X-ray confirms the diagnosis of an anterior shoulder dislocation of the glenohumeral joint without fracture. The core trainee on duty has approached you about relocating the shoulder, but is unsure about the sedation options available for this patient in the ED.

See Box 9.1 for a clinical summary of College of Emergency Medicine and Royal College of Anaesthetics sedation recommendations[1] and Box 9.2 for a clinical summary of sedation agents.

Box 9.1 Clinical summary of College of Emergency Medicine and Royal College of Anaesthetics sedation recommendations

Procedural sedation is a vital skill for the emergency physician. Many patients present requiring diagnostic and therapeutic procedures that benefit considerably from pharmacological sedation and as such, ED doctors are required to be familiar with a range of drugs and skills. The CEM and Royal College of Anaesthesia Working Party recommendations (2012) begin by reminding the clinician that 'sedation is a continuum at which a predetermined level is not always possible to maintain'.

Although there are many different sedative agents available to physicians, no single drug is 'perfect'. The ideal sedative would address the following:

- hypnosis
- anxiolysis
- amnesia
- be an anticonvulsant
- be safe in all age groups
- be non-cumulative
- be independent of renal and hepatic metabolism

(continued)

- have a rapid onset and offset times
- have no interactions with other drugs
- not produce respiratory or cardiovascular depression
- be cheap
- have no prolonged effect on memory or lasting psychological effect
- no long-term psychological effect

Benzodiazepines (BDZ) are the most widely used class of sedative drugs in emergency medicine and remain popular in the UK today, but are rarely used in Australasia, and North America. They provide hypnosis, amnesia, and anxiolysis. However they do not have any analgesic properties and therefore are commonly combined with an opioid.

The dose of the benzodiazepine should be adjusted based on a number of patient factors. Prior exposure to BDZs or a history of alcohol consumption will both increase the tolerance of the patient, meaning that a larger dose may have to be used. BDZs should be used in caution in the unwell or unstable patient as they can cause cardiovascular and respiratory depression and a key issue remains the unpredictable and depth and duration of sedation post procedure.

Data from College of Emergency Medicine and the Royal College of Anaesthetics: Safe sedation of adults in the Emergency Department. 2012.

Box 9.2 Clinical summary of sedation agents

Midazolam is the most commonly used BDZ in the ED for procedural sedation in the UK. It has variable solubility, being water-soluble at pH 4 but fat-soluble at pH 7. It is metabolized to 3 main metabolites: alpha 1-hydroxymidazolam, 4-hydroxymidazolam, and 1,4-hydroxymidazolam. These may accumulate if midazolam is given in large doses, or if the patient has renal or hepatic impairment

Sedative dose: initial dose 2–2.5 mg (0.5–1 mg in the elderly), with subsequent 1 mg incremental doses titrated to the required depth of sedation for procedural success

Propofol is commonly used as an intravenous anaesthetic induction agent, but is increasingly being used for procedural sedation. It acts on the GABA receptor complex and is metabolized by the liver to inactive metabolites. Its advantages lie in the fact that it has very rapid onset and offset times. However, it is also a potent depressant of the cardiovascular system and may cause significant hypotension, especially in patients with hypovolaemia or sepsis. The elimination half-life is variable but falls between 2–24 hours. However the clinical effect is much shorter than this due to the large volume of distribution of propofol, averaging 6–10 minutes

Sedative dose: 0.5–1 mg/kg

Ketamine acts by blocking N-methyl-D-aspartic acid (NMDA) receptors, resulting in dissociative anaesthesia. The advantage of ketamine for procedural sedation is the lack of cardiovascular or respiratory depressive effects. However, patients may experience unpleasant emergent phenomena as the effects wear off, such as auditory and visual hallucinations or delirium, which can be distressing, not only for the patient but also for their relatives and the treating physician.

Sedative dose: 0.5–2 mg/kg

Etomidate acts at the $GABA_A$ receptor and has an effect within 1 arm–brain circulation time (roughly 30 seconds). It is highly protein-bound and is metabolized in the liver to inactive metabolites. Although the half-life is about 75 minutes, the duration of its action is shorter (about 10 minutes) due to rapid redistribution. This, and the fact that it is cardiovascularly stable, means that it is useful as a sedative agent. The disadvantage of etomidate for procedural sedation is the fact that it can cause myoclonic activity, thus potentially making procedures (e.g. relocations) harder to perform.

Sedative dose: 0.1 mg–0.2 mg/kg

✪ **Learning point** American Association of Anaesthesiology (ASA) depths of sedation[2]

Minimal sedation—(Anxiolysis) where patients respond normally to verbal stimuli. Cognitive function may be impaired, however haemodynamics are unaffected.

(continued)

Moderate sedation—(known as conscious sedation) where consciousness is impaired but patients may respond to verbal response or tactile stimuli. Again, there is no loss of airway maintenance and no haemodynamic compromise.

Deep sedation—Patients cannot easily be roused and airway compromise may occur with inadequate ventilation. Cardiovascular function is mostly maintained.

General anaesthesia—No response to verbal or painful stimuli and loss of airway patency and ventilation with haemodynamic compromise requiring intubation and ventilation.

Dissociative sedation—Ketamine does not fit into these definitions and instead is defined as 'a trance like cataleptic state characterized by profound analgesia and amnesia, with retention of protective airway reflexes, spontaneous respirations, and cardiopulmonary stability.'

Data from American Society of Anesthesiologists. Practice guidelines for preoperative fasting and the use of pharmacologic agents to reduce the risk of pulmonary aspiration: application to healthy patients undergoing elective procedures. *Anesthesiology*. 1999; 90:896–905.

Clinical question: 'Is it in the best interest of the non-fasted patient to proceed with procedural sedation in the ED?'

As modern anaesthesia has developed, opinion regarding pre-procedural practice has also gone through many changes. Originally a 'nil-by-mouth from midnight' practice was adopted, but guidelines have subsequently become less strict due to a lack of supporting evidence. The ASA guidelines[3] currently recommend specific fasting times for patients prior to elective surgery, and these are widely accepted by the anaesthetic community.

In separate guidelines designed specifically to address the question of sedation by non-anaesthesiologists[2] the authors state: '[t]he literature does not provide sufficient evidence to test the hypothesis that pre-procedure fasting results in a decreased incidence of adverse outcomes in patients undergoing either moderate or deep sedation'.

The bottom-line recommendation is that: '[i]n urgent, emergent, or other situations in which gastric emptying is impaired, the potential for pulmonary aspiration of gastric contents must be considered in determining (1) the target level of sedation, (2) whether the procedure should be delayed, or (3) whether the trachea should be protected by intubation'.[3]

⊕ **Learning point** Continuum of depth of sedation: definition of general anaesthesia and levels of sedation/analgesia

Table 9.1 Spectrum of the depths of sedation

	Minimal sedation (Anxiolysis)	Moderate sedation/ Analgesia (conscious sedation)	Deep edation/ Analgesia	General Anaesthesia
Responsiveness	Normal response to verbal stimulation	Purposeful* response to verbal or tactile stimulation	Purposeful* response after repeated or painful stimulation	Cannot be roused, even with painful stimulus
Airway	Unaffected	No intervention required	Intervention may be required	Intervention often required

(continued)

Spontaneous ventilation	Unaffected	Adequate	May be inadequate	Frequently inadequate
Cardiovascular function	Unaffected	Usually maintained	Usually maintained	May be impaired

* Reflex withdrawal from a painful stimulus is not considered a purposeful response.

Because sedation is a continuum, it is not always possible to predict how an individual patient will respond.[4] Hence, practitioners intending to produce a given level of sedation should be able to intervene with patients whose level of sedation becomes deeper than initially intended.

Individuals administering 'Moderate sedation/Analgesia' (Conscious sedation) should be able to escalate treatment for patients who enter a state of 'Deep sedation/Analgesia', and similarly those administering 'Deep sedation/Analgesia' should be able to escalate interventions with tracheal intubation for patients who enter a state of 'General anaesthesia'.

Data from American College of Emergency Physicians, 'Clinical policy: procedural sedation and analgesia in the emergency department', Annals of Emergency Medicine, 2005, 45, pp. 177–196.

Certainly more relevant for emergency practitioners are the guidelines from CEM and the American College of Emergency Physicians. These state: '[t]here is insufficient evidence to determine absolute recommendations. Although recent food intake is not a contraindication for administering procedural sedation and analgesia, the emergency physician must weigh the risk of pulmonary aspiration and the benefits of providing procedural sedation and analgesia in accordance with the needs of each individual patient'.[5]

Researchers looking into risk factors for aspiration have often found it difficult to design good-quality, prospective studies due to the low incidence of aspiration in elective clinical practice. Green and Krauss[6] pooled data from 10 large studies conducted between 1980 and 1999 and found the overall incidence of aspiration to be 1 in 3420 and the incidence of aspiration mortality to be 1 in 125 109. Clearly such a low incidence of the primary outcome will make powering a study to show significance difficult. However there is a growing body of work that looks specifically at the risk of aspiration during procedural sedation. A summary of the pertinent studies is shown in Table 9.2.

Evidence[6,7,8] has suggested that there are a number of reasons to suppose that patients being sedated have a lower risk of aspiration than that reported within general anaesthesia, which are summarized here:

- Two-thirds of aspirations that occur during general anaesthesia happen during manipulation of the airway (i.e. intubation and extubation). These events of course do not feature during procedural sedation.
- Inhalational agents used during general anaesthesia are known to be emetogenic. These are not used during procedural sedation.
- Unconsciousness with resultant loss of airway reflexes is not the desired end point of procedural sedation. While it is acknowledged that sedation is a continuum, and practitioners must be prepared to deal with a patient who progresses from 'deep sedation' to 'general anaesthesia', the majority of patients should be able to maintain their own airway during emergency department sedation.
- The majority of emergency department procedural sedations are carried out in young and low-risk (i.e. ASA I/II) patients.
- Ketamine is often used for procedural sedation, which is known to preserve airway reflexes, thus lowering the risk of aspiration.

The ultimate decision of whether or not to proceed with procedural sedation in the emergency department requires careful balancing of the risks versus the benefits as assessed by addressing these points.

Table 9.2 Summary of larger studies investigating the association of vomiting/aspiration during emergency procedural sedation with fasting status

Author, date	Patient group	Outcomes	Key results	Study weaknesses
Agrawal[9] 2003 USA Single centre, prospective, observational	1014 consecutive paediatric patients requiring sedation in the ED	Relationship between fasting status and adverse events	396/905 patients were fasted as per ASA guidelines Vomiting: $n=15$ (1.5%) • associated with older age (median age 11.1 vs 5.3 years $p=0.03$) and Ketamine (OR 3.2; 95% CI 1.1–9.6 $p=0.04$) No aspirations No association between fasting status and adverse events • 8.1% patients who met fasting guidelines had adverse events vs 6.9% who were not fasted ($p=0.49$)	Incomplete data collection Not powered to detect significant difference in rate of vomiting +/– aspiration Single-centre study
Roback[10] 2003 USA Single centre, prospective, observational	2085 paediatric patients receiving parenteral sedation in the ED	Relationship between fasting status and adverse events	Median fasting time 5.1 hours (range 5 mins–32.5 hours) Vomiting: $n=156$ (7.5%) No significant difference in adverse events incidence based on duration of pre-procedural fasting No aspirations	No clear breakdown of numbers of patients fasted specifically as per ASA guidelines Incomplete documentation Observers not blinded to fasting status No power calculation
Campbell[11] 2005 Canada Retrospective case series	979 adult patients requiring procedural sedation in the ED	To assess the frequency of adverse events associated with procedural sedation	No cases of pulmonary aspiration	Single centre Sedation administered by Advanced Care Paramedics (ACPs)—possible external validity issues No documentation of incidence of vomiting
Cravero[12] 2006 USA Multi-centre, prospective, observational	30037 paediatric contacts requiring sedation/anaesthesia outside of the operating room	Demographics, complication rate	Vomiting: $n=142$ (incidence 47.2/10 000; 95% CI 39.8–55.7) Aspiration: $n=1$ (incidence 0.3/10 000; 95% CI 0.0–1.9) • patient had been fasted for > 8 hrs	Institutes self-selected Incomplete data collection All levels of sedation analysed together No indication given of relationship between fasting status and adverse events
Thorpe[13] 2010 England Systematic review	4657 adult cases and 17 672 paediatric cases requiring emergency procedural sedation 1954–2008	Association of fasting and aspiration during procedural sedation	Adults: 1 case report of pulmonary aspiration • 17 cases of vomiting during procedural sedation Paediatric: no reports of pulmonary aspiration	
Taylor and Bell[14] 2011 Australia Multi-centre Prospective, observational	2623 consecutive patients (adults and paediatric) requiring sedation in the ED	Demographics, complication rate	Vomiting: $n=34$ (1.6%; 95% CI 1.1–2.2) • univariate analysis suggested young age, low weight, and sedation with nitrous oxide or ketamine were significant risk factors • premedication with morphine or sedation with propofol or fentanyl was protective • fasting status was not significantly associated with vomiting Aspiration: $n=1$ (0.05%)	Low incidence of adverse effects therefore multivariate analyses were not appropriate meaning truly independent risk factors could not be determined Not a true consecutive sample Incomplete data collection)

Data from various sources (see references)

> ⊕ **Clinical tip** Reported risk factors for pulmonary aspiration
>
> Weighing the available evidence concerning procedural sedation and the risk of aspiration, the current strategy should involve:
> 1. Assessing the individual patient risk
>
> The ASA list a number of factors that they feel put patients into a higher risk category for aspiration:
> - Airway difficulties (e.g. difficult intubation, laryngospasm)
> - Emergency surgery
> - Advanced age (>70 years)
> - Higher ASA* physical status classification
> - Conditions predisposing to gastro-oesophageal reflux (e.g. oesophageal disease, pregnancy, hiatus hernia, peptic ulcer disease, gastritis, bowel obstruction, ileus, elevated intracranial pressure)
>
> 2. Assessing the timing and nature of last oral intake
> 3. Assessing the urgency of the procedure
> 4. Determine the predicted length and depth of sedation required

Answer

Fasting is not an absolute requirement for patients requiring procedural sedation in the ED. For this patient who has altered sensation in the axillary nerve distribution, performing the relocation remains the priority.

> ⑥ **Expert comment**
>
> The issue of whether or not to offer procedural sedation to patients who have not been fasted for the times recommended for general anaesthesia is a daily conundrum for the emergency physician. In a 2007 study including 404 ED sedations (282 unfasted) Bell et al noted no significant difference in the incidence of vomiting, apnoea, respiratory depression, suctioning or desaturation between fasted and unfasted patients. (Bell A, Treston G, McNabb C, et al *Emerg Med* Australis 2007;19:405–10). Similarly in a prospective observational study of over 1000 children Agrawal et al found no difference in adverse events between fasted and unfasten children (*Ann Emerg Med* 2003;42:636–46). Green et al have suggested that the clinician should balance the risks of aspiration against the risks of delayed procedural sedation (Green in *Ann Emerg Med* 2007;49:454–61). While there are no randomised trials of fasting in ED sedation current research suggests that in the fact non-fasted state offers no or only minimally increased aspiration risk in the ED setting and a recent ACEP statement suggests fasting is not a requirement for ED procedural sedation. Thus for critically unwell patients with tachyarrhythmias and haemodynamic compromise there is a clear need for urgent intervention and the issue is whether to secure the airway with rapid sequence induction and intubation or use procedural sedation. Both choices offer risks with the former requiring higher sedation doses with increased risk of cardiovascular collapse and the latter the risk of aspiration. The literature is clear that this risk is very small in the ED setting. For patients requiring joint manipulation the procedural is less urgent and a balanced assessment is made based upon the risks of aspiration and the risks of procedural delay; pain, increased swelling with muscle spasm making the procedure more challenging, and neurovascular compromise. In the upper limb alternatives such as ultrasound guided nerve blocks offer a simple alternative. Lower limb injuries allow the patient to be positioned at 30 degrees further improving respiratory mechanics and reducing the aspiration risk. Patients with non-urgent conditions that require non-ideal positioning, such as perianal abscesses, should wait or be referred to operating theatre.

Case progression

The nursing staff begin to prepare the bedside monitoring required and ask the junior doctor to help set up the ETCO2 monitoring system. The trainee helping you is unfamiliar with this request and enquires whether simple peripheral oxygen saturations would suffice during procedural sedation in the department. He rightly comments that the level of sedation should not reach a level to impair intrinsic airway control and thus wonders why anything more than simple bedside saturations are required.

Clinical question: Should ETCO$_2$ monitoring be routinely used during procedural sedation in the ED?

ETCO$_2$ monitoring is considered to be standard during general anaesthesia, acknowledging its unique use in the detection of hypoventilation of the patient. Although pulse oximetry is a useful way of detecting arterial desaturation, in the presence of a high FiO$_2$ the presence of hypoventilation may be masked.[10] By monitoring the ETCO$_2$ value, and also by analysing the shape of the waveform with each breath, it is possible to draw conclusions about the patient's respiratory effort on a breath-by-breath basis. Capnography via nasal cannulae is now widely available and many systems also have the advantage of combining ETCO$_2$ measurement with oxygen supplementation in the same device.

There are several studies investigating the relationship between ETCO$_2$ monitoring and the incidence of respiratory depression as quantified by a predefined fall in oxygen saturations on pulse oximetry (Table 9.3).

While there is evidence that ETCO$_2$ monitoring may be able to predict respiratory depression before pulse oximetry, especially given that it is considered best practice for patients to receive supplemental oxygen,[19,20] there is no clear evidence that this correlates to a clinically significant reduction in clinically relevant hypoxia or rhythm disturbances.

The current ASA guidelines for sedation by non-anaesthesiologists state that, '[m]onitoring of exhaled carbon dioxide should be considered for all patients receiving deep sedation and for patients whose ventilation cannot be directly observed during moderate sedation'.[2,3] The London Deanery indicates that all patients undergoing procedural sedation in the ED should have compulsory ETCO$_2$ monitoring (see Figure 9.1).

In addition, the recent 2012 College of Emergency Medicine guidelines on safe procedural sedation state that, '[c]apnography is also recommended at lighter levels of sedation; this is an emerging area of practice, and the use of capnography is expected to become routine'.

> **⊕ Clinical tip** Equipment recommendations for sedation
>
> An environment identical to that in which intubation and ventilation could occur
>
> Difficult airway equipment
>
> A trolley capable of being tipped head down
>
> Continuous high-flow oxygen with non-rebreath mask
>
> High-pressure suction with appropriate yanker catheters
>
> Monitoring: Pulse oximeter, ECG, NIBP, and continuous quantitative capnography
>
> 1000 ml bag of crystalloind fluids with giving sets

Pre-sedation checklist

Location: Resuscitation room					✓
Monitors	SpO2	End-tidal CO2	BP	ECG	
Equipment	Tiltable trolley	Airway trolley	Suction	Drugs drawn up and labeled	
Vascular access	IV Fluids				

Time first sedative given: **Time recovered:**

Drugs	1st Bolus	Aliquots	Aliquots	Total
1)				
2)				

Figure 9.1 London Deanery pre-sedation checklist.

Reproduced with permission from Health Education South London

Table 9.3 Summary of studies investigating the association of ETCO$_2$ and respiratory depression

Author, date, and country	Patient group	Study type	Outcomes	Key results	Study weaknesses
Burton[15] USA 2005	Convenience sample of adult and paediatric patients requiring procedural sedation in the ED 2l O$_2$ concurrently given	Prospective, single centre, observational, case series Physicians blinded to ETCO$_2$ values	Frequency of abnormal ETCO$_2$ readings (deviation of >10 mmHg from preprocedure, <30 mmHg or >50 mmHg) and the relationship to acute respiratory events	Study stopped early as interim safety check after 60 pts showed 60% of contacts (36/60) had abnormal ETCO$_2$ readings and 44% of these (16/36) had no other acute respiratory events observed. 33% pts (20/60) had an observed respiratory event and 85% (17/20) of these had abnormal ETCO$_2$ findings. 70% pts (14/20) had the abnormal ETCO$_2$ reading up to 4 mins before the respiratory event was observed	Convenience sample. Inability to record capnography (only capnometry) meant corroboration of observed waveforms later was not possible. Unclear re clinical significance of abnormal capnography in isolation
Deitch[16] USA 2010	Consecutive sample of patients > 18 yrs old suitable for propofol sedation. 3l O$_2$ concurrently given. 150 enrolled (18 lost due to > 35% data loss)	Prospective, randomized controlled, single-centre—randomized to standard monitoring+capnography or standard monitoring + blinded capnography	Whether ETCO$_2$ monitoring reduced the incidence of hypoxia (sats <93% for >15 s) by 15%. Intervention made on clinical ground or based on capnography	Similar incidence of respiratory depression (ETCO$_2$ > 50 mmHg, deviation of >10 mmHg from baseline or loss of waveform for >15 s), but significantly more hypoxia in group blinded to capnography (17 vs 27 pts, p=0.035, (95% CI = 1.3–33%). Resp depression was 100% sensitive for hypoxia (95% CI = 90–100%) and 64% specific (95% CI=53–73%). Median time between resp depression and onset of hypoxia = 60 s	Non-standard co-administration of opioids Higher than expected rate of hypoxia when compared to other studies Unclear re clinical significance of abnormal capnography in isolation

(continued)

Author, date, and country	Patient group	Study type	Outcomes	Key results	Study weaknesses
Lightdale[17] USA 2005	163 children having elective endoscopic procedures. Standardized monitoring in both arms with independent observers monitoring microstream capnography	Prospective, randomized, double-blind trial. Control group – independent observer indicated if $ETCO_2$ waveform absent for >60 s; intervention group -indication if absent waveform for >15 s	Primary outcome measure was pulse oximetry reading <95% for >5 s Secondary outcome measures were clinical suspicion of respiratory depression. Hypothesis was that acting on absent $ETCO_2$ waveform would decrease desaturation incidence	Those in the intervention arm were significantly less likely to have desaturation <95% for >5 s (11% vs 24%; p=0.03) 2 patients with desaturation did not lose their $ETCO_2$ waveform • all others had desaturation episode for mean time of 3.4 mins following initial loss of waveform. • no difference in time to desaturation between the 2 groups (p=0.4)	Randomized using sealed envelopes No documentation of inter rater reliability Under-powered (aiming for 174) No correlation between desaturation and clinically relevant outcome
Miner[18] USA 2002	74 adult patients undergoing procedural sedation in the ED	Prospective, observational, single centre	Evaluate the utility of $ETCO_2$ in detecting respiratory depression and whether it can be used o predict the level of sedation achieved	33 patients (44.6%) fulfilled at least one respiratory depression criterion Propofol caused less respiratory depression (p=0.008)	No control group. Small sample size No standardized method of sedation Definition of respiratory depression included $ETCO_2$ values, i.e. not independent Differences between different drugs secondary end point only; not powered to evaluate this

Data from various sources (see references)

Answer

ETCO$_2$ should be considered as standard in all patients undergoing procedural sedation in the ED.

> **⑥ Expert comment**
>
> Physiological monitoring is an essential part of safe procedural sedation. The environment for procedural sedation, as opposed to simple anxiolysis and analgesia, should be identical to that required for rapid sequence induction and intubation in the ED. This should include pulse oximetry, continuous 3- or 5-lead ECG, NIBP repeated every 3 minutes and ETCO$_2$.
>
> Some practitioners argue that supplementary oxygen is not required and as such, pulse oximetry is sufficient respiratory monitoring. However, most complications of procedural sedation are related to respiratory depression. Supplementary oxygen is cheap and safe in the patient group selected for ED-based procedural sedation. In this setting, hypoventilation is best detected by direct observation and ETCO$_2$. The addition of ETCO$_2$ reduces the time required to identify respiratory depression. No study has been powered to demonstrate improved safety of procedural sedation by using ETCO$_2$. It is a cheap intervention that provides evidence on both respiratory effort and cardiac output. Using this in procedural sedation also assists in developing skills at using ETCO$_2$ in cardiac arrest and in the monitoring of patients with reduced level of consciousness in the ED.

Case progression

You decide to continue with the procedure in the ED. A colleague has agreed to help with the procedure—you will be doing the sedation and she will reduce the shoulder. One of the ED nurses will also be with you to assist during the procedure. The patient is moved through to resus and you complete your pre-procedural checks. Your colleague asks what drug you will be using to sedate the patient.

You recently assisted in another procedural sedation where propofol was used with great success and no distress for the patient. You have previously completed 12 months of anaesthetics and are familiar with the use of propofol for general anaesthesia and suggest to the team that this would be your preferable option; however, both your trainee and the nursing staff politely question if this offers any advantage over midazolam, with which they are both familiar.

Clinical question: Can propofol be safely utilized by emergency physicians for procedural sedation in the ED?

Propofol has traditionally been used as an anaesthetic induction agent, although in recent years it has also been increasingly used for procedural sedation. It is the agent most commonly used in Australasia and North America. It has an excellent safety record when used by appropriately trained emergency physicians in a safe environment, as described in Table 9.4.

Based on this work, the American Society of Anesthesiologists (ASA) and the American Association of Nurse Anesthetists (AANA) released a joint position statement in 2004 regarding the use of propofol. It states that, '[w]henever propofol is

Table 9.4 Summary of key papers investigating the use of propofol in the ED

Author/Date	Patient group	Outcomes	Key results	Study weaknesses
Havel[19] 1999 USA Prospective, randomized, blinded	91 patients (aged 2–18) receiving sedation in the ED Propofol vs midazolam	Recovery times, degree of sedation and complication rates	Significantly quicker recovery times in the propofol group (14.9 mins+/–11.1 versus 76.4 mins+/–47.5; $p = <0.001$). No significant difference between adverse events rate	Not powered specifically to look at adverse events Study investigator not blinded to intervention Morphine also given to patients; iv lidocaine given to propofol group (pre-injection)
Taylor[20] 2004 Australia Multi-centre, prospective, randomized, blinded	86 patients requiring sedation for relocation of anterior shoulder dislocation in the ED	Time to awakening, ease of shoulder reduction and number of attempts	Significant shorter time to full wakefulness in the propofol group compared to midazolam (6.8 mins CI 5.5–8.1 vs 28.5 mins CI 20.9–36.1; $p = <0.001$) Fewer reduction attempts in the propofol group (1.3 CI 1.1–1.5 versus 1.8 CI 1.4–2.2; $p = 0.02$) No significant difference in adverse event rate between groups	More people and greater proportion of men in propofol group Not strict consecutive enrolment Difficulties blinding drug administration Some variables were measured subjectively e.g. body build
Burton and Miner[15] 2006 USA Multi-centre, prospective, observational	792 patients receiving propofol for procedural sedation in the ED	Assess the frequency of respiratory and cardiovascular events during sedation, and any relationship to patient descriptors	Oxygen saturations <90%*: n=61 (7.7%) Bag-valve ventilation*: n=31 (3.9%) Oral airway: n=2 (0.3%) Hypotension (SBP <100 mmHg or decrease in BP requiring IV fluids or another clinical intervention): n=28 (3.5%) Emesis: n=1 (0.1%) *Significantly associated with increased age No intubations, prolonged observation or hospital admissions	Variable sedation protocols across sites Relies on self-reporting No control group
Rex[21] 2009 USA Meta-analysis of published and unpublished data	646 080 cases of propofol sedation by non-anaesthetists for endoscopic procedures Worldwide	Safety profile Cost analysis (substituting anaesthetic- for endoscopist- delivered sedation)	11 patients required endotracheal intubation; 4 of these patients died (all ASA ≥3) Rate of bag-valve mask ventilation = 0.1%	Relied on self-reporting by individual centres Late occurring complications not tracked No standardization of sedation procedures
Taylor and Bell 2011[14] Australia Multi-centre prospective, observational	2623 consecutive patients (adults and paediatric) requiring sedation in the ED	Demographics, complication rate	Propofol use (alone/combination): n=1350. The use of propofol was a significant risk factor for having a respiratory event requiring an intervention (27.7%; $p = <0.001$), but was not a significant risk factor for having a hypotensive episode (1.7%; $p = 0.72$). Propofol was found to be protective for vomiting	Low incidence of adverse effects therefore multivariate analyses were not appropriate meaning truly independent risk factors could not be determined Not a true consecutive sample Incomplete data collection

Data from various sources (see references)

used for sedation/anesthesia, it should be administered only by persons trained in the administration of general anesthesia, who are not simultaneously involved in these surgical or diagnostic procedures. This restriction is concordant with specific language in the propofol package insert, and failure to follow these recommendations could put patients at increased risk of significant injury or death'.

This was followed in 2005 by the American College of Emergency Physicians (ACEP) clinical policy document on procedural sedation in the ED. This gives the Level B recommendation that, '[p]ropofol can be safely administered for procedural sedation and analgesia in the ED'.

Answer

Propofol is a safe and useful sedation agent in the ED when used by those competent at dealing with the potential adverse events that may arise. These adverse events include transient respiratory depression and hypotension, but in the vast majority of cases only require simple adjuncts and do not give rise to any long-term sequelae.

⓯ Expert comment

There is no ideal agent currently available for ED-based procedural sedation. The sedation agents in common use have changed over the past 2 decades. Benzodiazepines were commonly used in most Western countries, but in Australia and North America the vast majority of procedural sedations are performed using propofol and either opiate or ketamine analgesia, or ketamine supplemented by small doses of benzodiazepines. The potential advantages for both propofol and ketamine are speed of onset, reliability of sedation depth, deeper levels of sedation offered, and rapid off-set. A 2011–12 UK audit of over 400 patients across 3 large urban hospitals identified midazolam as the most commonly used sedation agent. It was used in 45% of sedations as compared to propofol (27%) and ketamine (19%). In this non-randomized observational study, propofol was associated with a significantly lower rate of a priori defined adverse events (including procedural failure) than other sedation agents ($p=0.008$). However, the safest drug combinations are those with which the operator is familiar and experienced.

The newest trend in sedation agents is to combine propofol and ketamine together in a syringe producing a solution with 5 mg/ml of each. The theory suggests that the cardiovascular depressive effects of propofol are balanced by ketamine and that ketamine provides analgesia in place of the previously used opiates. This may have a place in patients presenting to ED requiring urgent procedural sedation but data suggest there is no significant clinical advantage over propofol combined with an opiate, such as fentanyl, in terms of the rate of clinically significant cardiorespiratory depression. Many patients also attend ED and require imaging / investigations prior to having their procedure performed. In these cases a two-step approach first maximizing analgesia and then offering procedural sedation some time later may be the most pragmatic approach. This two-step approach may be associated with a reduction on adverse events.

A Final Word from the Expert

Procedural sedation is an essential skill for emergency physicians. It reduces the time patients are required to wait for many painful procedures, reduces the number of patients admitted to hospital, and reduces the burden on operating theatre. As such it combines improved quality of care with decreased costs or reduced length of stay. Procedural sedation should be undertaken in the same environment as induction of anaesthesia and tracheal intubation with trained personnel and in a fully monitored environment—that includes $ETCO_2$ and with supplementary oxygen.

Safe procedural sedation requires dedicated training and careful patient selection. There is no doubt as to the theoretical advantages offered by propofol and ketamine over benzodiazepines as sedation agents and this is supported by some safety and efficiency data. It is of credit to the speciality of emergency medicine that so much research has been performed and published around procedural sedation, so improving the safety and quality of care provided by our specialty.

References

1. College of Emergency Medicine and the Royal College of Anaesthetics: Safe sedation of adults in the Emergency Department. 2012.
2. American Society of Anesthesiologists. Practice guidelines for preoperative fasting and the use of pharmacologic agents to reduce the risk of pulmonary aspiration: application to healthy patients undergoing elective procedures. *Anesthesiology* 1999; 90:896–905.
3. American Society of Anesthesiologists. Practice guidelines for sedation and analgesia by non-anesthesiologists. *Anesthesiology* 2002; 96:1004–17.
4. American College of Emergency Physicians. Clinical policy: procedural sedation and analgesia in the emergency department. *Ann Emerg Med* 2005; 45:177–96.
5. Taylor, DM, Bell A, Holdgate A, *et al.* Risk factors for sedation-related events during procedural sedation in the emergency department. *Emerg Med Aus* 2011; 23:466–73.
6. Green SM, Krauss B. Pulmonary aspiration risk during ED procedural sedation: an examination of the role of fasting and sedation depth. *Acad Emerg Med* 2002; 9:35–42.
7. Raidoo DM, Rocke DA, Brock-Utne JG, *et al.* Critical volume for pulmonary acid aspiration: reappraisal in a primate model. *Br J Anaesth* 1990; 65:248–50.
8. Plourde G, Hardy JFL. Aspiration pneumonia: assessing the risk of regurgitation in the cat. *Can J Anaesth* 1986; 33:345–8.
9. Agrawal D, Manzi SF, Gupta R, *et al.* Preprocedural fasting state and adverse events in children undergoing procedural sedation and analgesia in a pediatric emergency department. *Ann Emerg Med* 2003 Nov; 42(5):636–46.
10. Roback MG, Wathen JE, Bajaj L, *et al.* Adverse events associated with procedural sedation and analgesia in a pediatric emergency department: a comparison of common parenteral drugs. *Acad Emerg Med* 2005 Jun; 12(6):508–13.
11. Campbell SG, Magee KD, Kovacs GJ, *et al.* Procedural sedation and analgesia in a Canadian adult tertiary care emergency department: a case series. *CJEM* 2006 Mar; 8(2):85–93.
12. Cravero JP, Blike GT, Beach M, *et al.* Incidence and nature of adverse events during pediatric sedation/anesthesia for procedures outside the operating room: report from the Pediatric Sedation Research Consortium. *Pediatrics* 2006 Sep; 118(3):1087–96.
13. Thorpe RJ, Benger J. Pre-procedural fasting in emergency sedation. *Emerg Med J* 2010 Apr; 27(4):254–61.
14. Taylor DM, Bell A, Holdgate A, *et al.* Risk factors for sedation-related events during procedural sedation in the emergency department. *Emerg Med Australas* 2011 Aug; 23(4):466–73.

15. Burton JH, Miner JR, Shipley ER, *et al*. Propofol for emergency department procedural sedation and analgesia: a tale of three centers. *Acad Emerg Med* 2006 Jan; 13(1):24–30. Epub 2005 Dec 19.

16. Deitch K, Miner J, Chudnofsky CR, *et al*. Does end tidal CO_2 monitoring during emergency department procedural sedation and analgesia with propofol decrease the incidence of hypoxic events? A randomized, controlled trial. *Ann Emerg Med* 2010 Mar; 55(3):258–64.

17. Lightdale JR, Goldmann DA, Feldman HA, *et al*. Microstream capnography improves patient monitoring during moderate sedation: a randomized, controlled trial. *Pediatrics* 2006 Jun; 117(6):e1170–8.

18. Miner JR, Martel ML, Meyer M, *et al*. Procedural sedation of critically ill patients in the emergency department. *Acad Emerg Med* 2005 Feb; 12(2):124–8.

19. Havel, CJ, Strait RT, Hennes H. A Clinical Trial of Propofol vs Midazolam for Procedural Sedation in a Pediatric Emergency Department. *Acad Emerg Med* 1999; 6:989–97.

20. Taylor DM, O'Brien D, Ritchie P, *et al*. Propofol versus Midazolam/Fentanyl for Reduction of Anterior Shoulder Dislocation. *Acad Emerg Med* 2005; 12:13–19.

21. Rex D, Deenadayalu V, Eid E, *et al*. Endoscopist-directed administration of propofol: a worldwide safety experience. *Gastroenterology* 2009; 137:1229–37.

22. Bell A, Taylor DM, Holdgate A, *et al*. Procedural sedation practices in Australian Emergency Departments. *Emerg Med Australas* 2011; 23:458–65.

23. Green, SM. Propofol in emergency medicine: further evidence of safety. *Emerg Med Australas* 2007; 19:389–93.

10 Atraumatic testicular pain

Oliver Spencer

Expert commentary Kambiz Hashemi

Case history

A 19-year-old man attends the ED with a painful left testicle. The pain started suddenly two hours earlier, and he currently scores the pain at 10 out of 10. Despite detailed history taking there is no history of trauma. He has no past medical history of note, takes no medications and has no allergies. He works as a scaffolder, smokes 10 cigarettes per day, and drinks socially at the weekends only. He is currently in a relationship and is monogamous.

Examination reveals an exquisitely tender raised right testicle, with a likely horizontal lie; the cremasteric reflex is tested for but is absent on the right side. Parental paracetamol and morphine are administered with minimal effect. You feel that the differential diagnosis includes acute testicular torsion, torsion of a hydatid cyst of Morgagni and epididymorchitis.

See Box 10.1 for a clinical summary of testicular torsion.

Box 10.1 Clinical summary of testicular torsion

Testicular torsion presents with an acute onset of diffuse testicular pain and tenderness and is due to twisting of the spermatic cord and blood supply to the ipsilateral testis.

In testicular torsion, the testicle is often raised and has a horizontal lie with the cremasteric reflex potentially decreased or absent.

Torsion occurs in 1 in 4000 males per year before 25 years of age.

65% of cases of torsion present between 12–18 years of age but can affect neonates and younger children. Torsion is rare after the age of 25.

The most common underlying cause is a congenital malformation known as a 'bell-clapper deformity'. This affects 1 in 125 males. In this condition, rather than the testes attaching posteriorly to the inner lining of the scrotum by the mesorchium, the mesorchium terminates early and the testis is free floating in the tunica vaginalis.

⭐ **Learning point** Acute scrotal pain

Acute scrotal pain is prioritized in the ED to minimize the chances of missing torsion. It must be remembered, however, that other causes exist and distinguishing features need to be sought.

Epididymitis—frequently develops from the spread of bacterial infection from the urethra or bladder, with sexually transmitted causes common. Manual elevation of the scrotum may relieve the pain from epididymitis (positive Prehn's sign) but not from a testicular torsion.

(continued)

Torsion of the testicular appendage—isolated tenderness of the superior pole of the testis. Signs include a palpable, hard, tender nodule of 2–3 mm in size, and blue discolouration can be visible known as 'the blue dot sign'.

Irreducible inguinal hernia—a patent tunica vaginalis allows herniation through the inguinal canal and then down the tract of the testes

Testicular haematoma/rupture—the clinical context of trauma is paramount and early exploration may again be needed.

Clinical question: Can the loss of the cremasteric reflex be used to confirm the diagnosis of testicular torsion?

To maximize the chance of successfully salvaging a torted testicle it is imperative to make an early diagnosis. You wonder whether any one particular sign, either by its presence or absence, could be considered diagnostic and therefore negate the need for further investigations. The absence of a cremasteric reflex and high position of the testis increase the likelihood of torsion.[1] The European Association of Urology quotes an absent cremasteric reflex as having a sensitivity of 100 % and specificity of 66 % for presence of testicular torsion. However, 3 of 31 patients with confirmed torsion in Murphy's series had a normal cremasteric reflex.[2] Kadish reported that 8 of 64 patients with epididymitis had an absent cremasteric reflex.[3]

> **✪ Learning point** Cremasteric reflex
>
> The cremasteric reflex is tested by lightly stroking the medial to superior part of the patient's thigh. The reflex utilizes both sensory and motor fibres from the genitofemoral nerves that originate from the L1 and L2 spinal roots. These nerves then initiate contraction of the cremaster muscle causing elevation of the ipsilateral testicle only.
>
> Loss of this reflex occurs in acute torsion but also in condition including epididymitis, upper and lower motor neurone disorders, L1 and L2 disorders, and injury to the nerve potentially during hernia repairs.

> **✚ Clinical tip** Torsion versus epididymitis
>
> **Table 10.1 Torsion versus epididymitis**
>
> | | Torsion | Epididymitis |
> |---|---|---|
> | Onset | Acute | Gradual |
> | Fever | Absent | Often present |
> | Cremasteric reflex | Absent | Usually present |
> | Scrotal lie of testis | Transverse and higher | Vertical and lower |
> | Prehn's Sign | No change in pain | Decrease in pain |
> | Dysuria | May be present | Often present |

> **✓ Evidence base** The cremasteric reflex in testicular torsion
>
> Beni-Israel *et al.* (2010):[1] performed a retrospective review of 523 children who presented to the ED with an acute scrotum. 17 had testicular torsion. Odds ratios with 95 % confidence intervals are detailed

(continued)

for symptoms and signs: abdominal pain OR 3.19 (95% CI 1.15–8.89); high position of testis OR 58.8 (95% CI 19.2–166.6); abnormal cremasteric reflex OR 27.77 (95% CI 7.5–100). Conclude abdominal pain, high position of testicle, and abnormal cremasteric reflex are associated with higher likelihood of torsion.

Murphy *et al.* (2006):[2] performed a retrospective review of 121 boys of less than 15 years of age. 113 had exploratory surgery. 31 had torsion; 9 required orchidectomy, 64 had a torted appendage, 12 epididymitis. Clinical findings: torted testis; pain 94%, swelling 80%, abnormal position 52%, blue dot 3%. Normal cremasteric reflex found in 3 of those who underwent orchidectomy. Torted appendage; pain 100%, swelling 23%, abnormal position 11%, blue dot 22%. Orchitis; pain 100%, swelling 100%, abnormal position 8%, blue dot 8%.

Kadish *et al.* (1998):[3] performed a retrospective review of 90 patients. 13 patients had testicular torsion; 100% absent cremasteric reflex, 23% tender epididymis, 38% scrotal oedema. 64 patients had epididymitis; 13% absent cremasteric reflex, 97% tender epididymis, 67% scrotal oedema.

Answer

There is no single sign that can be considered absolutely diagnostic for torsion. Absent cremasteric reflex and abnormal position/lie should though raise high clinical suspicion of testicular torsion.

> **❝ Expert comment**
>
> It should be remembered that a normal urinalysis does not exclude epididymitis. Similarly, an abnormal urinalysis does not exclude testicular torsion. The same rule can also apply to blood investigations with inflammatory markers such as CRP and ESR more often raised in epididymitis but not exclusively so.
>
> Although loss of cremasteric reflex is a useful sign in diagnosis of testicular torsion, its presence does not exclude the diagnosis and there are numerous case reports of normal cremasteric reflex in cases of testicular torsion.
>
> The diagnosis of torsion, as with many emergency presentations, relies upon the combination of history, examination, and point-of-care investigations to build a bigger clinical picture. Missing a torsion had significant consequences so the utmost care is needed.

Case progression

The urologist is contacted but states that he will be unable to review the patient for at least 1 hour as he is scrubbed in theatre. In the interim period he requests that an ultrasound scrotum and urinalysis are performed. The urinalysis is negative for blood, leucocytes, protein, ketones, and nitrates. One of your ED colleagues suggests you attempt a manual detorsion of the affected testicle as he believes this may help to relieve pain and potentially restore blood flow to the affected testicle, 'buying some time' before definitive intervention.

Clinical question: Is there a role for manual detorsion of a testicular torsion in the ED?

Traditionally, it has been taught that testicular torsion occurs in primarily a medial direction. In theory, provided adequate analgesia has been administered, then manual detorsion should be achieved by rotating the testicle in the lateral direction.

There are several case reports of this be successfully achieved in the literature and achieving relief of pain.[4,5]

Two retrospective case series have been published.[6,7] The residual torsion rate following a detorsion procedure ranging from 27–32 %. Dunn's paper reports the direction and degree of torsion rotation with 67 % rotating in a medial direction and 33 % in a lateral direction.[6] There was no difference between the left and right testicle. The degree of torsion rotation that can be found at the time of exploration in the operating theatre ranges from 180° to 1080°.[6]

Unless scrotal exploration is undertaken, it is not possible to know the direction or degree of torsion. Therefore if a procedure to try and untwist a suspected medial direction torsion was actually performed on a lateral direction torsion, this would increase the degree of torsion and further compromise blood flow to the testicle. As all these patients are going to undergo scrotal exploration one could argue that manual attempts to untwist a testicle are not justified as they could potentially worsen the problem.

✓ **Evidence base**   Manual detorsion in testicular torsion

Dunn (2008):[6] retrospective review of 200 males age 18 months to 20 years who underwent scrotal exploration. 186 records available. Torsion direction medial direction 67 %, lateral direction 33 %. No difference noted in direction of torsion between left and right testicles. Degree of torsion rotation ranged from 180° to 1080°. Manual detorsion attempted in 53 cases with residual torsion in 32 %.

Betts *et al.* (1983):[7] eight out of 11 cases of testicular torsion that attended an emergency department over the time period of 1 year were successfully untwisted. Doppler ultrasound used to document return of blood flow. All underwent subsequent fixation.

Answer

Attempted manual detorsion of a testicular torsion in the ED does not negate the need for urgent surgical exploration and testicular fixation.

ⓘ **Expert comment**

Manual detorsion is an old and well-documented technique, but safe only in expert hands. Although research has shown cases of successful detorsion with the 'open book' technique (rotation of medial to lateral), a caveat must exist as there remains the potential to exacerbate the degree of torsion as the direction of torsion is impossible to know clinically. It is also essential to confirm restoration of circulation to the testis following this procedure, something that is not always easy to do in the ED.

Although it may have a place for pre-operative management of such cases (to temporarily/partially restore blood flow), this technique has no place as primary management of testicular torsion and must not be considered an alternative to definitive exploration.

Case progression

The radiology department questions why the patient requires an ultrasound scan and vehemently suggests that if the clinical picture is one of torsion, a scan will not be able to rule out a torsion 100 %. You explain that you agree with this rationale but also that in the context of any potential time delay for surgery, it would

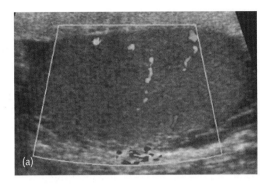

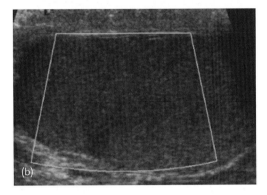

Figure 10.1 Ultrasound image of testicular torsion.

Reproduced from MJ Darby *et al.*, *Oxford Handbook of Medical Imaging*, 2012, Figure 16.20, page 255, with permission from Oxford University Press.

be advantageous to have a colour Doppler performed. The scan is conducted and unable to delineate any blood flow in the left testis (see Figure 10.1).

Clinical question: Is surgical exploration still warranted if an ultrasound demonstrates blood flow in the testicular artery?

Ultrasound has been used for the last 40 years to investigate the acute scrotum and diagnose conditions including torsion, epididymitis, orchitis, hydroceles, and tumors. The main rationale that clinicians use is to distinguish between inflammation and infarction and there are numerous observational studies that quote sensitivities ranging from 63 % up to 100 % in diagnosing testicular torsion with ultrasound. A combination of both gray-scale imaging and colour Doppler are commonly utilized. Caution must be taken though, as there are reports of blood flow being demonstrated on Doppler ultrasound with subsequent necrotic testes being removed at scrotal exploration.[8]

> ➕ **Clinical tip** Ultrasound findings for torsion[14]
>
> - Decreased or absent blood flow (initially venous then arterial flow)
> - Heterogeneous and hypoechoic echogenicity of the testicle
> - Enlarged testicle and epididymis secondary to congestion
> - 'Whirlpool pattern'—spiral twist of the spermatic cord
> - Hydrocele
> - Oedema of the scrotal wall
>
> Data from Datta *et al.* Torsion / Detorsion. *Ultrasound Quarterly.* 2011; 27:2: 127–128.

> ✪ **Learning point** European Association of Urology Guidelines—Paediatric Acute Scrotum[12]
>
> Doppler ultrasound is useful to evaluate an acute scrotum for testicular torsion, with a sensitivity of 63.6–100 % and a specificity of 97–100 %, and a positive predictive value of 100 % and negative predictive value 97.5 %.
>
> (continued)

The use of Doppler ultrasound may reduce the number of patients with an acute scrotum undergoing scrotal exploration, but it is operator-dependent and can be difficult to perform in pre-pubertal patients.

Doppler may also show a misleading arterial flow in the early phases of torsion and in partial or intermittent torsion: persistent arterial flow does not exclude testicular torsion.

Scintigraphy and, more recently, dynamic contrast-enhanced subtraction MRI of the scrotum also provide a comparable sensitivity and specificity to ultrasound.

These investigations may be used when diagnosis is less likely and if torsion of the testis still cannot be excluded from history and physical examination. This should be done without inordinate delay for emergent intervention.

Data from 12 European Association of Urology Guidelines http://www.uroweb.org/gls/pdf/19_Paediatric_Urology.pdf

---

✔ Evidence base Ultrasound in testicular torsion

Prando (2009) emphasized that ultrasound findings in torsion are crucially dependent on the length of time, the degree of rotation of the torsion that has occurred, and the tightness of the vessel compression. Caution is encouraged as the torted testis can show a normal sonographic appearance for the first 2–4 hours.[9]

Dudea (2010) highlighted that at greater than 360° degree rotation, ultrasound may demonstrate no blood flow, confirming the diagnosis.[10] Conflicting opinions exist at 180° rotation as venous flow stops but arterial flow is still present, therefore torsion can still be occurring whilst blood flow is demonstrated on Doppler.[10]

Arce (2002) suggested that attention should focus upon the spermatic cord rather than the testis. They were able to demonstrate that rotation of the spermatic cord can be demonstrated by ultrasound in 100% of patients in a small series of six consecutive patients.[11]

Answer

Testicular torsion can still occur whilst blood flow is demonstrated by ultrasound.

Case progression

The urologist reviews the patient and he is transferred directly to the operating theatre and scrotal exploration confirms a left testicular torsion. This is successfully untwisted and the testicle preserved. The patient has an uneventful recovery and is discharged the following day.

See Box 10.2 for future advances in this area.

Box 10.2 Future advances

A small study (25 patients) has been published reporting Interleukin-6 (IL-6) levels are significantly higher in epididymitis than testicular torsion.[13] Levels of Interleukin-1 and creatinine phosphokinase–MM were not found to be significantly different between testicular torsion and epididymitis.

Using a cut-off value of IL-6 >1.41 pg/ml, the positive predictive value of IL-6 in diagnosing epidiymitis was 78.6%. The negative predictive value of IL-6 in diagnosing testicular torsion was 100%.

The authors identify that one cannot draw definitive conclusions due to the small size of the study. The other limiting factor that will apply to using any serological marker in diagnosing or excluding a diagnosis of torsion is the time taken to perform the test and obtain a result.

A Final Word from the Expert

Missing a potential testicular torsion will always remain on the list of the ED clinician's 'never, events' with the given mantra of 'time being testicle'. As such, all presentations with testicular pain should rapidly be brought to a clinician's attention, and an early assessment performed with emergent mobilization of specialists and theatre if torsion is clinically suspected.

Many EDs have moved away from utilizing formal ultrasound in their patient pathways. Although the urologists may consider the investigation in equivocal cases, the caveat exists that flow can still be demonstrated in a partial torsion and as such exploration is still warranted.

Early referral pathways need to be defined and a multi-specialty approach essential to ensuring safe and timely management of the acute scrotum.

References

1. Beni-Israel T, Goldman M, Bar Chaim S, *et al*. Clinical predictors for testicular torsion as seen in the pediatric ED. *Am J Emerg Med* 2010; 28:7869.
2. Murphy F, Fletcher L, Pease P. Early scrotal exploration in all cases is the investigation and intervention of choice in the acute paediatric scrotum. *Pediatr Surg Int* 2006; 22:413–16.
3. Kadish H, Bolte R. A retrospective review of pediatric patients with epidiymitis, testicular torsion, and torsion of testicular appendages. *Pediatrics* 1998; 102:73–6.
4. Harvey M, Chanwai G, Cave G, Manual testicular detorsion under propofol sedation. *Case Reports in Medicine* 2009; 1687.
5. Mrhac L, Zakko S, Mohammed SJS, *et al*. Redistribution the sign of successful testicular detorsion. *Clin Nucl Med* 1997; 22:502.
6. Dunn JP. Manual Detorsion of the testicle. *N Z Med J* 2008; 121:82.
7. Betts JM., Norris M, Cromie WJ, *et al*. Testicular detorsion using Doppler ultrasound monitoring. *J Pediatr Surg* 1983; 18:607–10.
8. Allen TD, Elder JS. Shortcomings of color Doppler sonography in the diagnosis of testicular torsion. *JUrol* 1995; 154:1508–10.
9. Prando D. Torsion of the spermatic cord: the main gray-scale and doppler sonographic signs. *Abdom Imaging* 2009; 34:648–61.
10. Dudea S, Ciurea A, Chiorean A, *et al*. Doppler applications in testicular and scrotal disease. *Medical Ultrasonography* 2010; 12:43–51.
11. Arce J, Cortes M, Vargas JC Sonographic diagnosis of acute spermatic cord torsion Rotation of the cord: a key to the diagnosis. *Paediatr Radiol* 2002; 32:485–91.
12. European Association of Urology Guidelines <http://www.uroweb.org/gls/pdf/19_Paediatric_Urology.pdf>
13. Rivers KK, River EP, Stricker HJ, *et al*. The clinical utility of serological markers in the evaluation of the acute scrotum. *Acad Emerg Med* 2000; 7:1069–72.
14. Datta V, Dhillon G, Voci S. Torsion/Detorsion. *Ultrasound Quarterly* 2011; 27:2:127–8.

11 Pretibial laceration

Neel Bhanderi and Fleur Cantle

Expert Commentary Balj Dheansa

Case history

An 80-year-old lady presents to you in minors after having caught her right shin on a table leg 3 hours ago. She has 2 wounds to her anterior tibial surface, one is a simple linear wound and the other has a skin flap. She is mobilizing with a walking stick and is accompanied by her husband.

She has a history of type 2 diabetes mellitus, peripheral vascular disease, and hypertension, and is taking metformin, gliclazide, and amlodipine, with no known drug allergies.

See Box 11.1 for a clinical summary of pretibial laceration.

Box 11.1 Clinical summary of pretibial laceration

Attendance to ED with pretibial lacerations has been estimated to be as high at 5.2%;[1] however, the incidence may be higher as many injuries are managed in the community.

Pretibial lacerations are commonly seen in elderly females with multiple comorbidities such as peripheral vascular disease, diabetes, and cardiac failure. The complex physiology of this patient group not only influences wound healing but also the ability to rehabilitate.

The combination of complex medical needs and the relatively poor blood supply to the shin[2] means relatively trivial wounds may lead to significant morbidity.

The aim of any wound management is to reduce the risk of infection, encourage healing, and provide the best cosmetic outcome for the patient whilst causing minimal distress.

Skin-flap lacerations are prone to poor wound healing due to the decreased blood supply to the flap. A good outcome is not necessarily ensured by approximating the skin flap to skin.

Expert comment

With the increasing autonomous practice and extension of the role of the emergency nurse practitioner, it is possible that doctors working in the ED are becoming deskilled in the assessment and treatment of wounds. This is problematic as frequently their input will be sought if the wound is particularly complex or requires referral on to plastic surgery. It is therefore essential that they remain up-to-date regarding current evidence and practice.

Learning point Assessment and classification of pretibial wounds

Pretibial lacerations incorporate a range of injuries from small, superficial lacerations to full thickness degloving injuries. It is important to assess the wound fully in the first instance as this will influence the first aid care delivered and the ongoing management.

There is no universally accepted classification system for these injuries. An example of one such system is outlined in Table 11.1. See Figures 11.1, 11.2, 11.3, and 11.4 for images of each type.

(continued)

Table 11.1 Dunkin classification of pretibial injuries[3]

Type	Description
I	Laceration
II	Laceration or flap with minimal haematoma and/or skin-edge necrosis
III	Laceration or flap with moderate to severe haematoma and/or necrosis
IV	Major degloving injury

Suffix i denotes infection
From *Journal of Wound Care*. Copyright © 2003 MA Healthcare Ltd. Reproduced by permission of MA Healthcare. Dunkin C, Elfleet D, Ling CA et al., 'A step-by-step guide to classifying and managing pretibial injuries', *Journal of Wound Care*, 12, 3, pp. 109–111.

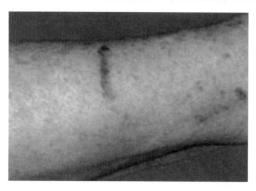

Figure 11.1 Type 1 laceration.

From *British Journal of Nursing*. Copyright © 2008 MA Healthcare Ltd. Reproduced by permission of MA Healthcare Ltd. Beldon P, 'Classifying and Managing pretibial lacerations in older people', *British Journal of Nursing*, Tissue viability supplement Vol 17 No 11.

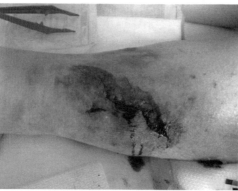

Figure 11.2 Type 2 laceration.

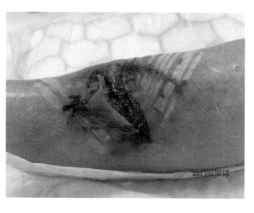

Figure 11.3 Type 3 laceration.

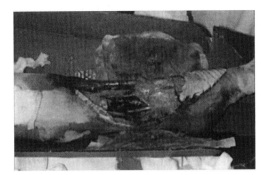

Figure 11.4 Type 4 laceration.

From *British Journal of Nursing*. Copyright © 2008 MA Healthcare Ltd. Reproduced by permission of MA Healthcare Ltd. Beldon P, 'Classifying and Managing pretibial lacerations in older people', *British Journal of Nursing*, Tissue viability supplement Vol 17 No 11.

> **+ Clinical tip** First aid for pretibial lacerations
>
> Whilst the patient is awaiting full assessment it is recommended that the wound be covered in moist, saline-soaked gauze[4] to prevent the flap drying out and shrinking.
>
> Patients should have their pain assessed at triage using a validated score as recommended by the College of Emergency Medicine[5] before any intervention is performed. Oral analgesia can be complimented by entonox.

> **Expert comment**
>
> It is essential to assess wounds carefully to get the best results. Appropriate assessment will allow the best method for managing a wound to be chosen. All wounds should be assessed for skin viability, presence of haematoma or active bleeding, skin loss (as opposed to skin retraction), and skin quality. Viable skin has an intact blood supply but it may be difficult to assess if it is bruised. Viable skin may blanch or bleed from the skin edge. If in doubt it may be best to give skin the benefit of the doubt. Skin retraction may be identified by gently pulling on the skin edges to redrape it and correctly position it. This may only be possible after complete evacuation of any haematoma.

Case progression

On initial assessment of the patient she appears quite comfortable. You remove the wet gauze and consider the wound; it appears quite dirty and requires irrigation.

Clinical question: Does sterile saline significantly reduce the risk of bacterial infection compared with tap water, when irrigating simple lacerations?

See Table 11.2.

Table 11.2 Evidence base for irrigation of wounds with sterile saline and tap water

Author and date	Design, subjects, and intervention	Main results
Fernandez (2002)[6]	Systematic review of trials which compared the cleansing of wounds with saline and other solutions 11 trials found: 7 comparing water and normal saline 3 comparing cleansing with no cleansing 1 comparing procaine spirit with water	The use of tap water to cleanse acute wounds was associated with a lower rate of infection than saline (OR 0.52, 95% CI 0.28–0.96)

Data from Fernandez R, Griffiths R, Ussia C, 'Water for wound cleansing', *Cochrane Database Systemic Reviews*, 2002, 4, CD003861.

> **Expert comment**
>
> Most plastic surgery and burns services now use running water and showers as a routine method of wound cleansing. Not only is it easy, cheap, and accessible, but the larger volumes used help with debridement and decolonization. It also allows a level of patient input. However, it is important, as with any procedure, to ensure the patient has adequate analgesia to ensure that the procedure is effective.

Answer

There is no evidence that using tap water to cleanse wounds increases the infection rate, and some evidence it reduces it.

Case progression

Following irrigation you consider the wound. There is clot adherent to the skin flap and the wound is actively bleeding. The skin appears pale and you are not certain if there is skin loss or if the skin is under tension from the clot as there is a large gap between the skin edge of the flap and the skin on the lower leg.

Any organized clot or haematoma which sits between the skin flap and the base of the wound will prevent healing as it will increase tension in the wound and may compromise the blood supply to the flap.[7] It has also been postulated that fat necrosis may be mediated by free radicals from haemolysed red blood cells[8] within the haematoma. It has been suggested that any haematoma can be removed in the emergency department using local anaesthetic and a Yankauer suction catheter[9] connected to wall suction. The technique involves using any overlying laceration as an entry port or making a stab incision if the wound is not broken. The suction catheter is then moved to and fro within the haematoma to break up the clot and allow its removal, and the cavity is then irrigated with normal saline. It is argued that the performance of such a procedure within the ED reduces the chance of pressure necrosis of the overlying skin but that it also negates the need for an emergency procedure under anaesthetic and therefore allows full work-up of the patient should a skin graft be necessary.

An alternative technique which has been described for traumatic subcutaneous heamatomas (not specifically in the pretibial region),[10] suggests using a 50-ml syringe connected to a 16-gauge cannula. The cannula is inserted into the haematoma at an oblique angle. The plunger is pulled back until a 10-ml syringe can fit between the withdrawn plunger and syringe base. This creates continuous high-pressure suction. The cannula and syringe is then pulled back and forward into the haematoma, breaking it up and draining it. This technique has the advantage of not requiring or creating a large entry point; however, the small calibre of the cannula means complete removal is unlikely.

> **❝ Expert comment**
>
> Often pretibial haematomas are well organized and adherent by the time patients present. The overlying skin may not be viable but adjoining tissue may also be at risk. The methods described earlier may be effective but it is essential to give adequate analgesia and use local anaesthesia to ensure the patient is not distressed. If the skin is already breached then running water may help remove the haematoma. If pain is not controlled then regional or general anaesthesia should be employed. It is essential to remove all haematoma and to stop any bleeding as otherwise it will re-accumulate (see Figure 11.5a and 11.5b).

Case progression

The haematoma is removed, but once the flap is laid down over the wound there is still a 6 mm gap between the 2 skin edges. You consider whether you should attempt to bridge the gap with sutures or adhesive tapes or leave the flap in the current position and apply a dressing to the wound.

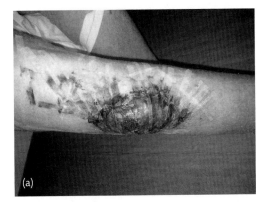

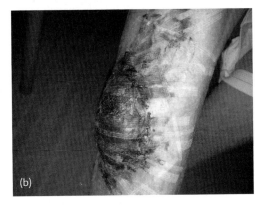

(a)

(b)

Figure 11.5 Skin under tension following closure with an inadequately evacuated haematoma.

⑥ Expert comment

In my practice, I thoroughly evacuate any haematoma, stop any bleeding (with pressure or with bipolar diathermy—sutures can be used if diathermy is not available), and then debride any obviously severely damaged tissue. I then replace the skin to close the wound as best as possible. A good dressing using non-adherent materials will protect the wound to allow healing. Sutures and steristrips rarely provide any further support and may cause undue tension or blistering and may also cut through tissue.

Clinical question: In pretibial lacerations in which the flap fails to meet with the skin edge, is it better to use sutures, adhesive tapes, or simply dress the wound?

See Table 11.3. The potential problems caused by suturing skin-flap lacerations was raised in the 1970s,[11,12] however closure of such wounds with sutures still occurs in the ED,[1] sometimes with disastrous consequences. To date, only one randomized controlled trial has looked specifically at the comparison of sutures or closure with adhesive tapes.

Table 11.3 Evidence base for wound closure in pretibial lacerations

Author and date	Design, subjects, and intervention	Main results
Sutton (1985)[13]	Prospective randomized trial of ED patients with linear or flap pretibial lacerations randomized to closure with adhesive strips or sutures. 76 patients completed 1 year follow-up	Significantly more necrosis seen in patients with flap lacerations closed with sutures ($p < 0.05$). Significantly slower healing in patients with flap lacerations treated with sutures ($p < 0.025$)

Data from Sutton R, Pritty P, 'The use of sutures or adhesive tapes for the primary closure of pretibial lacerations', *British Medical Journal*, 1985, 290, 6842, pp. 1627.

Answer

From this small, single-trial, adhesive tapes are preferred for primary closure of pretibial lacerations.

The difficulties these wounds present with regards to closure has led some to suggest novel methods of management;[14] for example, the use of adhesive tapes laid parallel to wound edges prior to closure with deep reinforced sutures followed by a gentle localised compression dressing. This technique negates the dead space in the wound and prevents tearing of fragile skin. A sample of 147 patients was studied. The average healing time was 26 days for the 112 patients with flap lacerations, and 16 days for the 35 linear laceration patients, which was reported to be shorter than the time quoted in the contemporary literature. This work, however, has not been reproduced or validated.

In the work by Dunkin *et al.*[3] the authors recommended the following algorithm for the management of pretibial lacerations according to initial classification (see Figure 11.6).

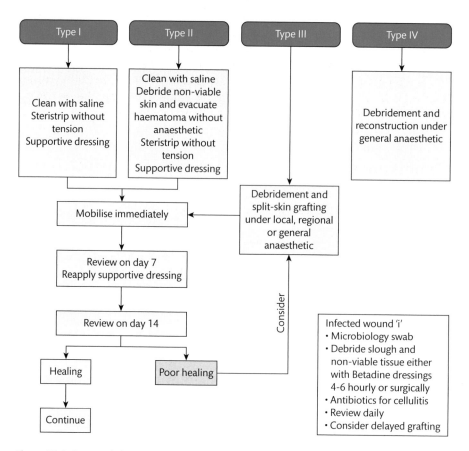

Figure 11.6 Suggested algorithm for the management of pretibial lacerations

From *Journal of Wound Care*. Copyright © 2003 MA Healthcare Ltd. Reproduced by permission of MA Healthcare. Dunkin C, Elfleet D, Ling CA *et al.*, 'A step-by-step guide to classifying and managing pretibial injuries', *Journal of Wound Care*, 12, 3, pp. 109–111.

Case progression

You decide to attempt to approximate the wound with adhesive strips. The patient is admitted to the observation ward for a multidisciplinary team assessment and pain control. On the observation ward, the nursing staff ask about what the instructions are for wound care and mobilization and what attention the wound will require on discharge.

Non-adherent dressings are recommended and although it has been found that dry dressings and paraffin-gauze dressings are used,[1] neither are ideal as they both cause trauma on removal, and paraffin dressings are thought to allow the migration of granulating cells through the dressing leading to prolonged inflammation and troublesome removal.[15] In a retrospective analysis[16] of 88 patients with grade 1 or 2 pretibial lacerations all treated with a silicon-coated dressing alone, 83 % were healed by day 8. One of the advantages of such dressings is that they can remain in place for 1 week. It has also been suggested[17] that the direction of the flap be drawn on the dressing so as the dressing can be removed in that direction in order to cause minimal disturbance. Some authors[18] recommend 'gentle compression' to assist in the prevention of oedema which may lift the flap and delay healing; this should be applied with caution in those with peripheral vascular disease and a history of smoking.

Patients should be mobilized straight away. The risks of keeping this patient group immobilized with bed rest are greater than any benefit it may confer to wound healing. In a recent meta analysis[19] which considered bed rest versus early mobilization following skin grafting for pretibial lacerations, no difference was demonstrated in split-skin graft healing between patients mobilized early compared to patients admitted to hospital for post-operative bed rest at either 7 (OR 0.86 CI 0.29–2.56) or 14 days (OR 0.74 CI 0.31–1.79). There was no difference in post-operative haematoma, bleeding, graft infection, or donor-site healing between the comparison groups.

Case progression

The patient is discharged home the next day with analgesia and a temporary care package. A week later the district nurse calls you to say that she has come to review the wound but she is concerned about how it appears and she thinks it might be infected. You advise the patient to return to the department. When the patient returns it is apparent that the flap has lifted from the base and appears necrotic and there is surrounding erythema. You are concerned that the patient should have been referred to a plastic surgeon at initial presentation.

Clinical question: What is the evidence for early skin grafting in pretibial lacerations?

See Table 11.4. Skin grafting, whether performed early or late, is usually performed by plastic surgeons under general anaesthetic. Disadvantages of this are the risks associated with a general anaesthetic in this often frail group, the necessity to transfer patients to another unit, and the creation of an additional wound in the donor site. These factors may be considered barriers to early plastic surgical involvement. In a survey of A&E departments,[1] it was found that 19 out of 22 emergency medicine consultants would refer to a plastic surgeon if they felt the wound was severe or not healing, and anecdotally this is still the practice in many departments today.

> **⑥ Expert comment**
>
> Early mobilization is routine for such injuries whether they have been dressed or skin-grafted. However, it is important to note that caution needs to be applied for those lacerations crossing a joint. Patients should also be reminded to elevate their legs when resting to avoid oedema.

It has been shown that the performance of early skin grafting under local anaesthetic in the ED by a surgeon is possible[20] with good results. In this study at 3 weeks 23 out of 25 achieved 100 % initial skin-graft take. However this requires a surgeon competent in the harvesting of skin grafts to be available together with the space and support staff required for such a procedure within the emergency department. To date there has only been 1 study comparing primary excision and grafting with conservative treatment.

Table 11.4 Evidence base early grafting in pretibial lacerations

Author, date, and country	Design, subjects, and intervention	Main results
Haiart et al. (1990)[21]UK	25 patients with pretibial lacerations randomized to either primary excision and grafting or defatting and steristrips Prospective randomized trial Healing time and length of hospital stay	A significant difference in healing time. 13.2 days for primary grafting and 40.7 days for defatting ($t=3.29$, $p <0.01$) No difference in hospitalization time

Data from Haiart DC, Paul AB Chalmers R et al., 'Pretibial lacerations: a comparison of primary excision and grafting with "defatting the flap"'. British Journal of Plastic Surgery, 1999; 43(3) pp. 312–314.

Answer

Pretibial injuries which result in flap lacerations should be treated by primary excision and grafting which can be easily carried out under local anaesthetic.

While this one study suggests improved healing rates in early grafted injuries, it is unlikely that plastic surgery units will accept all injuries and we will still need to be considerate about which wounds we refer immediately or arrange for specialist follow-up.

> **❝ Expert comment**
>
> The decision to skin graft a pretibial laceration should be made by someone competent to perform the procedure. Clinicians competent in the procedure require a suitable theatre environment to perform such surgery and suitable equipment. Modern practice usually requires meshing of the skin to increase the area covered and to reduce post-operative haematoma formation while larger skin grafts are probably best taken with a powered dermatome. Diathermy equipment should be available to help stop bleeding. Such facilities are not usually available in the ED, and hence performing the procedure within the department is unlikely to be feasible. Advice from the plastic surgery team should be sought if in doubt.
>
> The choice of anaesthetic may be influenced by the size of the injury and the premorbid condition of the patient. In addition to local anaesthetic and general anaesthetic, one can also consider regional anaesthetic. Areas greater than 15 × 10 cm may be difficult to manage under local anaesthetic.

> **★ Learning point** Criteria for referral to a plastic surgeon
>
> Pretibial lacerations are common and although there are no agreed national or specialty guidelines for referral for skin grafting, the following groups should be considered for review by the plastic surgery team:
>
> - Large haematoma with active bleeding
> - Skin loss greater than 15 cm^2
> - Complex flap or multiple skin lacerations
> - Large areas of non-viable skin

As in all healthcare matters, prevention is better than cure and it is likely that the prevention of pretibial lacerations would be considered in any falls prevention programme, but at present no studies have considered assessing a prevention policy although they have been proposed.

> **⊕ Clinical tip** Skin tear risk prevention[16]
>
> There are a number of interventions which have been suggested which may prevent pretibial lacerations. The skin on the pretibial region is thin and therefore at risk of injury and hence the use of emollients, stockings, or special leg protectors may provide some protection. There are environmental considerations which may reduce the risk of falls such as ensuring good lighting and sensible placement of furniture. Sharp areas of furniture or bed frames should be upholstered in soft material. Such measures, together with education of the elderly population and those who care for them may reduce such injuries and therefore the complications associated with them.
>
> Data from Meuleneire, F, 'Using a soft silicone-coated net dressing to manage skin tears', *Journal of Wound Care*. 2002; 11:(10) pp. 365–369.

A Final Word from the Expert

Pre-tibial lacerations can have a significant effect on patients and can take a very long time to heal. Early effective treatment can reduce healing time, reduce risks of infection, and allow patients to return to normal activity sooner. It is essential to assess patients effectively and liaise with the plastic surgery team to identify those who would most benefit from surgery as early as possible.

References

1. Davis A, Chester D, Allison K, *et al.* A survey of how a regions A and E units manage pretibial laceration. *J Wound Care.* 2004; 13(1):5–7.
2. Haertsch PA. The blood supply to the skin of the leg: a post-mortem investigation. *Br J Plast Surg* 1981; 34(4):470–77.
3. Dunkin C, Elfleet D, Ling CA, *et al.* A step-by-step guide to classifying and managing pretibial injuries. *J Wound Care* 2003; 12(3):109–11.
4. Cole E. Wound Management in the A and E Department. *Nurs Stand* 2003; 17(46):45–52.
5. Guideline for the management of pain in adults. London: College of Emergency Medicine, 2010. <http://www.collemergencymed.ac.uk/asp/document.asp?ID=4681>
6. Fernandez R, Griffiths R, Ussia C. Water for wound cleansing. Cochrane Database Syst Rev. 2002; (4):CD003861.
7. Bradley L. Pretibial lacerations in older patients: the treatment options. *J Wound Care* 2001; 10(1):521–3.
8. Angel MF, Naraymann MD, Swartz WM, *et al.* The etiological role of free radicals in haematomainduced flap necrosis. *Plast Reconstr Surg* 1986; 77(5):795–803.
9. Karthikeyan GS, Vadodaria S, Stanley PR. Simple and safe treatment of pretibial haematoma in elderly patients. *Emerg Med J* 2004; 21(1):69–70.
10. Chami G, Chami B, Hatley E, *et al.* Simple technique for evacuating traumatic subcutaneous haematomas under tension. *BMC Emergency Medicine* 2005; 5:11.
11. Tandon SN, Sutherland AB. Pretibial lacerations. *Br J Plast Surg* 1973; 26(2):172–5.
12. Crawford BS, Gipson M. The Conservative management of pretibial lacerations in elderly patients. *Br J Plast Surg* 1977; 30(2):174–6.

13. Sutton R, Pritty P. The use of sutures or adhesive tapes for the primary closure of pretibial lacerations. *Br Med J* 1985; 290(6842):1627.
14. Silk, J. A new approach to the management of pretibial lacerations. *Injury* 2001; 32(5):373–6.
15. Hollingworth H. The management of patients' pain in wound care. *Nurs Stand* 20(7):65–6.
16. Meuleneire, F. Using a soft silicone-coated net dressing to manage skin tears. *J Wound Care* 2002; 11(10):365–9.
17. Ratcliff CR, Fletcher KR. Skin tears: a review of the evidence to support prevention and treatment. *Ostomy wound manage* 2007; 53(3):32–4.
18. Bradley L. Pretibial lacerations in older patients: the treatment options. *J Wound Care* 2001; 10(1):521–3.
19. Southwell-Keely J, Vandervord J. Mobilisation versus Bed Rest after Skin Grafting Pretibial Lacerations: A Meta-Analysis. *Plast Surg Int* 2012; 2012: article ID 207452. <http://dx.doi.org/10.1155/2012/207452>
20. Shankar S, Khoo CT. Lower limb skin loss: simple outpatient management with meshed skin grafts with immediate mobilization. *Arch Emerg Med* 1987; 4(3):187–92.
21. Haiart DC, Paul AB, Chalmers R, *et al.* Pretibial lacerations: a comparison of primary excision and grafting with 'defatting the flap'. *Br J Plast Surg* 1990; 43(3):312–4.

12 Complex wrist fractures

Evan Coughlan and Sam Thenabadu

ⓘ **Expert commentary** John Ryan

Case history

A 42-year-old previously fit right-hand dominant man presents to the ED 2 hours after a mechanical fall onto his outstretched arm whilst working in his office. He initially describes his pain as 7 out of 10, but after paracetamol and codeine at the triage, and entonox whilst waiting for you, he tells you that the pain has reduced to a pain score of 4.

Examination reveals an obviously deformed tender distal left wrist, but thankfully no other associated injuries to the elbow or shoulder in particular. His range of movement at the wrist remains minimal but you feel this is limited by the pain and swelling more than the fracture positions. Close examination of the median, ulnar, and radial nerves does NOT reveal any obvious parasthesiae in a particular distribution, however, the patient describes episodically feeling 'some tingling' in all his fingers. There are no overlying wounds so you are confident that this is a closed fracture.

A radiograph is performed and demonstrates a Volar Barton fracture as seen in Figure 12.1. You contact the on-call orthopaedic junior doctor who, having reviewed the images on the X-ray image computer system, advises you to manipulate the wrist with 'whatever analgesia and anaesthesia you are familiar with' to prevent a potential evolving median nerve injury. He concludes that the wrist can then be placed in a plaster cast, and the patient safely discharged to the orthopaedic fracture clinic as an outpatient.

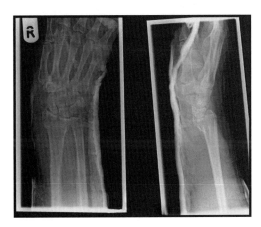

Figure 12.1 Radiograph of a Volar Barton's fracture.

See Box 12.1 for a clinical summary of wrist fractures.

Box 12.1 Clinical summary of wrist fractures

Fractures of the distal forearm are a frequent presentation to EDs with a prevalence of 9/10000 in men and 37/10000 in women aged more than 35 years.[1] As with all fractures, a proportion of these require manipulation within the emergency department.

Colles' fracture: an extra articular fracture of the radius within 2.5 cm of the wrist with a characteristic dorsally angulated 'dinner-fork' deformity of the metaphysis, with or without an associated ulnar styloid fracture. The classic mechanism is the fall on outstretched arm classically in an osteoporotic middle-aged or elderly woman.

Smith's fracture: an extra articular fracture of the distal radius with the metaphysis displaced volarly and tilted into posterior angulation—often referred to as a reverse Colles'. This mechanism occurs frequently from a backwards fall on the palm of an outstretched hand.

Volar Barton fracture: this is an intra-articular fracture of the distal radius, which involves the volar margin of the carpal surface and is associated with dislocation of the radiocarpal joint. These fractures also usually occur from a fall onto an outstretched arm, leading to dorsiflexion stress, during which the volar radiocarpal ligaments avulse the volar lip of the radius from the metaphysis.

You are uncomfortable with this management plan due to the nature of the fracture and the age of the patient, and are unsure whether a fracture that is displaced in the volar direction instead of the dorsal direction runs more risk of a median nerve palsy.

> **❝ Expert comment**
>
> The younger the patient, the greater the need to ensure as adequate a reduction as possible for a distal radius fracture. This is particularly important in a fracture sustained to the wrist of the dominant arm. Overall however, many reductions in the ED are surprisingly satisfactory, particularly among the older population with thin wrists. For Colles' fractures, a disimpaction followed by the locking position of flexion and ulnar deviation is not uncommonly the only reduction that is required. In adolescents with metaphyseal/epiphyseal involvement, the reduction often locks in easily as with a joint reduction. This makes the ED environment suitable as a one-stop-shop to manage such a fracture, with subsequent elective follow-up in an outpatient facility.
>
> More complex fractures, however, will most likely come to surgery. The reality remains, however, that in modern emergency healthcare, and increasingly in the future, out-of-hours specialty emergency care is becoming less and less available unless limb- or life-threatening. Pain relief, appropriate splinting, and procedures to minimize median nerve compression become in these circumstances the remit of the emergency physician.

Clinical question: Does early manipulation of wrist fractures reduce the risk of developing median nerve injury?

Median nerve palsy is a recognized complication of a fracture of the distal radius. The first documented case was described by Gensoul in 1836 in a traumatic injury to the median nerve noticed in the autopsy of a young girl who died from tetanus after an open fracture of her distal radius. During this procedure, the median nerve was found caught between the ends of the fractured radius.[2] (See Figure 12.2).

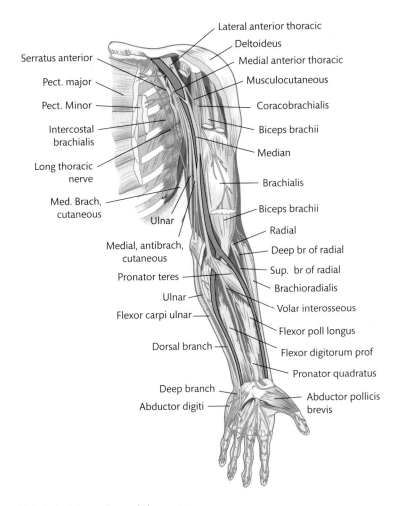

Lateral anterior thoracic
Deltoideus
Medial anterior thoracic
Musculocutaneous
Coracobrachialis
Biceps brachii
Median
Brachialis
Biceps brachii
Radial
Deep br of radial
Sup. br of radial
Brachioradialis
Volar interosseous
Flexor poll longus
Flexor digitorum prof
Pronator quadratus
Abductor pollicis brevis

Serratus anterior
Pect. major
Pect. Minor
Intercostal brachialis
Long thoracic nerve
Med. Brach, cutaneous
Ulnar
Medial, antibrach, cutaneous
Pronator teres
Ulnar
Flexor carpi ulnar
Dorsal branch
Deep branch
Abductor digiti

Figure 12.2 Path of the median and ulnar nerve.

This figure was published in *Gray's Anatomy*, Henry Gray, Figure 816, p. 938, Copyright 1918, with permission from Elsevier.

In 1933, Abbott and Saunders classified median nerve injuries into four groups:[3] primary injury, secondary injury, late or delayed involvement, and injuries associated with treatment—(a) acute palmar flexion and (b) reduction. Although this is the quoted classification, in practice it is easier to divide them into primary or secondary and the time of onset (acute, subacute, or late).[4] Primary median nerve injury is uncommon[9] and in general most traumatic nerve injuries are caused by compression. Endoneural oedema within a noncompliant perineurium leads to increased pressure within the nerve and hence damage. Factors such as swelling and position of reduction are associated with acute or subacute median nerve dysfunction. Delayed median neuropathy can occur months to years after the initial injury and are associated with persistent displacement, malunion, callus, and perineural scarring.

In primary injury, early surgical repair is advocated. In secondary injury, treatment varies depending on the cause. Primary injury can be differentiated from secondary as symptoms develop immediately and do not evolve. In acute secondary median neuropathy prompt treatment prevents persistence of symptoms,[10] and fractures should be reduced quickly and without excessive force.[9,11]

Although there is no clear evidence that a particular fracture type is more associated with median nerve injury, there is some evidence that more comminuted fractures may be associated with a higher incidence, irrespective of fracture type.[4,5] As such, early reduction of these fractures by manipulation and either external fixation or internal fixation would intuitively be an appropriate method of reducing pressure around the median nerve.

Position of immobilization seems the most directly associated factor in the development of median nerve symptoms. There is a correlation between fractures immobilized in a flexed and ulnarly deviated position and development of median nerve dysfunction. The pressure in the carpal tunnel is lower in the neutral position.[3,5–7] Several reports exist that suggest that using a haematoma block may also increase pressure around the median nerve and potentially lead to median nerve problems;[5,9,12] however, this has not been supported in larger literature reviews of haematoma blocks.[15,18,20–22]

Answer

There is no evidence specifically pertaining to Volar Barton fractures. There is limited evidence that in patients with distal radial fractures who have median nerve symptoms, prompt reduction of displacement may prevent persistent symptoms.

> **❝ Expert comment**
>
> Volar Barton-type fractures are less common than the Colles'-type fracture. Acute median nerve injuries are uncommon in clinical practice with distal radial fractures despite the large number of distal fractures we see. It would be disconcerting to be asked to consent to a randomized control trial on early versus delayed management of a significantly displaced distal radial fracture if one arm of the study was adequate immediate pain relief, so it is unlikely that we are ever going to have this piece of definitive work to guide us. Without high-level evidence though, it seems prudent to reverse the deformity as early as possible provided the emergency physician is competent and he or she can provide this therapy within the time constraints of delivering care in a modern ED.

Case progression

After discussing the radiographs with another ED colleague, a decision is made to manipulate this patient's fractured wrist. You are aware of 2 methods within your ED for providing the necessary analgesia for manipulation of distal radial fractures (Bier's block and hematoma block), but are unsure as to which is the most appropriate to use for this patient.

> **✚ Clinical tip** Bier's block–CEM Guidelines (2010)
>
> The performance of a Bier's block is becoming less common in UK EDs; however, the College guidelines have been developed to outline the key aspects of performing this regional anaesthesia to
>
> (continued)

endeavour to deliver better anaesthesia and analgesia. Bier's blocks should only be conducted in an ED where the following essential elements are available and conducted:

- A well-lit, fully equipped area with resuscitation equipment immediately available.
- A minimum of 2 practitioners present throughout, with 1 solely responsible for airway and resuscitative measure.
- A double pneumatic tourniquet cuff is available and inflated and tested for 5 minutes prior to the procedure.
- The cuff should be inflated for a minimum of 20 minutes and maximum of 45 minutes with clear documentation.
- Prilocaine 0.5 % (3 mg/kg) is the recommended drug used without any added adrenaline. Lignocaine or bupivocaine are not recommended.

Clinical question: Does a haematoma block or a Bier's block provide the best method of analgesia for reduction of distal radius fracture?

Displaced wrist fractures are common in the ED. The method of reduction of these wrist fractures has changed over time. In 1989, 33 % of reductions were with Bier's block, 44 % with general anaesthesia, 13 % with sedation, and a mere 7 % with haematoma block.[12] In a survey in 1995, haematoma blocks were being used with increasing frequency (33 %), whereas general anaesthesia (24 %) and sedation (7 %) were less common. The frequency of the use of Bier's block for reduction had remained unchanged (33 %).[13]

There have been 5 studies looking at this clinical question and a Cochrane review conducted. In all the studies, Bier's block has been associated with less pain than haematoma block.[19–23]

Abbaszadegan et al. found that the better anaesthesia and muscle relaxation with Bier's block allowed for easier manipulation and hence a more successful reduction. An improved radiological reduction in patients who had intravenous regional anaesthesia was also noted by Kendall et al. and Wardrope et al. Cobb et al. found that there was no difference in the adequacy of result between the two methods.

Kendall et al. noted more re-manipulations in the group treated with haematoma block due to an inadequate initial reduction. Abbaszadegan noted the re-displacement between groups was of the same magnitude, but also commented that 4 of the fractures in the local anaesthesia group displaced to such a degree after 10 days that re-reduction and external fixation of the fractures had to be performed.

There were no complications of either method cited by Cobb or Kendall. Abbaszadegan described 4 cases of median nerve palsy, divided evenly between both methods.

The duration of each procedure was similar in Cobb et al. Kendall noted that the time between examination of the patient and administration of the anaesthetic was significantly higher in the Bier's block group but that the overall transit time was no different. Wardrope et al. noted that a haematoma block was quicker to perform.

> ✓ **Evidence base** Haematoma block or Bier's block
>
> All papers in this area look at local and regional anaesthesia in Colles' fractures.
>
> - Carley (1998):[17] Bier's block is preferable to haematoma block for the reduction of uncomplicated Colles' fractures in the elderly
> - Handoll et al (2002):[16] Cochrane review which concluded that there was some indication that haematoma block provides poorer analgesia than Bier's block and that as such can hamper reduction.

Answer

Bier's block should be used where available in preference to haematoma block to reduce distal radial fractures.

Case progression

Unable to find the necessary cuff for the Bier's block, a decision is made to perform a haematoma block. Knowing the higher risk of requiring repeated attempts to acquire an adequate reduction with a haematoma block, the emergency physician wonders if ultrasound can be used in some way to improve the success of manipulation.

Clinical question: Can ultrasound be used to improve manipulation of distal radial fractures?

Ultrasound use in the manipulation of fractures allows the benefit of a real-time dynamic assessment of fracture position without the need for ionizing radiation as seen in Figure 12.3. The paediatric population in particular may benefit from this modality. Along with keeping the paediatric ED journey as 'fear free' as possible, the reduction in number of radiographs required is clearly a bonus to the growing child. Studies in this area have been small but have generally been encouraging in their results. However, ultrasound is very operator dependent and this may limit its usage.

Several non-randomized studies of variable sizes exist.[24-30] In general these studies suffer from small numbers, lack of randomization, and a control group. Success of reduction varies from 83–100 % in these studies. Chinnock *et al.*

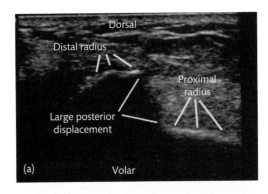

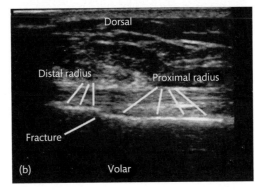

Figure 12.3 Ultrasound image of a distal radius fracture.

found no significant difference between the success rate of reduction under ultra-sound guidance and a historical control group.[29] Ang *et al.* found an improve-ment in success rate from 91 % in historical controls to 98.4 % with the use of ultrasound.[28]

Answer

There is some evidence that ultrasound could be used for guiding manipulation of distal radius fractures but the evidence is not of sufficient quality for recommenda-tion and further research is required.

⊘ Evidence base Ultrasound for manipulation of distal radial fractures

Brahm *et al* (2011): randomized single-blinded study of adult patients with a distal radial fracture. 47 patients were enrolled in the study, 27 randomized to have ultrasound guided reduction, and 20 to standard reduction. Three of the patients assigned to the control group had an ultrasound-guided reduction. An intention to treat analysis was performed. They found no difference in the adequacy of reduction, time of reduction, or in the number of patients who subsequently required operative repair. One patient in the standard group needed a repeat reduction in the ED.[31]

⑪ Expert comment

In recent years ultrasound is being used with increased frequency in EDs. For some time it had been used successfully in Europe although coverage was scant in the English-language publications. Its use has now advanced beyond the initial FAST and increasingly emergency physicians are utilizing ultrasonography for central line insertion, hepatobiliary disease assessment, and tendon assessment, to name just a few applications.

Its use in guiding the reduction of forearm fractures has the benefit of being a point-of-care diagnostic test. It can indicate the need for further reduction or correction of a manipulation where required while a patient or her arm arm is sedated/anaesthetised without recourse to a supplementary procedure involving re-anaesthetizing or re-sedation where the initial manipulation is unsatisfactory.

(continued)

Examining in ultrasound use has become a mandatory part of the Fellowship of the College of Emergency Medicine; however, its extended use beyond FAST will require significant numbers of faculty within the specialty competent to instruct and its varied uses in musculoskeletal trauma will mean that a department is not likely always to have the expertise required. Logistically this has the potential to generate confusion when a patient presents who requires a distal forearm fracture manipulation, and the necessary skills to manage this clinical situation are not always available from within that department.

These difficulties are currently likely to restrict the widespread use of ultrasonography in complex forearm manipulation.

⊕ Clinical tip Manipulation techniques for Colles'-type radius fractures

The optimal correction of displacement and angulation is vital to ensure a return of function. Most ED clinicians will have their personal favourite techniques for reducing these fractures, but the principles if not the exact nuances remain the same.

Disimpaction of the impacted fracture segments is the first important stage and this can often be achieved by simple traction. One school of thought, however, is to exaggerate the fracture displacement direction by hyperextending the wrist then applying traction to disimpact the pieces. Application of palmar flexion and ulnar angulation will then return the wrist to the anatomical position.

In principal, a Smith's-type distal radius fracture could be reduced, utilizing the reverse approach to that discussed earlier with traction performed in wrist supination with a dorsal angulation force applied. The fracture, however, will still remain intrinsically unstable.

The application of the plaster cast is a time when the mobile fracture segments can move out of position, so a 'final moulding' is recommended as the plaster sets to ensure an acceptable position is maintained. The check X-ray is crucial and inadequate reduction position should mandate removal of the plaster and re-manipulation.

A Final Word from the Expert

Patients who have sustained a simple Colles' fracture commonly present to the ED. Management is easy to teach and the indication for reduction is easy to plot with angles, if not immediately clinically apparent. Methods used to manage these fractures are starting to evolve from the traditional Bier's block through haematoma block to procedural sedation.

The need for manipulation of more complex fractures such as a Volar Barton fracture—likely to proceed to surgery in due course anyway—is based more on the desire to minimize the potential for damage to the median nerve, although this in itself is a rather uncommon problem. Despite the evidence being thin that early reduction decreases the likelihood of median nerve damage due to compression, it is perhaps intuitive if not a basic tenet of orthopaedic trauma that as pain relief accrues from early reduction and immobilization, it is not unreasonable to proceed with this line.

The choice of analgesia for the procedure is varied. It is likely that 'fashion' driven by logistical issues will change the face of the procedure going forwards. It would not be chivalrous of emergency medicine to neglect new procedures and new tools in attempting to reduce the complications of managing a complex wrist fracture.

References

1. College of Emergency Medicine: Intravenous regional anaesthesia for distal forearm fractures (Bier's block). London: College of Emergency Medicine, March 2014.
2. Meadoff N. Median nerve injuries in fractures in the region of the wrist. *Calif Med* 1949; April; 70(4):252–6.
3. Abbott LC. Saunders JB de CM. Injuries of the median nerve in fractures of the lower end of the radius. *Surg Gynaecol Obstet* 57:507–16.
4. Dennison DG. Median nerve injuries associated with distal radius fractures. *Techniques Orthop* 21(1):48–53.
5. Dresing K, Peterson T, Schmit-Neuerburg KP. Compartment pressure in the carpal tunnel in distal fractures of the radius: a prospective study. *Arch Orthop Trauma Surg* 1994; 113:285–9.
6. Bauman TD, Gelberman RH, Mubarak SJ, *et al.* The acute carpal tunnel syndrome. *Clin Orthop* 1981; 156:151–6.
7. Gelberman RH, Hergenroeder PT, Hargens AR, *et al.* The carpal tunnel syndrome: a study of carpal tunnel pressures. *J Bone Joint Surg* 1981; 63A: 380–3.
8. Gelberman RH, Szabo RM, Mortensen WW. Carpal tunnel pressures and wrist position in patients with Colles fractures. *J Trauma* 1984; 24:747–9.
9. Cooney WP III, Dobyns JH, Linscheid RL. Complications of Colles' fractures. *J Bone Joint Surg* 1980; 62A:613–19.
10. Kongsholm J, Olerud C. Carpal tunnel pressure in the acute phase after Colles' fracture. *Arch Orthop Trauma Surg* 1986; 105(3):183–6.
11. Kozin S, Wood M. Early soft-tissue complications after fracture of the distal part of the radius. *J Bone Joint Surg* 1993; 75A:144–53.
12. Cassebaum WH. Colles' fracture. A study of end results. *JAMA* 1950; 143:963–5.
13. Hunter JB, Scott MJL, Harries SA. Methods of anaesthesia used for reduction of Colles' fractures. *BMJ* 1989; 299:1316–17.
14. Kendall JM, Allen PE, McCabe SE. A tide in the management of an old fracture. *J Accid Emerg Med* 1995; 12:187–8.
15. Case RD. Haematoma block – a safe method of reducing Colles' fractures. *Injury* 1985; 16:469–70.
16. Handoll HHG, Madhok R, Dodds, C. Anaesthesia for treating distal radial fractures in adults. *Cochrane Database of systematic reviews*, Issue 3.
17. Carley S. Haematoma block versus intravenous regional anaesthesia in Colles' fractures. *J Accid Emerg Med* 1998; 15(4):229–30.
18. Abbaszadegan H, Jonsson U. regional anaesthesia preferable for Colles' fracture. Controlled comparison with local anesthesia. *Acta Orthop Scand* 1990; 61(4):348–9.
19. Cobb AG, Houghton GR. Local anaesthetic infiltration versus Bier's block for Colles' fracture. *BMJ* 1985; 291:1683–4.
20. Cobb AG, Houghton GR. Comparison of local anaesthetic infiltration and intravenous anaesthesia in patients with Colles' fracture. *J Bone Joint Surg* 1985; 67(5):845.
21. Kendall JM, Allen P, Younger P, *et al.* Haematoma block or Bier's block for Colles' fracture reduction in the accident and emergency department—which is best? *J Accid Emerg Med* 1997; 14(6):352–6.
22. Wardrope J, Flowers M, Wilson DH. Comparison of local anaesthetic techniques in the reduction of Colles' fracture. *Arch Emerg Med* 1985; 2(2):67–72.
23. Walter-Larsen S, Christophersen D, Fauner M, *et al.* Intravenous regional analgesia compared to infiltration analgesia in the reduction of distal forearm fractures. *Ugeskrift for Laeger* 1998; 150(32):1930–2.
24. Chern T, Jou I, Lai K, *et al.* Sonography for monitoring closed reduction of displaced extra-articular distal radius fractures. *J Bone Joint Surg* 2002; 84A(2):194–203.

25. Chen L, Kin Y, Moore C. Diagnosis and guided reduction of forearm fractures in children using bedside ultrasound. *Paediatr Emerg Care*, 2007; 23(8):528–31.
26. Wong CE, Ang AS, Ng K. Ultrasound as an aid for reduction of paediatric forearm fractures. *Int J Emerg Med*, 2008; 1:267–71.
27. Patel DD, Blumberg SM, Cain EF. The utility of bedside ultrasound in identifying fractures and guiding fracture reduction in children. *Paediatr Emerg Care* 2009; 25(4):221–5.
28. Ang S, Lee S, Lam K. Ultrasound-guided reduction of distal radius fractures. *Am J Emerg Med* 2010; 28:1002–8.
29. Chinnock B, Khaletskiy A, Kuo K, *et al.* Ultrasound-guided reduction of distal radius fractures. *J Emerg Med* 2011; 40(3):308–12.
30. Majeed M, Mukherjee A, Paw R. Ultrasound-guided hematoma block and fracture reduction: a new way to go forward. *Critical Care* 2010, 14(S1):P269.
31. Brahm J, Turner J. A randomised controlled trial of Emergency Department ultrasound-guided reduction of distal radius fractures. *Annals Emerg Med* 2011: 58(4);S230–1.

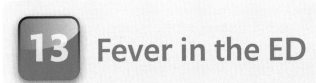

Fever in the ED

Chidi Ejimofo and Sam Thenabadu

❝ Expert commentary Beth Christian

Case history

A 35-year-old Afro-Caribbean man attends the ED with a letter from his GP stating that he has had a recurrent headache, abdominal pain, and fever for the past 3 weeks since returning from a 2-month trip 'looking for a wife' in West Africa. During his trip, he self-medicated with over-the-counter chloroquine whenever he felt unwell, along with occasional herbal medications provided by a village elder.

He has attended his GP practice 2 days earlier, and the referral letter confirms that the GP has ruled out possible malaria having sent blood for microscopy and rapid diagnostic testing (RDT) which was negative. He has no medical history of note, is not on any regular medications and is fully immunized. He has been resident in the UK for the past 7 years, and prior to that lived in West Africa.

On examination, he is appears unwell but is in no acute distress. His general observations are as follows: HR 98 bpm, BP 137/93 mmHg, RR 28 breaths/min and an oral temperature of 39.8°C. In view of his temperature, the triage nurse has already given him paracetamol 1 g orally and placed a request for 'routine bloods'.

See Box 13.1 for a clinical summary of malaria.

Box 13.1 Clinical summary of malaria

A common and lethal febrile illness caused by infection of red blood cells (RBCs) by protozoa of the genus Plasmodium that it is a notifiable disease in the UK.

Four species of Plasmodium typically infect humans; *P. falciparum*, *P. vivax*, *P. ovale*, and *P. malariae*. A fifth, primate malaria species *P. knowlesi* is an emerging cause of malaria in South East Asia.[1]

Human transmission is via the bite of infected female, night-feeding Anopheles mosquitoes.

In 2009 it was present in 108 countries and territories, causing 225 million cases and an estimated 781 000 deaths.[2] In the UK, between 1500 and 2000 people are diagnosed with malaria each year with 10–20 deaths.

P. falciparum causes most malaria deaths worldwide, and accounts for 75% of all cases in the UK.[4,5]

Between 2005 and 2009, 73% of cases diagnosed in the UK were patients born in Africa or South Asia.[3]

The usual incubation period of *P. falciparum* is 10–14 days; most patients will present within a month of exposure. Other forms of malaria may, however, be latent for up to a year afterwards, so detailed travel histories remain paramount.

❝ Expert comment

Fever in the ED covers a broad spectrum of conditions from infancy to geriatrics. It is helpful to categorize by age and risk factors, with special categories for the returned traveller, drug-induced pyrexia, and environmental conditions.

(continued)

Fever in the returned traveller should be considered as a specific entity on its own requiring a different style of history taking, differential diagnosis and investigation. It is vital to know not only which country a patient has visited but also exactly where they have been. e.g. rural settings versus 5-star hotels.

Fever in a returned traveller due to malaria is a relatively common presentation to UK EDs, but may not be so for EDs elsewhere so it is vital for a clinician to appreciate the patient's total population and where he/she tends to visit for holidays family and business.

A keen clinician should take a detailed history and then be prepared to investigate and to repeat investigations as necessary until the patient improves.

Clinical question: Do rapid diagnostic tests (RDTs) improve our ability to rule out malaria in the non-immune traveller?

Malaria cannot be safely diagnosed or excluded on clinical grounds alone.[4] Light microscopy of a blood films is regarded as the 'field standard' against which the sensitivity and specificity of other diagnostic methods must be assessed;[6,7] however one negative blood sample does not exclude a diagnosis of malaria.

In the UK the Health Protection Agency recommends '[w]here malaria is suspected blood films should be examined every 12 to 24 hours for 3 days whilst other diagnoses are also considered'.[4] Even after 3 negative films, if malaria is still considered a possible diagnosis, expert advice should be sought from a specialist in tropical or infectious diseases.

Most malaria cases are found in countries where cost-effectiveness of healthcare is a major concern, and there are limited resources for the provision of laboratory equipment and the training of personnel. The development of RDTs was initially to address these concerns and the World Health Organisation (WHO) recommended their use in situations where good quality microscopy was unavailable.[8] Despite this, RDTs are presently being used alongside light microscopy to diagnose malaria in non-endemic countries such as the UK.[9]

An additional difficulty is the absence of an agreed standard RDT for use in the UK.[9] Current RDTs vary in their compliance with WHO-proposed technical characteristics for RDTs,[10] but common weaknesses include decreased sensitivity in parasitaemias $< 0.002\%$ (< 100 parasites/µl), poor speciation of non-*falciparum* parasites, and an inability to differentiate sexual stages from asexual stages of the parasites. A meta-analysis of available research showed no advantage of RDTs over expert microscopy of sequential blood films in ruling out malaria. As such RDTs are still recommended as a diagnostic adjunct to microscopy.

✅ Evidence base RDTs in malaria?

Marx et al. (2005)[11] carried out a systematic review and meta-analysis of 21 test accuracy studies to determine the ability of different RDTs to rule out malaria in non-immune patients with suspected malaria. They found that for *P. falciparum*, HRP-2-based tests were more accurate than parasite LDH-based tests: negative likelihood ratios were 0.08 and 0.13 respectively ($p=0.019$ for the difference). However, for non-falciparum species the negative likelihood ratios were increased; 0.24 (*P. vivax*) and 0.66 (*P. malariae* or *ovale*). Furthermore, RDT performance dropped markedly for parasite

(continued)

densities <100 parasites/µl (negative likelihood ratio 0.33 [95% CI=0.22–0.50]) compared to densities >100 parasites/µl (negative likelihood ratio 0.07 [95% CI=0.03–0.17]).

Stauffer et al. (2009)[12] conducted a prospective multi-centre study comparing the diagnostic performance of an FDA-approved HRP-2-based RDT to microscopy. They found the RDT to have superior accuracy for all forms of malaria: negative likelihood ratios were 0.03 and 0.15 respectively (p=0.003). However, the study compared the RDT to a single blood film rather than the standard of 3 films. In addition it did not address the performance at low parasite densities.

Answer

At present there is no conclusive evidence that RDTs improve our ability to rule out a diagnosis of malaria in the non-immune traveller.

Case progression

On reviewing the patient you find him to be in no acute distress. He does, however, have a low-grade pyrexia (37.8 °C) but states that his headache and abdominal pain have resolved. Physical examination reveals normal neurological and cardiovascular systems. On respiratory examination he remains tachypnoeic (22 breaths/min) but auscultation is unremarkable. You note he has non-tender submandibular lymph nodes, but ENT examination reveals no obvious pathology. Abdominal examination reveals splenomegaly and bilateral non-tender inguinal lymphadenopathy.

Given the persistent pyrexia and headache allied with a history of foreign travel you decide to screen the patient for pyrexia of unknown origin. LFTs, blood cultures, thick and thin blood films for malaria, urinalysis, urine microscopy and culture, and a chest X-ray are all ordered. The earlier ordered investigations reveal the following results:

- Haemoglobin 10.9 g/dL
- White cell count 2.6×10^9/L
- Neutrophil count 1.2×10^9/L
- Platelet count 107×10^9/L
- U&E and glucose within normal limits

> ✪ **Learning point** Fever of unknown origin
>
> The classic definition of pyrexia of unknown origin (PUO) derives from a case series of 100 patients[13] and requires a temperature greater than 38.3 °C on several occasions, a fever lasting longer than 3 weeks, and a failure to reach a diagnosis despite 1 week of inpatient investigation. The strict classic definition of PUO helps to prevent common and self-limiting conditions (usually viral) from being included as PUO.
>
> Viral illnesses will typically resolve within 2 weeks of onset.[14] Four patient categories, based on their potential aetiology, have been proposed for PUO: classic, nosocomial, immune deficient, and HIV-associated.[15] In addition, the classical definition of PUO has been revised to reflect these categories; the criteria have been adjusted to include an evaluation of at least three days in hospital, 3 outpatient visits, or 1 week of outpatient testing.[14]

Another member of the ED team expresses concern over the patient's low white cell count, and questions whether the level of neutropenia could indicate sepsis or other causes of immunocompromise, thus mandating admission of the patient.

Clinical question: Does neutropenia mandate admission in all PUO patients?

Neutropenia is defined as a decrease in circulating neutrophils in the non-marginal pool.[16] These are only 4–5% of the total body neutrophil stores, as the majority are to be found in the bone marrow. The absolute neutrophil count (ANC) is used to gauge the severity of neutropenia. It is calculated by multiplying the total white blood cell count by the percentage of neutrophils (including band forms) and is measured in cells per microlitre of blood; an ANC of < 1500 cells/µL is felt to define neutropenia.[17] The risk of contracting a bacterial infection rises with the severity of neutropenia.

However, the most common form of neutropenia in the world is benign ethnic neutropenia, found in 25–50% of persons of African descent as well as several Middle Eastern ethnic groups.[18] These individuals do not have an increased susceptibility to infection despite having a persistently low ANC. This diagnosis may be appropriate in patients from these ethnic backgrounds who lack a history of susceptibility to infection and are unremarkable on physical examination.

> ✔ **Evidence base** How valid is the ANC definition of neutropenia?
>
> Hsieh *et al.* (2007)[19] performed a population-based, cross-sectional study to determine differences in neutrophil counts in the US population according to ethnicity, age, sex, and smoking status. They found that relative to white participants, black participants had lower leukocyte counts (mean difference, 0.89 × 109 cell/L; P <0.001), lower neutrophil counts (0.83 × 109 cell/L; P <0.001), and similar lymphocyte counts (0.022 × 109 cell/L; P=0.36). The prevalence of neutropenia (neutrophil count <1.5 × 109 cell/L) was 4.5% among black participants compared to 0.79% among white participants.
>
> Grann *et al.* (2007)[20] studied the prevalence and severity of neutropenia among women in 6 ethnic groups. Having enrolled 263 women aged 20–70 years with no diagnosis of cancer, they found an association between their ethnicity and their median WBC (P=0.006) and ANC (P=0.0001). Of the 12 women in the study with neutropenia (defined as an ANC=1500), all were of African or Caribbean descent.

Answer

The classic definition of neutropenia is based on normative data in Caucasian populations. Benign ethnic neutropenia can be considered a normal variant, as it confers no clinical disadvantages[18] and thus does not always mandate admission.

See Table 13.1 for a classification of fever of unknown origin.

> ⊕ **Clinical tip** Assessment of neutropenia
>
> The risk of infection in neutropenia rises significantly when the ANC falls below 0.5×10^9 cell/L. Common findings in neutropenic patients include:
>
> - Low-grade pyrexia
> - Painful swallowing, pain in the oral cavity or recurrent mouth ulcers
> - Painful and /or swollen gums
> - Multiple recurrent skin abscesses
> - Recurrent ear and sinus infections
> - Peri-rectal discomfort
> - Non-specific respiratory symptoms (cough, shortness of breath)
>
> Benign ethnic neutropenia should only be diagnosed in otherwise healthy patients who do not have repeated or severe infections.

Table 13.1 Classification of fever of unknown origin

Category of PUO	Definition	Common aetiologies
Classic	Temperature >38.3 °C Duration > 3 weeks Evaluation of at least 3 outpatient visits or 3 days in hospital	Infection, malignancy, collagen vascular disease
Nosocomial	Temperature >38.3 °C Patient hospitalized 24 or more hours but with no fever on admission Evaluation of at least 3 days	*Clostridium difficile* enterocolitis, drug-induced, pulmonary embolism, septic thrombophlebitis, sinusitis
Immune deficient (neutropenic)	Temperature >38.3 °C Neutrophil count of 0.5×10^9/L or less Evaluation of at least 3 days	Opportunistic bacterial infections, aspergillosis, candidiasis, herpes virus
HIV-associated	Temperature >38.3 °C Duration of > 4 weeks for outpatients, > 3 days for inpatients HIV infection confirmed	Cytomegalovirus, *Mycobacterium avium-intracellulare* complex, *Pneumocystis carinii* pneumonia, drug-induced, Kaposi's sarcoma, lymphoma

Data from Durack DT, Street AC. Fever of unknown origin - re-examined and redefined. *Curr Clin Top Infect Dis.* 1991; 11:35-51.

⚙ Expert comment New infectious disease patterns

Increasingly we need to track the evolving international disease burdens and consider emerging infections such as SARS in 2008–09, and now novel coronavirus which came from the Middle East. Again, a detailed travel itinerary should alert the clinician as to the risk of a patient returning with such an infection. These new infections have a much greater significance for the health community due to the potential for epidemics. Vigilance, universal precautions, and notification of patients presenting with such illnesses will be vital in containing spread.

Case progression

On further questioning, the patient admits to having had unprotected sexual intercourse with different partners on his trip. You now feel that the patient requires admission as he is neutropenic and the source of the fever has not been determined. The additional historical information provided suggests several possible causes of PUO (see Table 13.2). Unhappy with this line of questioning, the patient self-discharges.

Table 13.2 Differentials of PUO

Infections	Neoplasms	Autoimmune conditions	Miscellaneous
• Tuberculosis	• Lymphomas	• Rheumatoid arthritis	• Drug-induced fever
• Abdominal abscesses	• Chronic leukaemias	• Rheumatic fever	• Factitious fever
• Pelvic abscesses	• Metastatic cancers	• Systemic lupus erythematosus	• Non-infective hepatitis
• Dental abscesses	• Renal cell carcinoma	• Polymyalgia rheumatica	• Deep vein thrombosis
• Subacute infective endocarditis	• Hepatoma	• Temporal arteritis	• Sarcoidosis
• Osteomyelitis	• Colon carcinoma	• Inflammatory bowel disease	• Complications from cirrhosis
• Prostatitis	• Pancreatic carcinoma	• Adult Still's disease	• Unknown
• Sinusitis	• Sarcomas		

(continued)

Infections	Neoplasms	Autoimmune conditions	Miscellaneous
• CMV infection • Epstein-Barr virus infection • HIV • Q fever • Toxoplasmosis • Brucellosis	• Myelodysplastic syndromes	• Reiter's syndrome • Polyarteritis nodosa	

> **❝ Expert comment** HIV and PUO
>
> HIV should be considered as part of the differential diagnosis for many of our patients who have a PUO. The fever may be as a result of a sero-conversion illness in a patient with a new HIV infection or pre-existing immunosuppression may lead to the emergence of old favourites such as TB.
>
> HIV testing should be performed in patients presenting to the ED who have features suggestive of PUO or immunocompromised infection. Patients should have a relevant history taken regarding their risk for HIV as an initially negative test may require repeat testing if the patient's exposure was recent.
>
> CEM recommends that HIV testing should be performed in the ED providing there is a clinical suspicion that the patient may have an HIV-related condition or if the local prevalence of HIV infection within the local community is high (2/1000).
>
> As with many tests ordered in the ED where the results are not available immediately and the patient is to be sent home, there must be an appropriate local hospital system in place to ensure the test result is reviewed by a responsible clinician who will inform the patient of the result and counsel as necessary regarding the next steps in their care.
>
> I would caution any ED clinician considering HIV testing for a patient he/she intends on discharging home from the ED when there is not an appropriate follow-up service available. In those circumstances, the patient's GP may be a better clinician to take over the responsibility of counselling and arranging testing.

The following day he re-attends with his headache having returned along with 2 further episodes of high-grade fever associated with sweating and rigors. The thick and thin blood films performed the previous day identify *Plasmodium falciparum* with a parasitaemia of 1%. Other than mildly deranged LFTs, all other investigations are unremarkable. The patient asks you for tablets to take at home as he has had malaria several times in the past while in West Africa and never required admission.

Clinical question: Can *P. falciparum* malaria be treated on an outpatient basis in the UK?

You are aware that UK malaria treatment guidelines[5] call for the admission of all *P. falciparum* malaria patients. However, you know that in uncomplicated *P. falciparum* malaria the recommended management is with oral antimalarials. You wonder if you can discharge the patient on these.

> **✪ Learning point** WHO Malaria severity criteria (1990 and 2000)
>
> • Cerebral malaria
> • Severe anaemia—haematocrit <15% or Hb <5g/L
> • Renal failure—<400ml/24 hrs
>
> (continued)

- Pulmonary oedema and ARDS
- Hyopglycaemia—<2.2 mmol/l
- Circulatory failure—systolic BP <70 mmHg
- Abnormal bleeding / DIC
- Repeated generalised convulsions
- Acidosis—<7.25 or HCO3 <15 mmol/l
- Macroscopic haemoglobinuria
- Impaired consciousness
- Hyperparasitaemia—>5% parasitaemia
- Hyperbilirubinaemia—>43

Data from World Health Organization, 'Severe falciparum malaria', *Transactions of the Royal Society of Tropical Medicine & Hygiene*, 2000, 94, 1, pp. 1–90.

✅ **Evidence base** Can uncomplicated *P. falciparum* safely be managed on an outpatient basis?

Bottieau *et al.* (2007)[21] carried out a 5-year prospective cohort study enrolling all patients diagnosed with *P. falciparum* malaria. Patients that were non-vomiting, had parasitaemias <1% and exhibited none of the World Health Organisation 2000 criteria of severity were offered ambulatory treatment. None of these 214 patients consequently developed any malaria-related complications. However, 10 were later admitted (5 for vomiting, 4 for persistent fever and parasitaemia, and 1 for a recrudescence).

Melzer *et al.* (2009)[22] carried out a literature review on the outpatient treatment of falciparum malaria in developed countries and presented local data from the UK. Out of 142 cases of *P. falciparum* malaria, 78 were eligible for outpatient management (adult, non-pregnant, parasitaemias <2%, no WHO 2000 criteria of severity). Only 52, however, received outpatient management, and of these 15 were then lost to follow-up. The authors concluded that a large UK-based safety study or randomized trial was required before outpatient management could be recommended.

Answer

While there are studies that suggest that the outpatient management of uncomplicated *P. falciparum* is safe in selected cases, further work needs to be done. At present all *P. falciparum* cases in the UK should be admitted for further management.

The patient finally accepts your advice and is admitted to the ward, having been started on oral quinine 600 mg 8-hourly and doxycycline 200 mg daily.

❝ Expert comment

Uncomplicated malaria should be manageable as an outpatient even if *P. falciparum* is diagnosed, providing the ED and medical team have a clear clinical guideline to follow, including the management of unplanned re-attendances.

In most cases, intravenous rehydration, paracetamol, and observing the patient for up to 6 hours, enables the ED team to observe the patient's clinical improvement and be confident that the infection is uncomplicated. It is essential that the first dose of antimalarials is taken whilst in hospital and the patient retained for long enough to ensure that is not vomited up.

It is considerably more difficult trying to make this clinical decision within a 4-hour time limit. Having access to a short-stay ward is vital to enabling safe early discharge from hospital for patients requiring ongoing anti-malarial treatment. It is not admission avoidance, but it will reduce length of hospital admission from a standard 2–3 days to a less than 12-hour admission.

Once discharged from hospital, the patient should have a medical review arranged within 72 hours by the medical/infectious disease team, and be provided with clear written instructions as to if and when they should re-attend.

> ⊗ **Learning point** The other malarias
>
> *P. knowlesi*—This is an emerging cause of malaria, accounting for up to 70% of cases in certain parts of South East Asia.[23] Morphologically it is very similar to *P. malariae* and has been misdiagnosed as such on blood films. Unlike *P. malariae* however, it replicates every 24 hours, leading to hyperparasitaemia, severe disease, and possible fatalities (similar to *P. falciparum*).
>
> *P. knowlesi* should be considered in all patients coming from South East Asia, especially if diagnosed with '*P. malariae* hyperparasitaemia' by blood films. Such patients should be treated intensively in the same manner as *P. falciparum*.

A Final Word from the Expert

This topic covers an important area that many doctors find problematic to manage. Patients often present after hours when lab testing may be more restricted and the fear of missing a serious illness is high. The presentation of a returned traveller raises the difficulties a clinician can have in taking an adequate travel history, including risk factors for HIV disease, which in this case provoked the patient to self-discharge.

The prevalence of HIV disease is on the rise in inner-city areas of the UK and areas of higher migrant settlement. Whilst the ED is not an ideal environment to perform HIV screening, we may need to take the public health lead of doing such testing opportunistically when patients attend our EDs for other reasons. The same patient population at risk of having HIV is over-represented as ED attenders and may often have minimal contact with primary care.

In my opinion, the PUO patient requires a decent period of observation to witness them when afebrile and 'well' between their fever spikes. Without witnessing this interlude, one cannot be sure that there is nothing more sinister at hand. Short-stay admissions are a safe and efficient alternative to a standard inpatient stay, and should be considered for a number of our common ED presentations including the case in question.

References

1. Cox-Singh J. Plasmodium knowlesi malaria in humans is widely distributed and potentially life threatening. *Clin Infect Dis* 2008; 46(2):165–71.
2. World Health Organisation. World Malaria Report 2010. <http://www.who.int/malaria/world_malaria_report_2010/en/index.html>
3. Health Protection Agency. *Malaria-Epidemiological Data*. <http://www.hpa.org.uk/Topics/InfectiousDiseases/InfectionsAZ/Malaria/EpidemiologicalData/>
4. Chiodini PL, Hill D, Laloo DG, *et al. Guidelines for malaria prevention in travellers from the United Kingdom*. London: Health Protection Agency, 2007 <http://www.hpa.org.uk/webc/HPAwebFile/HPAweb_C/1203496943523>
5. Laloo DG, Shingadia D, Pasvol G, *et al.* UK Malaria treatment guidelines. *Journal of Infection* 2007; 54:111–21.
6. World Health Organisation. Guidelines for the treatment of malaria, Second Edition. <http://whqlibdoc.who.int/publications/2010/9789241547925_eng.pdf>
7. Moody A. Rapid diagnostic tests for malaria parasites. *Clin Microbiol Rev.* 2002; 15:66–78.
8. World Health Organisation. The use of malaria rapid diagnostic tests, Second Edition. 2006. <http://www.wpro.who.int/NR/rdonlyres/A30D47E1-1612-4674-8DF8-FCA031CDB9BA/0/Reduced_web2_MalariaRDT_20062ndedition.pdf>

9. Chilton D, Malik AN, Armstrong M, *et al*. Use of rapid diagnostic tests for diagnosis of malaria in the UK. *J Clin Pathol* 2006; 59:862–6.

10. World Health Organisation. Malaria diagnosis—new perspectives. Report of a joint WHO/USAID informal consultation 25–27 October 1999. 2000. <http://www.wpro.who. int/NR/rdonlyres/0CCB6282-EBFD-47C1-B8B4-4186E684DD3E/0/NewPersectives.pdf>

11. Marx A, Pewsner D, Egger M, *et al*. Meta-Analysis: Accuracy of rapid tests for malaria in travellers returning from endemic areas. *Ann Intern Med* 2005; 142:836–46.

12. Stauffer W, Cartwright C, Olson D, *et al*. Diagnostic performance of rapid diagnostic tests versus blood smears for malaria in US clinical practice. *Clin Infect Dis* 2009; 49(6):908–13.

13. Petersdorf RG, Beeson PB. Fever of unexplained origin: report on 100 cases. *Medicine* (Baltimore) 1961; 40:1–30.

14. Dykewicz MS. Rhinitis and sinusitis. *J Allergy Clin Immunol* 2003; 111(suppl 2):5520–9.

15. Durack DT, Street AC. Fever of unknown origin—re-examined and redefined. *Curr Clin Top Infect Dis* 1991; 11:35–51.

16. Watts RG. Neutropenia. In: Lee GR, Foerster J, Lukens J, *et al*. (eds). *Wintrobe's Clinical Hematology*, Tenth Edition. Baltimore, MD: Lippincott, Williams & Wilkins, 1999, pp. 1862–8.

17. Boxer LA, Blackwood RA. Leukocyte disorders: quantitative and qualitative disorders of the neutrophil, part 1. *Pediatr Rev* 1996; 17:19–28.

18. Haddy TB, Rana SR, Castro O. Benign ethnic neutropenia: what is a normal absolute neutrophil count? *J Lab Clin Med* 1999 Jan; 133(1):15–22.

19. Hsieh M, Everhart JE, Byrd-Holt D, *et al*. Prevalence of Neutropenia in the U.S. Population: Age, Sex, Smoking Status, and Ethnic Differences. *Ann Intern Med* 2007; 146:486–92.

20. Grann VR, Bowman N, Wei Y, *et al*. Ethnic neutropenia among women of European, African, and Caribbean backgrounds. *JCO*, 2007 ASCO Annual Meeting Proceedings Part I. Vol 25, No. 18S (June 20 Supplement), 2007: 6587.

21. Bottieau E, Clerinx J, Colebunders R, *et al*. Selective ambulatory management of imported falciparum malaria: a 5-year prospective study. *Eur J Clin Microbiol Infect Dis* 2007 Mar; 26(3):181–8.

22. Melzer M, Lacey S, Rait G. The case for outpatient treatment of Plasmodium falciparum malaria in a selected UK immigrant population. *J Infection* 2009 Aug; 59(4):259–63.

23. McCutchan TF, Piper RC, Makler MT. Use of Malaria Rapid Diagnostic Test to Identify Plasmodium knowlesi Infection. *Emerg Infect Dis* 2008 Nov; 14(11):1750–2.

Tricyclic antidepressant overdose

Shwetha Rao and Emma Townsend

ⓘ **Expert Commentary** Paul Dargan

Case history

An 18-year-old female presents at 10 p.m. having taken 15 tablets of amitriptyline (150 mg tablets) 30 minutes earlier. The tablets belonged to her mother and she took them intentionally after an argument with her boyfriend.

She denies co-ingestion of other drugs or alcohol. She has no past medical history, no regular medications, and no allergies. She has presented via ambulance with her best friend. No treatment has been given by the ambulance crew, and her initial observations are as follows: T 36.2, P 105, RR 17, BP 90/40, SpO_2 99 % on air, GCS 14. The ambulance ECG strip shows a sinus tachycardia.

See Box 14.1 for a clinical summary of tricyclic overdose.

Box 14.1 Clinical summary of tricyclic overdose

- Tricyclic antidepressants (TCAs) are associated with a much greater risk of acute toxicity and fatality when taken in overdose compared to other antidepressants.
- Death rates in England 1993–2004 per million prescriptions of antidepressants were 10 times higher in TCAs than all other antidepressants.[1]
- The commonest TCA taken in fatal overdose is dosulepin (dothiepin) which, along with amitriptyline, has been shown to have comparatively greater risk of toxicity than other TCAs.
- TCAs are rapidly absorbed from the gastrointestinal tract and undergo first-pass metabolism. They are highly protein-bound and have a large but variable volume of distribution (15–40 L/kg). They are metabolized by hepatic enzymes and excreted by the kidneys; they have a long half-life, generally greater than 24 hours (the half-life of amitriptyline is 31 to 46 hours).
- TCAs exhibit their toxic effects through 4 main pharmacological mechanisms:

  1. Anticholinergic action
  2. Inhibition of norepinephrine and serotonergic reuptake at nerve terminals
  3. Direct α-adrenergic blockade
  4. Membrane stabilizing effect on the myocardium by blockade of the cardiac and neurological fast sodium channels

---

Case progression

As she has presented to you within an hour of ingestion you consider if any method of gastric decontamination would be appropriate for her.

> ⊗ **Learning point** Gastric decontamination in tricyclic overdose
>
> Gastric decontamination is the process of removal of recently ingested poison to help reduce its absorption. It can potentially be achieved using the following procedures:
>
> - Gastric lavage
> - Activated charcoal
> - Whole bowel irrigation
> - Naso-gastric aspiration
> - Use of emesis and cathartics—these are not recommended in routine practice anymore
>
> The pharmacokinetics of TCAs are altered in overdose of a large quantity of the drug. Gastrointestinal absorption may be delayed because of inhibition of gastric emptying and entero-hepatic recirculation may prolong the final elimination. The concentration of unbound tricyclic (free in the plasma) may also increase if the overdose causes respiratory depression resulting in a respiratory acidosis and/or in the context of a metabolic acidosis, both of which will reduce protein binding.

The UK College of Emergency Medicine guideline working group[2] performed a short-cut systematic review of the choice of gastric decontamination in tricyclic overdose and concluded that activated charcoal could be used within the first hour of ingestion and was safe when the patient was not obtunded or was intubated. Gastric lavage could be considered only in patients who are intubated.[2,3] Other decontamination methods such as ipecac-induced emesis or whole-bowel irrigation are not recommended in TCA poisoning.

> ❝ **Expert comment**
>
> There are no data to suggest that gastric lavage improves outcome in patients with TCA poisoning and there is a risk of significant complications including increasing absorption by pushing tablets into the small intestine and hypoxia/tachycardia increasing the risk of arrhythmias.[4] Gastric lavage should therefore not be used routinely in the management of the patient with TCA poisoning and if used should only be carried out by clinicians with appropriate training and expertise.[5]
>
> There are no data from clinical studies to demonstrate that activated charcoal has an impact on outcome in TCA poisoning. However, based on data from volunteer studies, it is reasonable to consider activated charcoal administration within 1–2 hours of a significant (> 3–4 mg/kg body weight) TCA overdose.[4]

Case progression

The patient is seen immediately in resus and is given activated charcoal but is reluctant to ingest it. The history remains unchanged, on examination her GCS remains 14 (E3, M5, V6), and her observations are similar. You gain intravenous access and send baseline blood tests including full blood count, renal/liver function tests, arterial blood gas, and request an ECG (see Figure 14.1).

Clinical question: What investigations can be used as markers of toxicity?

Petit *et al.* demonstrated in 1976 that in patients with a total tricyclic concentration greater than 1000 µg/l there was an increased incidence of seizures, coma, and cardiac arrest.[6] However, plasma tricyclic concentrations are not widely available and laboratory assays often lack sensitivity in detecting active metabolites.

Several studies have looked into the ECG abnormalities associated with TCA overdose and have found a strong correlation with plasma TCA concentrations.[6–9]

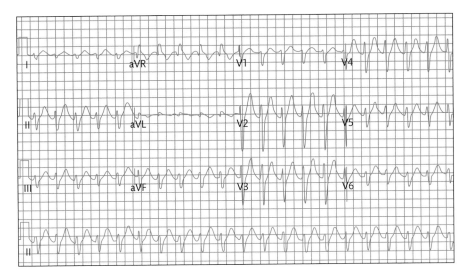

Figure 14.1 ECG changes seen in TCA overdose.

The ECG abnormalities seen in significant overdose include:[6-8,10,11]

- QRS width > 100 ms
- R wave > 3 mm in lead aVR (right axis deviation of the terminal 40 ms vector of the QRS complex in the frontal plane or the T 40 ms of the QRS axis)
- Brugada pattern and Bundle branch block patterns
- Prolonged QT

Bailey *et al.* (2004)[10] performed a meta-analysis of 18 studies of prognostic indicators to predict seizures, arrhythmia, and death in tricyclic overdose. These were reviewed systematically for the use of ECG or tricyclic concentration in predicting severity (see Table 14.1).

Table 14.1 The pooled sensitivity (Sen) and specificity (Spe) results for Bailey meta-analysis

Criteria	QRS width abnormality (QRS > 100 ms)	QTc > 430 ms	T40-ms axis	TCA concentration
Seizures	Sen−0.69 Spe−0.69	Non computable	Sen−0.50 Spe−0.72	Sen−0.75 Spe−0.72
Ventricular arrhythmias	Sen−0.79 Spe−0.46	Sen−0.78 Spe−0.56	Sen−0.33 Spe−0.71	Sen−0.78 Spe−0.57
Death	Sen−0.81 Spe−0.62	Sen−0.50 Spe−0.68	Sen−0.33 Spe−0.71	Sen−0.76 Spe−0.60

Data from Bailey B, Buckley NA, Amre DK. A meta-analysis of prognostic indicators to predict seizures, arrhythmias or death after tricyclic antidepressant overdose. *J Toxicol Clin Toxicol* 2004; 42(6):877-88.

Answer

The meta-analysis suggested that ECG and TCA concentration have similar accuracies but relatively poor performance for predicting complications associated with tricyclic overdose such as seizures, ventricular arrhythmias, or death. Nevertheless, an ECG should be recorded as part of the initial work-up in TCA overdose as although it is not a perfect marker of toxicity, ECG changes, when present, are likely to result from the toxic effect of the drug. Changes such as QRS widening, prolonged QT, R wave in aVR are therefore useful to predict complications and severity of the overdose.

> **❝ Expert comment**
>
> Although some studies suggest that plasma TCA concentrations can predict cardiovascular toxicity, TCA concentrations are not widely available. Patients with TCA poisoning can develop severe, life threatening complications within 1–6 hours of ingestion, and from a practical perspective, serial plasma TCA concentrations would never be available in a time frame to be able to guide bedside clinical management.
>
> Conversely, regular repeated 12-lead ECGs can provide a rapid and reliable tool to assess risk in patients with TCA poisoning. The presence of QRS prolongation, QTc prolongation, and/or right axis deviation of the T40 ms of the QRS axis should alert the clinician to an increased risk of arrhythmias and seizures. However, as noted earlier, these have moderate sensitivity and specificity and so it is important that they are interpreted in light of the overall clinical picture and that other factors such as acid-base status and level of consciousness are taken into account.
>
> The T40 ms axis is difficult to measure; however, when an abnormal terminal rightward axis is present, there will be a terminal R-wave in lead aVR (as shown in the ECG in Figure 14.1).

Case progression

The patient's observations are repeated and the nurse informs you that she is concerned about the deteriorating blood pressure.

T 36.2, P 115, RR 20, BP 80/35, SpO$_2$ 100 % on 10l, GCS 14.

A 1-litre bolus of 0.9 % sodium chloride has been given and the patient has been positioned head down.

Clinical question: When should sodium bicarbonate be used?

The use of sodium bicarbonate in the treatment of tricyclic toxicity was first reported in the 1970s (see Table 14.2). The mechanism of action is thought to be both through the hypertonic sodium load resulting in changes in TCA binding to the cardiac sodium channel and through changes in the acid-base status with relative alkalaemia resulting in greater TCA protein binding.[3,12,13]

Table 14.2 Evidence for the use of bicarbonate in TCA overdose

Study	Design, subjects, and intervention			Main results	
Animal study—McCabe[12] (1998)	• Randomized controlled animal study including 24 swines divided into 4 groups of 6 receiving an intervention for an induced toxicity of nortriptyline				
	Group	Intervention	Systolic BP	Mean QRS width	Surviving subjects
	1	Saline	54 ± 18 mmHg	144 ± 38 ms	1/6
	2	Sodium bicarbonate	85 ± 19 mmHg	105 ± 38 ms	2/6
	3	Hypertonic saline	134 ± 21 mmHg	80 ± 14 ms	5/6
	4	Hyperventilation	60 ± 12 mmHg	125 ± 46 ms	1/6

Data from McCabe JL, Cobaugh DJ, Menegazzi J, *et al.* Experimental tricyclic antidepressant toxicity: A randomized, controlled comparison of hypertonic saline solution, sodium bicarbonate and hyperventilation. *Ann Emerg Med* 1998; 32(3 ptl):329–33.

In this model, hyperventilation had a limited impact. Hypertonic sodium bicarbonate was effective and a greater effect was seen with hypertonic saline suggesting that both sodium loading and alkalinization have an impact.

(continued)

Study	Design, subjects, and intervention	Main results
Hoffman JR et al.[14] (1993) USA	• Retrospective cohort study • Included patients with moderate to severe toxicity admitted to ED or ICU • Sodium bicarbonate was infused as preferred treatment with aim to alkalinize to a pH 7.5	91 patients included of who 43 were admitted to ICU 20/21 patients with hypotension showed improvement 39/49 showed improved QRS width 40/85 showed improved CNS status
Koppell C[15] (1992) Germany	• Retrospective cohort study included 184 cases of overdose • 8 patients with cardiac disturbance • 100 mmol of sodium bicarbonate administered	4/8 patients treated reverted to sinus rhythm

Blackman *et al.* (2001)[16] conducted a systematic review of the effects of plasma alkalinization in TCA overdose. The review included 8 case reports and 4 case series which showed beneficial effects of bicarbonate therapy with resolution of ECG changes and hypotension. However, there have been no randomized trials in humans and the best evidence comes only from animal studies.

Answer

Despite limiting evidence in humans, sodium bicarbonate has been used in the correction of hypotension, arrhythmias, and ECG abnormalities in tricyclic overdose. When used, the aim should be to alkalinize the blood pH to 7.45–7.55.

> **☆ Learning point** Adjunctive treatments for the treatment of arrhythmias in TCA overdose
>
> In general, antiarrhythmic drugs especially the Class Ia and Ic drugs should be avoided due to their sodium channel blocking effect. The correction of hypotension, hypoxia, and acidosis will reduce the cardiotoxic effects of TCAs.[9]
>
> Foianini A et al.[17] reviewed articles that studied the use of phenytoin and lignocaine in the treatment of the cardiac toxicity induced by TCAs. They recommended their use only in cases where the cardiac arrhythmias or hypotension is refractory to treatment with sodium bicarbonate or hypertonic saline, or in which physiological derangement (e.g. severe alkalosis or hypernatremia) limits effective use of these primary strategies.
>
> Glucagon and magnesium sulphate have been used as adjuncts in treatment of cardiotoxicity and ECG abnormalities where sodium bicarbonate has been unsuccessful.[3,18]

Case progression

You decide to treat her with a bolus of 50 ml of 8.4 % sodium bicarbonate followed by an infusion of sodium bicarbonate. During treatment she has a generalized convulsion and the cardiac monitor continues to show a widened QRS. You discuss the case with ICU and they suggest considering the use of intralipid.

Seizures in TCA poisoning are usually self-limiting, but where treatment is necessary benzodiazepines are the treatment of choice,[3,18] Barbiturates are preferred as the second line in benzodiazepine-resistant seizures and phenytoin is best

❝ Expert comment

The evidence for the use of hypertonic sodium bicarbonate in TCA toxicity largely comes from in vitro and animal studies; however, the observational retrospective cohort studies in patients with TCA toxicity noted in Table 14.2 support its use.

Even in the absence of acidosis, alkalinization to an arterial pH of 7.45–7.55 with intravenous hypertonic (8.4%) sodium bicarbonate should be considered in patients with TCA toxicity who have:

• QRS duration greater than 120 msec
• arrhythmias
• hypotension resistant to fluid resuscitation

❝ Expert comment

Anti-arrhythmics should be avoided in patients with TCA toxicity. Hypertonic sodium bicarbonate is the first-line treatment for arrhythmias. Patients not responding to alkalinization should be managed with DC cardioversion and/or over-drive pacing.

avoided due to its potential to exacerbate arrhythmias in TCA toxicity. Patients with decreased conscious level and respiratory depression may require intubation.

Clinical question: In tricyclic overdose does intralipid help reverse cardiac instability (arrhythmias/hypotension/ECG abnormalities)?

Intra lipid emulsion (ILE), also described as 'lipid rescue', is a bolus of lipid emulsion; there are various theories on the mechanism of action of intralipid. One theory is that it may act as a 'lipid sink' to sequester lipophilic drugs such as local anaesthetics, hence reducing their availability for receptor binding. TCAs are lipophilic drugs and animal studies and case reports suggest they may have a role in the treatment of TCA poisoning (See Table 14.3).

Table 14.3 Evidence for the use of intralipid in TCA overdose

Study	Design subjects and intervention	Main results
Harvey M et al.[19]	Randomized controlled trial. 30 rabbits infused with clomipramine and induced hypotension treated with 0.9% normal saline, 8.4% sodium bicarbonate, and 20% intralipid	Mean difference in mean arterial pressure between Intralipid- and saline-solution-treated groups was 21.1 mm Hg (95% CI 13.5–28.7 mm Hg) and 19.5 mm Hg (95% CI 10.5–28.9 mm Hg) at 5 and 15 minutes, respectively. Mean difference in mean arterial pressure between Intralipid- and bicarbonate-treated groups 19.4 mm Hg (95% CI 18.8–27.0 mm Hg) and 11.5 mm Hg (95% CI 2.5–20.5 mm Hg) at 5 and 15 minutes
Human case reports		
Boegevig et al.[20] 2011	Case report—A 36 year old who presented after ingesting 5.25 g of dosulepin showed ECG changes and seizures improved with treatment of a ILE	
Bargeon et al.[21] 2012	Case report—54-year-old man with ingestion of 2.25 g of amitryptiline who had refractory hypotension after treatment with sodium bicarbonate and inotropes showed response after treatment with a bolus of 100 ml of 20% intralipid followed by an infusion	
Kiebard et al.[22] 2010	Case report—A 25-year-old lady who developed a cardiac arrest with a wide complex tachycardia which showed no response to conventional advanced life support and sodium bicarbonate improved with a intralipid emulsion and was discharged from hospital with no neurological sequelae	
Harvey et al.[23] 2012	Case report—51 year old who presented in shock after taking a multidrug self-poisoning and found to have a 43 mg/kg of amitriptyline, showed improvement in hypotension after a 100 ml bolus followed by a 400 ml infusion of intra lipid	
Hendron D[24] 2011	Case report—20 month old who showed no improvement with sodium bicarbonate therapy, had successful treatment with ILE with narrowing of the QRS complexes and rise in blood pressure	
Nair A[25] 2011	Case report—34 year old who developed seizures and cardiac arrest after a fatal tricyclic overdose revealed marked reduction in cardiovascular instability after commencement of intralipid 20% infusions with no further arrhythmias	

(continued)

Human case reports	
Al-Duaij N[26] 2009	Case report—A 52-yr-old lady with 6 g overdose of imipramine who showed initial response to advanced life support and sodium bicarbonate treatment developed delayed seizures and cardiac instability which responded only to reatment with ILE
Carr D[27] 2009	Case report—80-year-old man found with a GCS -3 after a fatal overdose of doxepin showed minimal response to conventional treatment with orogastric lavage and alkalinazation therapy upto a pH of 7.73 with sodium bicarbonate. He was treated with ILE which improved his ECG and hypotension within 2.5 hours of initiation of therapy

Data from various sources (see references)

Answer

ILE has shown good promise in 1 animal study of tricyclic overdose. No randomized trials have been performed in humans, however, several case reports describe successful resuscitation with ILE where sodium bicarbonate had been unsuccessful. If treatment with sodium bicarbonate and alkalinization to a pH of 7.45–7.55 fails to reverse signs of cardiac toxicity, it may be considered.

Case progression

The patient is transferred to the intensive care unit for invasive monitoring. After 24 hours the ECG has normalized and she has had no further fits. She is transferred to a ward for review by the psychiatric team.

ᏈᏈ Expert comment

There is currently limited evidence for the use of intralipid in the management of TCA toxicity and many of the case reports are constrained by insufficient information on the conventional therapies that were used prior to or alongside intralipid. One other important factor is that TCAs have long half-lives and therefore there is the potential for recrudescence of toxicity after intralipid therapy.

Currently intralipid therapy should only be considered in patients with severe toxicity, in particular ventricular arrhythmias, resistant to hypertonic sodium bicarbonate and other conventional therapy.

✛ Clinical tip Long-term outlook

The greatest risk of arrhythmias, convulsions, and death is in the first 8–12 hours after ingestion. Patients with severe tricyclic overdose who improve with early appropriate treatment generally have no evidence of any long-term neurological or other physiological sequel.[21,22,24,25,26]

A Final Word from the Expert

Tricylic antidepressant poisoning can be associated with severe and potentially life-threatening toxicity. Significant toxicity can occur with ingestions >3–5 mg/kg and life-threatening effects can be seen with ingestions of >10–15 mg/kg.

All patients with TCA toxicity should have a 12-lead ECG and be observed for a minimum of 6 hours with ECG monitoring. Patients who are asymptomatic with normal 12-lead ECG 6 hours after ingestion are not likely to develop toxicity.

Early advice from a poisons centre and/or clinical toxicologist should be considered in patients with significant TCA toxicity.

The 12-lead ECG is a useful tool for predicting risk in TCA poisoning, and the presence of QRS or QTc prolongation and/or a positive R-wave in aVR is associated with an increased risk of arrhythmias and convulsions.

Hypertonic sodium bicarbonate should be considered in patients with QRS >120 ms, arrhythmias, and/or hypotension resistant to fluid resuscitation. Anti-arrhythmics should *not* be used in TCA-related arrhythmias.

References

1. Morgan O, Griffiths C, Baker A, Majeed A. Fatal toxicity of antidepressants in England and Wales, 1993–2002. *Health Stat Q* 2004; 23:18–24.
2. Body R, Bartram T, Azam F, *et al*. Guidelines in Emergency Medicine Network (GEMNet): Guideline for the management of tricyclic antidepressant overdose. *Emerg Med J* 2011;28(4):347–68.
3. Kerr GW, McGuYe AC, Wilkie S. Tricyclic antidepressant overdose: a review. *Emerg Med J* 2001; 18(4):236–41.
4. Dargan PI, Colbridge MG, Jones AL. The Management of Tricyclic Antidepressant Poisoning: The Role of Gut Decontamination, Extracorporeal Procedures and Fab Antibody Fragments. *Toxicol Rev* 2005; 24 (3):187–94.
5. Benson BE, Hoppu K, Troutman WG, *et al*. Position paper update: gastric lavage for gastrointestinal Decontamination. *Clin Toxicol (phila)* 2013; 51(3):140–6.
6. Petit JM, Spiker DG, Ruwitch JF, *et al*. Tricyclic antidepressant plasma levels and adverse effects after overdose. *Clin. Pharmacol Ther* 1977; 21:47–51.
7. Boehnert MT, Lovejoy FH. Value of the QRS duration versus the serum drug level in predicting seizures and ventricular arrhythmias after an acute overdose of tricyclic antidepressants. *N Engl J Med* 1985; 313:474–9.
8. Thanacoody HK, Thomas SH. Tricyclic antidepressant poisoning: cardiovascular toxicity. *Toxicol Rev* 2005; 24(3):205–14.
9. Caravati EM, Bossart PJ. Demographic and electrocardiographic factors associated with severe tricyclic antidepressant toxicity: *J Toxicol Clin Toxicol*, 1991; 29(1):31–43.
10. Bailey B, Buckley NA, Amre DK. A meta-analysis of prognostic indicators to predict seizures, arrhythmias or death after tricyclic antidepressant overdose. *J Toxicol Clin Toxicol* 2004; 42(6):877–88.
11. Liebelt EL, Francis PD, Woolf AD. ECG lead aVR versus QRS interval in predicting seizures and arrhythmias in acute tricyclic antidepressant toxicity. *Ann Emerg Med* 1995; 26(2):195–201.
12. McCabe JL, Cobaugh DJ, Menegazzi J, *et al*. Experimental tricyclic antidepressant toxicity: A randomized, controlled comparison of hypertonic saline solution, sodium bicarbonate and hyperventilation. *Ann Emerg Med* 1998; 32(3 ptI):329–33.
13. Brown TCK, Barker GA, Dunlop ME, *et al*. The use of sodium bicarbonate in the treatment of tricyclic antidepressant-induced arrhythmias. *Anaesth Intensive Care* 1973; 1:203–10.
14. Hoffman JR, Votey SR, Bayer M, *et al*. Effect of hypertonic sodium bicarbonate in the treatment of moderate-to-severe cyclic antidepressant overdose. *Am J Emerg Med* 1993; 11(4):336–41.
15. Koppel C, Wiegreffe A, Tenczer J. Clinical course, therapy, outcome and analytial data in amitriptyline and combined amitriptyline/chlordiazepoxide overdose. *Hum & Exp Toxicol* 1992; 11(6):458–65.
16. Blackman K, Brown SGA, Wilkes GJ. Plasma alkalinization for tricyclic antidepressant toxicity: A systematic review. *Emerg Med (Freemantle)* 2001; 13(2):204–10.
17. Foianini A, Joseph Wiegand T, Benowitz N. What is the role of lidocaine or phenytoin in tricyclic antidepressant-induced cardiotoxicity? *Clin Toxicol (Phila)* 2010; 48(4):325–30.
18. TOXBASE online reference. <http://www.toxbase.org/Poisons-Index-A-Z/A-Products/Amitriptyline --------/>
19. Harvey M.; Cave G. Intralipid Outperforms Sodium Bicarbonate in a Rabbit Model of Clomipramine Toxicity. *Ann Emerg Med* 2007; 49(2):178–85.
20. Boegevig S, Rothe A, Tfelt-Hansen J, *et al*. Successful reversal of life threatening cardiac effect following dosulepin overdose using intravenous lipid emulsion. *Clin Toxicol* 2011; 49(4):337–9.

21. Bargeon JL, Brennan E, *et al*. Lipid rescue for tricyclic antidepressant toxicity: A case report. *Clin Toxicol* 2012; 50(7):584.

22. Kiberd MB, Minor SF. Lipid therapy for the treatment of a refractory amitriptyline overdose *CJEM* 2012; 14(3):193–7.

23. Harvey M. Cave G. Case report: Successful lipid resuscitation in multidrug overdose with predominant tricyclic antidepressant toxidrome; *Int J Emerg Med* 2012; 5(1):8.

24. Hendron D, Menagh G, Sandilands EA, *et al*. Tricyclic antidepressant overdose in a toddler treated with intravenous lipid emulsion *Pediatrics* 2011; 128(6):1628–32.

25. Nair A, Paul E, Protopapas M. Management of near fatal mixed tricyclic antidepressants and selective serotonin reuptake inhibitor overdose with intralipid 20% emulsion. *Anaesthesia and intensive care* 2013; 41(2):264.

26. Al-Duaij N, Lipid emulsion therapy in massive imipramine overdose. *Clinical Toxicol* 2009; 47(5)(460):710.

27. Carr D, Boone A, Hoffman RS, *et al*. Successful resuscitation of a doxepin overdose using intravenous fat emulsion (IFE). *Clin Toxicol* 2009; 47(7):710.

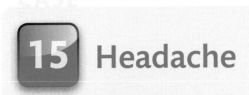

15 Headache

Katie McLeod

Ⓘ Expert commentary Andrew Hobart

Case history

A 58-year-old woman presents to the ED with a sudden onset history of headache and neck stiffness. The headache came on while walking to work 2 hours earlier, and she describes it as her worst-ever headache, akin to 'being hit over the back of the head'. She has vomited twice since. The headache has not been relieved by paracetamol and worsens when retching to vomit. There is no history of head injury, fevers, or visual disturbance.

She had migraines as a teenager, but these were different in nature and associated with flashing lights. Her only other past medical history is of hypertension that has been well controlled with amlodipine. Observations at triage reveal a temperature of 37.2 °C, pulse at 90 beats per minute and regular, BP 140/80mmHg. She was alert and orientated.

See Box 15.1 for a clinical summary of headaches.

Box 15.1 Clinical summary of headaches

Headache is a common presentation to the ED, making up around 1–2% of all attendances in the UK.[1]

The majority of headaches seen in the ED are benign in origin, but there are inevitably some serious pathological causes for headache, which need to be excluded; many of these can be distinguished by the history and examination, but others require further investigation. The pattern of the headache is particularly significant for primary headaches and other associated clinical features suggest a more significant pathology. A sound knowledge of the different types of headaches is essential for the ED clinician.

Classification of headaches[2,3]

Acute single episode

Meningitis
Encephalitis
Tropical illness, e.g. malaria
Subarachnoid haemorrhage
Sinusitis
Head injury

Acute recurrent attacks

Migraine
Cluster headache
Glaucoma
Recurrent (Mollaret's) meningitis
Trigeminal neuralgia

(continued)

Subacute onset

Giant cell arteritis
Chronic subdural
Space-occupying lesion
Carbon monoxide poisoning
Idiopathic intracranial hypertension

Chronic headache (>15 days/month for >3 months)

Tension headache
Chronically raised ICP
Medication misuse

Data from Oxford Handbook of Clinical Medicine 8th Edition. Longmore M, Wilkinson I, Davidson E, et al., and MacGregor, Steiner TJ, Davies PTG. British Association for the Study of Headache. Guidelines for All Healthcare Professionals in the Diagnosis and Management of Migraine, Tension-Type, Cluster and Medication-Overuse Headache. 3rd edition (1st revision); September 2010

✪ **Learning point** Symptoms suggestive of secondary headache—SIGN Guideline[4]

Secondary headaches are attributed to an underlying pathological condition. Red-flag features which should prompt referral for further investigation:

- New onset of, or change in, headache in patients who are aged over 50 years
- Thunderclap: rapid time to peak headache intensity (seconds–5 minutes)—same-day specialist assessment required
- Focal neurological symptoms (e.g. limb weakness, aura <5 minutes or >1 hour).
- Non-focal neurological symptoms (e.g. cognitive disturbance)
- Change in headache frequency, characteristics, or associated symptoms
- Abnormal neurological examination
- Headache that changes with posture
- Headache waking the patient up (N.B. migraine is the most frequent cause of morning headache)
- Headache precipitated by exertion or Valsalva manoeuvre (coughing, straining)
- Patients with risk factors for cerebral venous sinus thrombosis
- Jaw claudication or visual disturbance
- Neck stiffness
- Fever
- New-onset headache in a patient with a history of HIV infection
- New-onset headache in a patient with a history of cancer

This information is reproduced from SIGN Guideline 107 'Diagnosis and management of headache in adults' by kind permission of the Scottish Intercollegiate Guidelines Network. Scottish Intercollegiate Guidelines Network (SIGN). Diagnosis and management of headache in adults. Edinburgh: SIGN; November 2008. (SIGN Guideline 107). [cited 23 Jun 2014]. Available from URL: http://www.sign.ac.uk

---

❝ Expert comment Headaches in the ED

The incidence of serious underlying pathology in patients presenting to the ED with a headache has been estimated to be 1 in 10. By comparison, the incidence in neurology outpatient clinic is 1 in 100, and in primary care it is 1 in 1000. The majority of patients presenting with headache will have a normal clinical examination but this does not exclude serious pathology.

Headache is high on the list of presenting complaints for ED discharges that result in major clinical negligence claims.

The patient is in obvious distress with a pain score of 6/10 but has only had paracetamol thus far, so prior to further examination you decide to give some further analgesia. The diagnosis is still unclear, but you wonder which would be the most appropriate additional analgesia at this stage.

Clinical question: What is the best analgesia to administer for the headache?

It is important to provide symptom relief for patients in the ED but the choice of what is 'best analgesia' seems to vary between individual practitioners. Because of the broad scope of headache presentations to the ED, initially the likely diagnosis needs to be considered when prescribing to ensure administration of appropriate analgesia (see Table 15.1).

Table 15.1 Headache aetiologies and recommended treatment regimes

Type of headache	Population	Clinical features	Analgesia
Migraine	15% of adults at some time in their lives 3:1 Women:Men Late teens to 50s	May have aura for 15–30 mins followed by throbbing headache in <1 hour Nausea, vomiting, photophobia/phonophobia Triggers	Step 1: Aspirin 900 mg/6 h[5] or ibuprofen 400–600 mg[6] or other NSAID with prochlorperazine,[7] metoclopramide, or domperidone for nausea Step 2: Rectal analgesic such as Diclofenac 100 mg with antiemetic Step 3: Specific anti-migraine drugs triptans, e.g. sumatriptan 50 mg[8], aolmitriptan 2.5–5 mg, Ergotamine tartrate 1–2 mg
Tension-type headache	Up to 80% of the population 3% have chronic sub-type, >15/7 per month	Tight band or pressure around head. Symptoms may radiate to neck Tenderness to scalp Last 30 mins–7 days	Reassurance Aspirin 600–900 mg[9] NSAIDS[10] Prophylaxis: amitriptylline
Cluster headache	0.05% of the population	Typically twice every 24 hrs for 15–160 mins Clusters last 4–12 wks Rapid onset pain around one eye, unilateral headache	Oxygen 100%, 10–20 min[11] sumatriptan 6 mg s/c[12] zolmitriptan nasal spray Prophylaxis: verapamil prednisolone
Medication over-use headache	Up to 2% of the population Can affect children	Chronic headache May be related to mixed analgesics, particularly containing codeine	Withdrawal of medication, gradual if opiate. naproxen[13] Preventive medication: amitriptylline, gabapentin, valproate
Trigeminal neuralgia	Age >50 Around 14% are secondary to aneurysm, tumour, MS, chronic inflammation	Unilateral, in the trigeminal nerve distribution, typically mandibular or maxillary divisions Intense stabbing pain May be brought on by washing, eating, talking	Carbamazepine phenytoin gabapentin
Dental pain	All ages	Pain around teeth or jaw Worsened by chewing and heat/cold	Paracetamol NSAIDS Opioid analgesia Mefanamic acid
Glaucoma	Elderly, long-sighted (hypermetropic)	Aching pain develops rapidly around one eye Reduced vision Nausea and vomiting Fixed mid-dilated pupil	Acetazolamide 500-mg IV Topical β-blocker Topical steroid Anti-emetic Supine position

Data from various sources (see references)

⊘ **Evidence base** Analgesia for headaches

Migraine

A Cochrane review published in 2010 compiled data from randomized controlled trials treating migraine with 900/1000 mg aspirin compared to placebo or sumatriptan 50/100 mg, with or without metoclopramide.[5] 13 studies including a total of 4222 participants found that all active treatments were superior to placebo, with NNTs of 8.1, 4.9, and 6.6 for 2-hour pain-free, 2-hour headache relief, and 24-hour headache relief with aspirin alone versus placebo, and 8.8, 3.3, and 6.2 with aspirin plus metoclopramide versus placebo. Sumatriptan 50 mg was no better than aspirin alone for 2-hour pain-free and headache relief, but sumatriptan 100 mg was better than the combination of aspirin plus metoclopramide for 2-hour pain-free, but not for headache relief.

Tension-type headache

A double-blind, double-dummy, randomized parallel-groups comparative trial in the UK[9] comparing aspirin 500 mg and 1000 mg with paracetamol 500 mg and 1000 mg vs placebo showed that doses of aspirin at 500/1000 mg and paracetamol 1000 mg were statistically significant compared to placebo, despite a high placebo-response rate (54.5 %), whereas paracetamol 500 mg alone showed no benefit.

Cluster headache

A study conducted by the National Hospital for Neurology and Neurosurgery[11] looked at 109 adults in a double-blind, randomized, placebo-controlled, cross-over trial over a period of 4 cluster headaches. They compared high-flow oxygen over a 15-minute period at the onset of headache with high-flow air. The primary end point was to be pain-free or have adequate relief at 15 minutes. They found that 78 % with oxygen vs 20 % with air reached the primary end-point ($p < 0.001$) with no adverse events.

⊘ **Evidence base** NICE guideline for headache (2012)

The recommendations for analgesia have predominantly remained the same; however, in the treatment of acute migraine a triptan has been recommended as a first-line agent along with either paracetamol or an NSAID. Non-oral preparations of triptans should be administered if oral medication is not tolerated. For migraine prophylaxis topiramate and propranolol remain the current recommendation but further RCTs to assess the efficacy of amitriptyline and pizotifen have been suggested.

Other prophylactic treatments include acupuncture for tension-type headache and verapamil and ambulatory oxygen for recurrent cluster headache.

Data from CG150 'Headaches: Diagnosis and management of headaches in young people and adults', NICE Guidelines, 2012

Answer

Each potential aetiology has a different most effective treatment strategy. Identifying a likely differential diagnosis is important to avoid treating blindly and ineffectually.

❶ **Expert comment**

The relief of pain and suffering is one of the primary duties of the emergency physician and the provision of adequate analgesia should not be delayed until diagnosis is confirmed. If the clinical

(continued)

features suggest that a specific primary headache disorder is present, it is sensible to prescribe a treatment based on that diagnosis where feasible.

However many of the drugs recommended for primary headache disorders are not normally part of the standard ED pain-control ladder (e.g. aspirin) or may not be routinely stocked in the ED (e.g. gabapentin, triptans).

Another pitfall for the unwary is to assume that a response to a diagnosis-based therapy increases the probability of, or even confirms that diagnosis. This is not so as a systematic review by Pope *et al.* in 2008[14] found that 44% of patients with secondary headache responded to treatments such as anti-emetics and NSAIDS. The use of triptans resulted in an even higher response rate even in secondary headaches.

Case progression

On examination the patient was alert and orientated with a normal cardiovascular and respiratory examination. Neurological examination of the cranial and peripheral nerves was grossly normal with normal fundoscopy, pupils equal and reactive to light and the GCS remaining 15 throughout. There was some mild subjective neck stiffness; however, Brudzinski's and Kernig's signs were negative and there was no photophobia or rash.

Blood tests were ordered including FBC, renal profile, coagulation studies, and a decision to order a non-contrast CT head scan was taken. Co-codamol and ibuprofen were given for the headache, which gave some relief.

The CT head scan was reported by the neuro-radiologist as follows: 'There is no intracranial abnormality. If SAH is clinically suspected lumbar puncture will be needed to exclude the diagnosis'.

Subarachnoid haemorrhage

The infamous clinical presentation of 'the worst headache of my life' has long been taught to necessitate investigations to exclude a SAH. It has been argued that although there are features suggestive of SAH, none are specific enough and the concern is that cases will be missed if rigid rules are adhered to.

As emergency physicians it is imperative not to miss SAH given the associated morbidity and mortality, however, the diagnostic pathway includes an invasive LP and the level of clinical suspicion must be weighed up against possible complications from over-investigation.

Of patients presenting to the ED with acute headache, between 2% and 10% may be due to SAH. The majority of SAH is due to trauma, but aneurysmal SAH makes up around 85% of non-traumatic cases.[15]

A proportion of patients with SAH will have had a 'sentinel' or warning bleed in the preceding 30 days, resulting from an aneurysmal leak. A case-controlled study found that approximately 40% of patients admitted with SAH reported episodes of severe headache, compared with only 1 of 20 patients with cerebral infarction and none of 100 with a non-neurological disorder.[16]

A lot of work has been done to establish a clinical decision rule for the prediction of SAH from the clinical history and examination. A study conducted to determine high-risk clinical characteristics for SAH found that of the patients diagnosed 93.1 % complained of 'worst ever headache', 71.1 % complained of neck stiffness or pain, 58.6 % had vomiting and 23.1 % had onset during exertion.[17]

⊕ **Clinical tip** Classification of SAHs

Fisher

Grade 1—none evident
Grade 2—less than 1 mm thick
Grade 3—more than 1 mm thick
Grade 4—diffuse or intraventricular haemorrhage or parenchymal extension (see Figure 15.1)

Reproduced from Fisher C, *et al.*, 'Relation of cerebral vasospasm to subarachnoid hemorrhage visualized by computerized tomographic scanning', *Neurosurgery*. 6:1 pp. 1–9, Copyright 1980, with permission from the Congress of Neurological Surgeons.

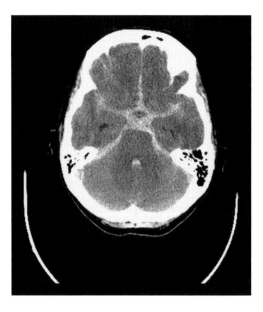

Figure 15.1 CT head—Grade 4 subarachnoid haemorrhage

Clinical question: In a neurologically intact patient with suspected SAH, is lumbar puncture still indicated following a normal non-contrast CT to rule out subarachnoid haemorrhage?

See Table 15.2 for evidence for performing LPs after CT.

Table 15.2 Evidence for performing LPs after CT

Author, date, and country	Patient group	Method	Results	Study strengths and weaknesses
Van der Wee[18] Jan 1989–Jan 1993,Department of Neurology, 2 university hospitals in the Netherlands	Acute headache, alert, no neurological deficit, CT performed within 12 hours after the onset of headache	CTs interpreted by a neuro-radiologist and 2 neurologists Patients with normal CT had LP >12 hrs after onset of headache	175 patients investigated, abnormal CT in 117 Of remaining 58, 2 had CSF xanthochromia Sensitivity of CT 98% (95% CI 94–99.8%)	No kappa value given for CT results between interpreters Good follow-up of data, few patients lost 79/175 patients had a ruptured aneurysm, possible spectrum bias
Morgenstern[19] Mar 1995–Jun 1996, Large Academic Hospital, Houston, TX	Triaged in ED with 'worst headache ever' or '10/10 severity'	Prospective study, recruited from ED triage. Neuro-radiologists blinded to study. Patients divided into groups on whether CT was >24 hrs or >24 hours from headache onset	170 patients eligible, 107 enrolled SAH on CT in 18, further 2/79 diagnosed on LP Sensitivity of CT 97.5%, (95% CI 91.2–99.7%)	63/170 patients not enrolled, 35 had no specified reason Prospective study, good follow-up of patients Sensitivity not calculated by the authors Small numbers, 10 patients refused LP
Gunawardena[20] Apr 1993–Sep 2000, Frenchay Hospital, Bristol	Admitted to neurology or neurosurgical units with suspected SAH Normal CT interpreted by neuro-radiologist No focal abnormal neurology	Retrospective case notes analysis	9/263 patients were found to have cerebral aneurysm following LP and a normal CT	The primary outcome was to assess the sensitivity of haem pigments for SAH CTs were all interpreted by a neuro-radiologist, may not be possible in smaller centres
Stefan A Dupont[21] Jan 1998–Jan 2008, Emergency Department, Rochester, MN	Alert, neurologically intact, non-traumatic 'thunderclap' headache, who had CT reported as normal and went on to LP	Retrospective analysis Patients had CT reported by radiologist/neuro-radiologist unblinded to clinical information. LP if reported normal	Of 4662 patients, only 152 fitted inclusion criteria 18 positive for xanthochromia, 13 had aneurysm on angio	Primary outcome is testing sensitivity of xanthochromia High proportion of late presentations (Mean time to CT 29.5 hrs, not skewed by outliers) No confidence intervals calculated
Perry[22] Nov 2000–Nov 2003, 2 tertiary care academic EDs in Canada	Patients aged >15 Headache or syncope with headache Alert, GCS 15/15 Headache reaching a maximum intensity in <1 hour	Prospective multicentre cohort study Patients enrolled at triage in ED	61/592 patients diagnosed with SAH 55 diagnosed on CT and 6 on LP Follow up carried out in 89.6% Strategy of CT and LP had 100% sensitivity for SAH (95% CI 94–100%)	60/592 patients lost to follow-up, which could change results considerably Many false positive LPs due to traumatic taps, but only patients with SAH confirmed on angiography were counted Patients were recruited from ED and treated with usual clinical care, so results should be reproducible
Byyny[23] Data collected Aug 2001–Dec 2004, US tertiary academic centre and referring hospital's ED	Patients identified from Radiology diagnostic coding, laboratory CSF samples, and SAH discharge diagnosis coding. Data split into groups depending on level of consciousness	Retrospective review of medical notes Patients were divided into 3 groups: Headache and normal conscious level, headache, and abnormal conscious level, no headache with abnormal conscious level	Of the group with headache and normal conscious level 78/87 patients diagnosed with SAH had a positive CT Sensitivity 90% (95% CI 81–95%)	Investigators not blinded, but notes were reviewed by 2 people and kappa values given Retrospective review of notes, so all reports reflect usual practice

(continued)

Author, date, and country	Patient group	Method	Results	Study strengths and weaknesses
Jeffrey J Perry[24] Data collected Nov 2000–Dec 2009, Emergency Departments of 11 tertiary teaching hospitals in Canada, 9 with neurosurgical units	Alert patients >15 years old with non-traumatic acute headache (maximum intensity in <1 hour) or syncope associated with headache, who had CT	Prospective multicentre cohort study, part of a larger study on a clinical decision rule for headache Patients identified in the ED	3132 patients enrolled, 926 had LP 240 diagnosed with SAH Overall sensitivity of CT 92.9% (95%CI 89–95.5%) If CT in within 6 hours of onset, sensitivity 100% (97–100%), specificity 100% (99.5–100%)	Sample size calculation Robust follow-up method Incidence of SAH twice as high in <6-hours group. Not mentioned in paper or explanation given Visual inspection for xanthochromia may lead to different detection rates Equivalent mix of general/neuro radiologists Study did not interfere with clinical decision-making

Data from various sources (see references)

Key clinical evidence

The largest and most comprehensive research to-date addressing the question was published in the BMJ in 2011.[24] A multi-centre prospective cohort study was carried out in Canada between 2000 and 2009. 3132 were enrolled, of whom 240 had confirmed SAH. The sensitivity of CT was found to be 100% (95% CI 97.0–100%) in those imaged <6 hours from onset of headache, which reduced to 85.7% (95% CI 78.3–90.9%) if imaged at >6 hours.

All current international guidelines still recommend LP following a normal non-contrast CT in all cases. The most recent of these were compiled by the American Heart Association and published online in Stroke in May 2012.[25]

Answer

Current research and guidelines from the College of Emergency Medicine[1] and the Scottish Intercollegiate Guidelines Network[4] still recommend LP following a normal CT scan in ALL patients regardless of quality and timing of the CT scan performed.

> **❝ Expert comment**
>
> Technology for CT scanning has developed rapidly since the technique was invented by Geoffrey Hounsfield in 1972. Multiple-slice acquisition and image-enhancement software mean that the 'resolution' of CT images gets better and better every year. Clinical research studies may be effectively out of date by the time they are published as the imaging technique used has been superseded.
>
> Bayesian logic would suggest that in patients with a 10% pre-test probability of subarachnoid haemorrhage, if CT scanning is 98% sensitive, the residual post-test probability of the condition is 0.15%. Due to the potentially catastrophic result of a second bleed, patients and their physicians may feel that further investigation is still merited to further reduce the chances of missing such a diagnosis. However, if sensitivity of early scanning using the latest technology approaches 100% and we choose to investigate patients with less than 10% pre-test probability, a normal CT may become a rule-out test for SAH.
>
> However, before we abandon the automatic lumbar puncture after a negative CT for lone acute sudden headache, we need to take other issues into account.
>
> The patient with a low pre-test probability may be more likely to have had a smaller volume bleed. It can be demonstrated that very small amounts of blood will not change the radio-density of CSF enough to be detected by CT of any slice thickness.
>
> The reported sensitivity for SAH of CT scanners depends not only on the technology used but also on the level of training, subspecialty, and setting of the reporting radiologist. The reliability of a report from a registrar using a laptop from home may be less than that of a consultant neuro-radiologist sitting using a full high-resolution workstation in a darkened room.

Case progression

A lumbar puncture is performed showing no evidence of xanthochromia and the headache is now slowly subsiding with analgesia. You have excluded SAH, but the patient is very keen to know what caused the headache and puzzled as to why you do not have a diagnosis despite the invasive and high-dose radiation imaging you have performed.

Clinical question: Which other diagnoses may present as severe sudden onset headaches?

Ruling out subarachnoid haemorrhage is an important clinical step in patients with sudden onset headache due to the significant morbidity and mortality, but SAH only accounts for approximately 10 % of these presentations. If the CT and LP are both normal there is still no diagnosis reached. Patients are concerned about being discharged home and want a definitive answer to the aetiology of the headaches.

> ✔ **Evidence base** Diagnostic outcomes for thunderclap headache
>
> See Table 15.3 for diagnostic outcomes for thunderclap headache.

Table 15.3 Diagnostic outcomes for thunderclap headache

Paper and date	Number	Criteria looked at	Follow-up period	Outcomes
Perry (2008)[22]	592	Non-traumatic acute headache Normal neurological examination Recurrent headache excluded	3 years	Benign headache 46.5 % Migraine 26.4 % SAH 10.3 % Viral illness 6.9 % Post-coital headache 2.5 % Musculoskeletal 1.4 % Syncope 1.2 %
Perry (2011)[24]	3132	Non-traumatic acute headache Normal neurological examination Excluded Headache >14/7 Recurrent headache	6 months	Benign headache 55.9 % Migraine 20.1 % SAH 7.7 % Viral illness 2.9 % CVA/TIA 2.1 % Post-coital headache 1.8 % Sinusitis 1.1 % Syncope 1.1 %
Boesiger and Shiber[26]	177	Adults presenting to the ED with headache who had CT and LP for investigation of SAH	3 months to 1 year	Unspecified headache 53 % SAH 3.4 % Migraine 9 % Meningitis 8 % Syncope 8 %
O'Neill[27]	116	Patients referred for CT with clinically suspected SAH	Inpatient records reviewed	SAH 21.5 % Unspecified headache 19 % Migraine 9.5 % Cerebral infarct 7.8 % Viral illness 6.9 % Seizure/epilepsy 4.3 % Drug/alcohol 2.6 %

(continued)

Expert comment

Ruling out subarachnoid haemorrhage is not the only diagnostic need in the investigation of the lone acute sudden headache. Some of the mimics of SAH require diagnosis and treatment. For example, cerebral venous sinus thrombosis can present with thunderclap headache; clinical examination may be unremarkable and CT reported as normal. Whilst a non-traumatic LP in such a case will be negative for blood and xanthochromia, a raised opening pressure could give a clue to the diagnosis.

Paper and date	Number	Criteria looked at	Follow-up period	Outcomes
Landtblom[28]	137	Patients attending the ED with sudden onset headache within 10/7 and an onset to maximum intensity of <10 seconds. All patients had CT and LP	12 months	SAH 16.7% Cerebral infarction 3.6% Intracerebral haemorrhage 2.2% Aseptic meningitis 2.9% Cerebral oedema 0.7% Sinus thrombosis 0.7% Unspecified benign headache, figures not given

Data from various sources (see references)

Answer

Although sudden onset thunderclap headaches immediately make the ED clinician look to rule out SAH, in over 50% of cases a diagnosis of non-specific benign headaches is reached, the next leading cause is attributed to migranous headaches. See Box 15.2 for future advances.

⊙ Learning point Cardiac manifestations of SAH[29]

Cardiac manifestations of SAH probably occur in over 50% of patients with the pathophysiology thought to be overstimulation of the myocardium by catecholamine release during or shortly after SAH.

During the acute stage, 50–100% of patients will demonstrate ECG changes. The most common are ST segment and T wave changes, U waves, and QTc prolongation.

4–8% of patients will have malignant arrhythmias including ventricular tachycardia (VT), torsade de pointe, and asystole. Predictors of arrhythmia are increasing age, severity of neurological injury, ECG changes on arrival to ED, and a history of arrhythmia. The treatment of tachyarrhythmias with β-blockers needs to be balanced against the likelihood of reducing cerebral blood flow.

The most severe manifestation is neurogenic stunned myocardium (NSM), causing reduced left ventricular function, reduced cardiac output, and cerebral blood flow. This is generally reversible and should respond to inotropes.

Data from Behrouz R, Sullebarger JT, Malek AR. Cardiac manifestations of subarachnoid haemorrhage. Expert Rev. Cardiovasc Ther 2011; 9(3):303–7.

Box 15.2 Future advances

The combination of MRI/MRA seems to be the best non-invasive diagnostic technique, but invasive angiography is still the neurosurgical gold standard. At present hospital resources do not allow for this modality but perhaps this will provide a less invasive definitive investigation in the future.

A Final Word from the Expert

The management of headaches in the ED presents a number of challenges. Considered a relatively trivial presentation by some, there is a surprisingly high prevalence of significant secondary headache disorders, yet there may be precious few clues as to which patients harbour serious pathology.

After careful history taking and clinical examination the mainstays of further investigation involve either expense and high-radiation exposure (CT), or discomfort and risk of morbidity (LP).

For these reasons the emergency physician must strive to limit the exposure of patients to such investigations without missing the life-threatening diagnoses.

References

1. Ferguson C. Guideline for the management of lone acute severe headache for the College of Emergency Medicine. London: College of Emergency Medicine, December 2009.
2. Longmore M, Wilkinson I, Davidson E, *et al.* Oxford Handbook of Clinical Medicine Eighth Edition. Oxford: Oxford University Press, 2010.
3. MacGregor, Steiner TJ, Davies PTG. British Association for the Study of Headache. Guidelines for All Healthcare Professionals in the Diagnosis and Management of Migraine, Tension-Type, Cluster and Medication-Overuse Headache. Thirrd edition (1st revision). Hull; British Association for the Study of Headache, September 2010.
4. Diagnosis and management of headache in adults, Scottish Intercollegiate Guidelines Network—Edinburgh: SIGN, November 2008.
5. Kirthi V, Derry S, Moore RA, *et al.* Aspirin with or without an antiemetic for acute migraine headaches in adults. *Cochrane Database Syst Rev* 2010; 4:CD008041.
6. Kloster R, Nestvold K, Vilming ST. A double-blind study of ibuprofen versus placebo in the treatment of acute migraine attacks. *Cephalalgia* 1992; 12:169–71.
7. Sharma S, Prasad A, Nehru R, *et al.* Efficacy and tolerability of prochlorperazine buccal tablets in treatment of acute migraine. *Headache* 2002; 42:896–902.
8. Pfaffenrath V, Cunin G, Sjonell G, *et al.* Efficacy and safety of sumatriptan tablets (25 mg, 50 mg and 100 mg) in the acute treatment of migraine: defining the optimum doses of oral sumatriptan. *Headache* 1998; 38:184–90.
9. Steiner TJ, Lange R, Voelker M. Aspirin in episodic tension-type headache: placebo controlled dose-ranging comparison with paracetamol. *Cephalalgia* 2003; 23:59–66.
10. Lange R, Lentz R. Comparison of ketoprofen, ibuprofen and naproxen sodium in the treatment of tension-type headache. *Drugs Exp Clin Res* 1995; 21:89–96.
11. Cohen AS, Burns B, Goadsby PJ. High-flow oxygen for treatment of cluster headache: a randomized trial. *JAMA* 2009; 302(22):2451–7.
12. Law S, Derry S, Moore RA. Triptans for acute cluster headache. *Cochrane Database of Systematic Reviews* 2010, Issue 4. Art. No.: CD008042. doi: 10.1002/14651858.CD008042.pub2
13. Dodick DW. Clinical practice. Chronic daily headache. *N Engl J Med* 2006; 354:158–65.
14. Pope JV, Edlow JA. Favorable response to analgesics does not predict a benign etiology of headache. *Headache* 2008; 48:944–50.
15. Van Gijn J, Kerr RS, Rinkel GLE. Subarachnoid haemorrhage. *Lancet* 2007; 369:306–18.
16. Verweij RD, Wijdicks EFM, van Gijn J. Warning headache in aneurysmal subarachnoid hemorrhage. *Arch Neurol* 1988; 45:1019–20.

17. Perry JJ, Stiell IJ, Sivilotti ML, *et al.* High risk clinical characteristics for subarachnoid haemorrhage in patients with acute headache: prospective cohort study. *BMJ* 2010; 341:c5204

18. Van der Wee N, Rinkel GJ, Hasan D, *et al.* Detection of subarachnoid haemorrhage on early CT: is lumbar puncture still needed after a negative scan? *J Neurol Neurosurg Psych* 1995; 58:357–9.

19. Morgenstern LB, Luna-Gonzales H, Huber JC, *et al.* Worst headache and subarachnoid haemorrhage: prospective, modern computed tomography and spinal fluid analysis. *Ann Emer Med* 1998 Part 1; 32(3):297–304.

20. Gunawardena H, Beetham R, Scolding N, *et al.* Is cerebrospinal fluid spectrophotometry useful in CT scan-negative suspected subarachnoid haemorrhage? *EurNeurol* 2004; 52: 226–9.

21. Dupont SA, Wijdicks EF, Manno EM, *et al.* Thunderclap headache and normal computed tomographic results: value of cerebrospinal fluid analysis. *Mayo Clin Proc* 2008; 83(12): 1326–31.

22. Perry JJ, Spacek A, Forbes M, *et al.* Is the combination of negative computed tomography result and negative lumbar puncture result sufficient to rule out subarachnoid haemorrhage? *Ann Emer Med* 2008 51; 6:707–13.

23. Byyny RL, Mower WR, Shum N, *et al.* Sensitivity of noncontrast cranial computed tomography for the emergency department diagnosis of subarachnoid haemorrhage. *Ann Emer Med* 2008; 51(6):697–703.

24. Perry JJ, Stiell IG, Sivilotti ML, *et al.* Sensitivity of computed tomography performed within six hours of onset of headache for diagnosis of subarachnoid haemorrhage: prospective cohort study. *BMJ* 2011; 343:d4277.

25. Sander Connolly E, Rabinstein AA, Carhuapoma JR, *et al.* Guidelines for the management of aneurysmal subarachnoid haemorrhage: A guideline for healthcare professionals from the American Heart Association/American Stroke Association. *Stroke* 2012; 43(6):1711–37.

26. Boesiger BM, Shiber JR. Subarachnoid haemorrhage diagnosis by computed tomography and lumbar puncture: are fifth generation CT scanners better at identifying subarachnoid haemorrhage? *JEM* 2005; 29(1):23–7.

27. O'Neill J, McLaggans, Gibson R. Acute Headache And Subarachnoid Haemorrhage: A Retrospective Review Of CT And Lumbar Puncture Findings. *SMJ* 2005; 50(4):151–3.

28. Landtblom A-M., Fridriksson S, Boivie J, *et al.* Sudden onset headache: a prospective study of features, incidence and causes. *Cephalalgia* 2002; 22:354–60.

29. Behrouz R, Sullebarger JT, Malek AR. Cardiac manifestations of subarachnoid haemorrhage. Expert Rev. *Cardiovasc Ther* 2011; 9(3):303–7.

16 Self-harm

Fleur Cantle

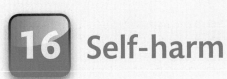

 Expert commentary Sean Cross

Case history

A 23-year-old woman is brought to the ED by her friend in the early hours of the morning having made very deep lacerations to both wrists with a razor blade. She was bleeding on arrival and pressure bandages have been applied. She is heavily under the influence of alcohol but she is able to give you a relatively coherent story. Initially she is calm, however, as you take a more detailed history she becomes obviously distressed, as it emerges that she has just split up with her partner of several months the night before. On reviewing her medical records you see that she has presented at least 20 times before to your department following previous episodes of self-harm by cutting and one previous episode of overdose, but this was several years ago. The patient has agreed to speak with you although the conversation is not the easiest and she is answering your questions with very short replies only. The staff tell you not to spend too much time with her as 'she is here all the time'.

See Box 16.1 for a clinical summary of self-harm.

Box 16.1 Clinical summary of self-harm

Defining self-harm is not easy. Traditionally it is seen as those people who present with an overdose or a self-inflicted laceration, but it could also been seen as including a range of other presentations where self-inflicted harm occurs as a result of the choices people make, such as alcohol-related presentations, eating disorders, or a whole range of other risk-taking behaviours.

NICE[1] defines self-harm as 'self-poisoning or self-injury irrespective of the purpose of the act'.

Even if one restricts the definition to include only those specific acts of immediate self-injury, it is still a common presentation to EDs in the UK with over 200 000 estimated presentations each year.[2]

Acts of self-harm which present to the ED are perhaps the tip of the iceberg, with much higher rates taking place in the community, 1 study reporting a self-harm rate of 13.2% of 15 and 16-year-old pupils.[3]

It is wrong to see the majority of cases as an attempt at suicide as they are not.[4] As such, past definitions of all such cases as 'suicide attempts' or 'parasuicide' are not helpful.

The motivations behind self-harm can be varied but often include a mix of reasons which some find difficult to understand, such as a dysfunctional coping mechanism at times of stress, impulsivity or control issues, or a need to self-injure to gain a sense of release or relief.

The 'non-understandability' of many of these motivations and the use of unhelpful and pejorative labels such as 'attention-seeking' can be at the root of difficulties between services and patients reported in service-user literature.[5].

Self-harm is not a psychiatric diagnosis; it is an act or behaviour. The cohort of people who present with self-harm will represent a heterogeneous population in terms of ICD-10 diagnoses. Depressive disorders, personality disorders, and substance misuse disorders are common.[8] However, crisis presentations without any sign of mental disorder are also common.

Case progression

The patient overhears the staff being dismissive about her presentation. She becomes angry and is abusive to the doctor.

> ✪ **Learning point** Attitudes of clinical staff to patients who self-harm
>
> There have recently been 2 systematic reviews published which have considered staff attitudes to patients who self-harm.
>
> **Taylor et al. (2009):**[7] considered the attitudes of service users who self-harm towards clinical service in 31 international papers. Generally service users reported negative experiences. Patients who had self-harmed reported feeling they were treated differently from other patients in the ED. They attributed this to the fact they had self-harmed.[8] Service users felt ED staff were unconcerned with their mental health but focused on the physical problem.[9] It was reported that their experience would be improved by increased and improved communication from staff and increased patient participation in decision making[10] and increased empathy towards those who self-harm.[9]
>
> **Saunders et al. (2012):**[11] This review considered the attitudes of clinical staff to people who self-harm in 74 international papers. It reported negative attitudes and feelings of irritation, anger, frustration, and helplessness. More hostile attitudes were found towards those who self-harm compared to those with physical illness, in one study this was found to be 49.3% compared to 2.5% for those with other diagnoses.[12] Emergency staff were less likely than other staff to feel sympathy for people who self-harm, made fewer attempts to make people feel secure, and were less likely to view those who repeatedly harm themselves as being at greater risk of subsequent suicide.[13]

> ❝ **Expert comment**
>
> Studies such as this suggest that that the experiences of service users who self-harm are poor and the attitude of staff in many cases is unacceptable and does not meet the needs of these patients. This may in part be reflective of lack of training into the complex communication skills required in such cases but may also indicate how difficult staff members find it to feel empathy in such situations. Complex presentations, requiring time to engage, do not sit well with quality indicators.
>
> Challenging many of these prevailing ideas in our EDs is important. Training and supervision can help, particularly focusing on why self-harm behaviours can elicit such strong feelings. However, continually linking back either to the need for care and compassion or to the bigger picture of mortality outcomes discussed later in this case is a key part of providing responsible clinical leadership in the ED.

Case progression

The ED doctor who is completing the initial assessment manages to calm the patient down and continues to take a history of the circumstances of the injury. During this assessment it is decided to undertake an assessment of 'risk'. The doctor remembers learning the 'SAD PERSONS' score.

Clinical question: How should this patient's risk be assessed by the doctor?

The concept of risk in this population refers not only to the risk of repetition of the act but also to the risk of the completion of a more serious act leading to increased morbidity or mortality. Deeming a patient 'high risk' may mandate greater input from acute psychiatric services and possible interventions to reduce the completion of further acts. Studies show that around 15 % of people who present with self-harm will do so again within the year, and that up to 40 % will do so at some point.[14]

In addition, the rate of completed suicide in this cohort is markedly elevated from the background population. Up to 1 % of people who attend an ED with self-harm will engage in an act of completed suicide within a year. This puts the rate at up to 100× the background population. For this reason the NICE guidelines[1] recommend that all patients who self-harm should be assessed for 'risk' although it is suggested that this assessment be completed by 'specialist mental health professionals' and not the ED team.

There are a variety of actuarial assessment instruments that may be used to assess the risk, looking to identify those risk factors that are seen as static (non-changeable) and dynamic (those which can be changed). Some instruments also look for a range of indicators of seriousness associated with the actual act, such as whether the person was alone or whether they wrote a note, for example. The highest quality assessments will also include a range of psycho-therapeutic interventions such as insight building or problem solving and are usually drawn from cognitive behavioural therapy (CBT) models. Attempts to construct a follow-up package tailored for the patient should occur. For example, if there is a mental disorder present, how best to treat and manage this through use of medication or talking therapy in the medium term. The NICE guidelines stress that if a standardized risk-assessment scale is used to assess risk, it should be used to identify high-risk patients and not low-risk patients who can be discharged without the offer of services.

⊗ **Learning point**   Modified SAD PERSONS scale

For the modified SAD PERSONS scale[15] see Table 16.1.

Table 16.1 Modified SAD PERSONS scale

S: Male sex	1
A: Age < 19 or > 45	1
D: Depression or Hopelessness	2
P: Previous suicidal attempts or psychiatric care	1
E: Excessive ethanol or drug use	1
R: Rationale thinking loss	2
S: Single, widowed, or divorced	1
O: Organized or serious attempt	2
N: No social support	1
S: Stated future intent	2
May be safe to discharge (depending on circumstances	0–5
May require psychiatric consultation	6–8
Probably requires hospital admission	> 8

Reproduced from Robertson and Clancy, Oxford Handbook of Emergency Medicine Fourth Edition, 2010, Table 14.2, page 614, with permission from Oxford University Press

Whilst such scales are commonly used in the ED, a recent longitudinal analysis[16] of 566 people concluded that neither the SAD PERSONS score nor the modified SAD PERSONS score accurately predict future suicide attempts. They are very useful for giving a snapshot of the seriousness of this event at this time, but should not be a substitute for a full psychiatric assessment where resources allow.

❝ Expert comment

NICE guidance states that every person presenting with self-harm should be offered a psycho-social assessment;[1] however, the literature suggests this may not always be the case,[17] There is significant variability across the country in how easily this can occur. One study found that these occurred in approximately 60% of cases.[18] Some EDs have 24-hour mental health liaison services on site whilst others have an on-call non-resident or next day service. The psycho-social assessment has several functions: to go into greater detail regarding the circumstances of the self-harm, and to conduct a risk assessment and needs assessment for the patient to determine the seriousness of the event and its appropriate immediate and longer-term management. All clinical encounters to some degree involve a doctor making judgements about risk. ED doctors will undoubtedly have views about patients who present with self-harm; however, thorough risk assessments, and taking into account all factors including the impact of a patient's ongoing mental state need to be done carefully and properly as part of a psycho-social assessment.

Case progression

Initially your patient agreed to stay in the department and await the psychiatric liaison team. However, something appears to have occurred which has resulted in her becoming more distressed and she has told the nursing staff that she is leaving. You have been asked by the charge nurse to return to speak with her quickly because she was overheard having a heated discussion on her mobile phone and looked as though she was starting to get her things together. You go and speak to her and she informs you she has to leave and doesn't want any further help.

✛ Clinical tip Patients at risk of absconding

In patients who are high risk for absconding from the department such as those with a high suicide risk or drug and alcohol dependence,[19] prior to a full history, examination, and risk assessment being performed it is sensible to have documented details of their description (e.g. clothing and distinguishing features). Careful consideration should also be given to whether such patients require a cannula as it would be necessary for you to recall the patient via the police if you were concerned about the patient's safety if they had a cannula in situ. Guidance on what do when a patient absconds from the ED has been published by the College of Emergency Medicine.[20]

Clinical question: Can a patient who has self-harmed self-discharge prior to a risk assessment and review by the psychiatric team?

It is vital that your patient receives a full assessment and management of her physical and psychological situation. At this point there are a series of 'unknowns' that need to be addressed properly. If she is pressing to leave before you can fully address these, you must make an assessment of the capacity of the person's ability to make this decision.

Healthcare professionals in England and Wales have 2 major legal frameworks within which to act to restrict someone's liberty and insist that they stay in a hospital: the Mental Health Act (1983) (MHA),[21] and the Mental Capacity Act (2005) (MCA).[22]

The MCA can be used to insist on a patient remaining in hospital if criteria are met for determining whether a person lacks the capacity to make the 'task-specific' decision on whether to leave the hospital. The MCA defines the possibility of coming to this conclusion based on the presence of 'an impairment of, or a disturbance in the functioning of the mind or brain'.

This is obviously a very broad definition and in this particular case *may* include such things as the toxic effects of the overdose, alcohol or other drugs, or even an aroused emotional state.

There are 5 key principles underlying the subsequent assessment in relation to a specific event—in this case the capacity to make the decision to leave. These are summarised in this Learning point.

If capacity is deemed not to exist, it is quite clear that the Act expects you as clinician to attempt to build it. This is an important point in cases such as this. A common fear is that you only have 2 options: allow the patient to go or physically restrain. However, an ED-based study assessing whether the capacity was present in a decision about a simple treatment intervention saw a marked increase in capacity by the simple use of an information sheet.[7] It is an important reminder of the need to take time and care over this issue by speaking with your patient, attempting to build capacity through use of more information, gaining help from friends or relatives, and trying to enable to patient to see the importance of remaining in hospital.

This examination must be undertaken carefully and the process clearly documented using this language of the MCA. The capacity assessment is happening over 1 issue—in this case, whether the patient has the capacity to decide to leave the department. If you determine that she does not, you have the legal ability to restrict liberty by acting in her best interests. Should this course of action be undertaken, the clinical assessment must be kept under continual review as the situation will change and evolve, and therefore the best interests of the patient will also change and evolve.

> **✪ Learning point** 5 key principles of the Mental Capacity Act
>
> - A presumption of capacity
> - Maximizing decision-making capacity
> - The freedom to make unwise decisions
> - One must always act in a patient's best interests
> - The least restrictive option should be pursued

> **✪ Learning point** The capacity assessment
>
> When conducting your capacity assessment you must determine whether the patient is able to:
>
> 1) Understand the information given
> 2) Retain that information
> 3) Use and weigh the information
> 4) Communicate back to you the decision made

Case progression

Just before the patient leaves her sister arrives. She is able to calm the patient down and highlights to the patient that she has not had her wounds tended to and that they are still bleeding. After leaving them for 20 minutes to talk, the patient appears much calmer and agrees to stay.

> **⊕ Clinical tip** NICE management of injuries sustained by self-harm[1]
>
> For the management of uncomplicated injuries caused by self-cutting, NICE recommends that tissue adhesive should be recommended as first-line treatment in wounds of 5 cm or less, unless the service user requests adhesive strips.
>
> It is also suggested that clinicians may consider offering advice regarding self-management of superficial injuries. However, this may not be appropriate for all service users and is dependent on the patient making a clinical assessment of his/her injury.
>
> Self-harm: short-term treatment and management: understanding NICE guidance—information for people who self-harm, their advocates and carers, and the public (including information for young people under 16 years). London: National Institute for Clinical Excellence, 2004.
>
> Data from Self-harm: short-term treatment and management: understanding NICE guidance—information for people who self-harm, their advocates and carers, and the public (including information for young people under 16 years). London: National Institute for Clinical Excellence. 2004.

Clinical question: Can we intervene in the ED to prevent repetition of self-harm and lower the risk of suicide?

Attempting to reduce repetition rates successfully is a common way of assessing the success of an intervention in this area. However, the evidence base is not strong. A variety of different kinds of talking therapies have been shown to positively impact on the repetition rate. In particular, CBT[23] has a growing evidence base, but other kinds of therapies including brief psychodynamic interventions have also been suggested.[24] Many of these studies point towards a 'problem-solving' approach being of significant use. This has face validity when considering that you wish to change the likelihood of a person making the same choices—to engage in an act of self-harm—when similar pressures or circumstances come around again. The offer of some form of psychotherapy should be made according to recent guidance.[25] However, in order for any talking therapy can take place, it is necessary for a person to engage with services somewhere. There is evidence that 'did-not-attend' rates for onward referral to follow-up are very high. One study in adolescents demonstrated an improvement by significantly increasing the rate of subsequent engagement by deployment of a standardized 'therapeutic assessment' in the ED at the time of the self-harm assessment.[26] Extension of this to adults may be one way forward. In addition, an array of evidence pointing to 'nudge-'type interventions such as postcard or mobile telephone follow-up reducing the repetition rates have been put forward.[27,28] Generic roll-out of these has not been recommended in a recent large-scale review of the evidence, although targeting of particular sub-groups may still be warranted and remains an area of research.

One theme to emerge from all kinds of research in this area—from telephone follow-up to sitting down with a therapist—is the necessity for engagement. Given what we know about the risks involved at a group level, it is important to be thinking in terms of these when assessing and managing your patient at the individual level. It is undeniable that there is an array of challenges in managing these presentations well in the ED, but if engagement is a key to better management in the community, there is significant face validity to the argument that this should start in the ED.

Case progression

A review by the mental health liaison services found the patient to be more open to the possibility engagement after leaving the hospital. She did not wish to have an onward referral to mental health services but was open to seeing a primary care counsellor. A telephone conversation between the mental health liaison team and the GP facilitated this.

A Final Word from the Expert

There are many challenges in dealing with self-harm presentations, not least the way in which ED services and mental health services work together. Understanding the role we all play in the bigger system is important in helping to achieve a good result by constantly focusing on the patient's best interests. Addressing the dreadful rates of associated repetition and completed suicide is important. The solution to a problem of repeat ED attendance is unlikely to be found in the ED itself. However, moving forward from this rather banal statement is difficult, as it requires emergency unscheduled services to understand and potentially engage with a host of community services. Mental health liaison teams can be extremely important in facilitating this. Attempting to speak with GPs, mental healthcare coordinators, or substance misuse key workers can sometimes be of significant help—if enormously time-consuming—in attempting to find the right package for every patient. Recent changes to quality indicator targets in England and Wales may be a significant driver in helping to improve this.

References

1. Self-harm: short-term treatment and management: understanding NICE guidance—information for people who self-harm, their advocates and carers, and the public (including information for young people under 16 years). London: National Institute for Clinical Excellence, 2004.
2. Hawton K, Bergen H, Casey D, *et al.* Self-harm in England: a tale of three cities. Multicentre study of self-harm. *Soc Psychiatry and Psychiatr Epidemiol* 2007; 42(7):513–21.
3. Hawton K, Rodham K, Evans E, *et al.* Deliberate self-harm in adolescents: self-report survey in schools in England. *BMJ* 2002; 325(7374):1207–11.
4. Hawton K, James A. Suicide and deliberate self-harm in young people. *BMJ* 2005; 330(7496):891–4.
5. Taylor TL, Hawton K, Fortune S, *et al.* Attitudes towards clinical services among people who self-harm: systematic review. *Br J Psychiatry* 2009; 194(2):104–10.
6. Haw C, Hawton K, Houston K, *et al.* Psychiatric and personality disorders in deliberate self-harm patients. *Br J Psychiatry* 2001; 178(1):48–54.
7. Taylor T, Hawton K, Fortune S, *et al.* Attitudes towards clinical services among people who self-harm: systematic review *Br J Psychiatry* 2009 194(2):104–10.
8. Horrocks J, Hughes J, Martin C, *et al.* Patient experience of hospital care following self-harm—A qualitative study. University of Leeds 2005.
9. Brophy, M. Truth Hurts: Report of the National Enquiry into self-harm among young people. London: Mental Health Foundation, 2006.
10. Bywaters, P, Rolfe A. A look beyond the scars. Understanding and responding to self-injury and self-harm. London: NCH. 2002.
11. Saunders K, Hawton K, Fortune S, *et al.* Attitudes and knowledge of clinical staff regarding people who self-harm: A systematic review. *J Affect Disord* 2012; 139(3):205–16.
12. Creed FH, Pfeffer JM. Attitutes of house physicians towards self-poisoning patients. *Med Educ* 1981; 15(5):340–5.
13. Suokas J, Lonngvist J. Work stress had negative effects on the attitudes of emergency personnel towards patients who attempt suicide. *Acta Psychiatr Scand* 1989; 79(5):474–80.
14. Zahl DL, Hawton K. Repetition of deliberate self-harm and subsequent suicide risk: long-term follow-up study of 11,583 patients. *Br J Psychiatry* 2004; 185:70–5.
15. Wyatt JP, Illingworth RN, Graham CA, *et al. Oxford Handbook of Emergency Medicine*, Fourth Edition. Oxford: Oxford University Press, 2012.
16. Bolton JM, Spiwak R, Sareen J. Predicting suicide attempts with the SAD PERSONS scale: a longitudinal analysis. *J Clin Psychiatry* 2012; 73(6):e735–41.
17. Olfson M, Marcus SC, Bridge JA. *Arch Gen Psychiatry* 2012; 69(1):80–8.
18. Kapur N, Murphy E, Cooper J, *et al.* Psychosocial assessment following self-harm: results from the multi-centre monitoring of self-harm project. *J Affect Disord* 2008; 106(3):285–93.
19. Mental Health and Drug and Alcohol Office, Mental Health for Emergency Departments—A reference Guide. Sydney: NSW Department of Health, 2009.
20. CEC Best Practice guideline—The Patient who Absconds (May 2013). <http://www.collemergencymed.ac.uk/Shop-Floor/Clinical%20Guidelines/Clinical%20Guidelines/default.asp>

21. Code of practice: Mental Health Act 1983. London: TSO, 2008.

22. Mental Capacity Act 2005: code of practice. London: TSO, 2007.

23. Slee N, Garnefski N, van der Leeden R, *et al*. Cognitive-behavioural intervention for self-harm: randomised controlled trial. *Br J Psychiatry*: 2008; 192(3):202–11.

24. Guthrie E, Kapur N, Mackway-Jones K, *et al*. Randomised controlled trial of brief psychological intervention after deliberate self-poisoning. *BMJ* 2001; 323(7305):135–8.

25. Kendall T, Taylor C, Bhatti H, *et al*. Longer-term management of self-harm: summary of NICE guidance. *BMJ* 2011; 343:d7073.

26. Ougrin D, Zundel T, Ng A, *et al*. Trial of Therapeutic Assessment in London: randomised controlled trial of Therapeutic Assessment versus standard psychosocial assessment in adolescents presenting with self-harm. *Arch Dis Child* 2011; 96(2):148–53.

27. Carter GL, Clover K, Whyte IM, *et al*. Postcards from the EDge project: randomised controlled trial of an intervention using postcards to reduce repetition of hospital treated deliberate self-poisoning. *BMJ* 2005; 331(7520):805.

28. Vaiva G, Ducrocq F, Meyer P, *et al*. Effect of telephone contact on further suicide attempts in patients discharged from an emergency department: randomised controlled study. *BMJ* 2006; 332(7552):1241–5.

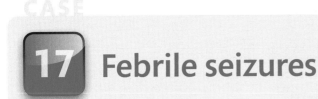

17 Febrile seizures

Rhys Beynon

ℹ **Expert commentary** Ian Maconochie

Case history

A 20-month-old female attends the paediatric ED by ambulance with a generalized tonic–clonic seizure. The seizure started 10 minutes ago at home. The child was given 15 litres of oxygen per minute via a non re-breathe mask and a single dose of rectal diazepam (5 mg) by the local ambulance service. She has not been unwell at all and her parents have not detected a fever, however in the ED her temperature is 39.5 °C.

She has no significant past medical history, is not on any medications, and is fully immunized. She has a 7-year-old brother who had a single febrile seizure when he was 2 years old.

See Box 17.1 for a clinical summary of febrile seizure.

Box 17.1 Clinical summary of febrile seizure

- One in 25 children will have at least one febrile seizure.
- One in 3 of those with febrile seizures will have recurrent seizures.
- Children rarely develop their first seizure before 6 months or after 3 years.
- Between 2% and 5% of all children have 1 or more febrile seizure by the age of 5 years.[1]
- Febrile convulsions commonly start in the second year of life. Children are at greatest risk between 6 months and 3 years of age, however the age of onset has been reported to vary from as young as 2 months to 7 years and 9 months.[2] The general agreement is that they commonly occur between 6 months and 6 years.[3]

Clinical question: How should the seizures be controlled in a child with a febrile convulsion?

The management of a child with febrile seizures should follow the Advanced Paediatric Life Support Algorithm for seizures (Figure 17.1).[4] This algorithm is a product of the work of the Status Epilepticus Working Party in 2000.[5]

The aim is to stop the seizure as soon as possible. Most febrile seizures stop within 5 minutes; however, any seizure that lasts longer than 10 minutes is at a high risk of lasting up to 30 minutes.[6] The aim of treating a prolonged seizure is to prevent brain injury. As a seizure continues it also becomes progressively more difficult to stop,[7,8] therefore the best way of terminating a seizure is with early initiation of treatment. The general agreement is that drugs should be administered when seizures have a duration of 5 minutes or more.[9]

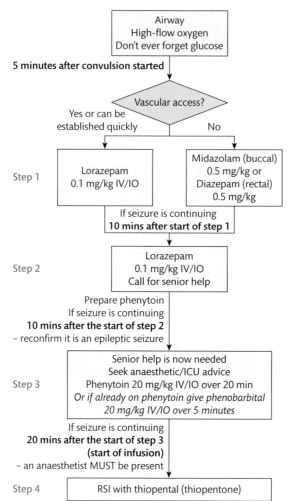

Figure 17.1 Treatment algorithm for the fitting child.

Reproduced from The Advanced Life Support Group, *Advanced paediatric life support: the practical approach, 5th edition*, published by Wiley, Copyright © 2010, John Wiley, and Sons.

⊕ **Clinical tip** Hypoglycaemia

The mnemonic continues as 'DEFG': don't ever forget glucose. It is appropriate to check the capillary blood glucose at the initial assessment, as hypoglycaemia is an important and easily correctable cause of prolonged seizures.[4]

The amount of glucose given is usually 2 mls/kg of 10% glucose followed by an infusion containing glucose.[4]

✪ **Learning point** Causes of seizures in childhood

Febrile seizures are a common condition seen in the ED. It is, however, important to consider alternative causes for seizures in children. These would include:[4,9]

- Acute electrolyte imbalance—hypoglycaemia, hypocalcaemia, hyponatraemia, and hypomagnesaemia
- Cerebral infection—meningitis or encephalitis
- Drug overdose, toxins, and poisons.
- Idiosyncratic drug reaction
- Acute head injury
- Hypoxia / anoxia
- Seizures secondary to pre-existing neurological abnormality, including CNS malformations, previous brain injury, and cerebral palsy
- Cerebrovascular accident
- Systemic hypertension
- Epilepsy
- Metabolic diseases
- Subarachnoid haemorrhage (uncommon)

The algorithm should be followed as outlined in Figure 17.1 and until the seizure has terminated.

Step 1 and 2

Benzodiazepines are the first-line drugs for treating seizures. The preferred administration of drugs is via the IV route as it offers superior onset of action, bioavailability, and efficacy.[7,10]

IV lorazepam is usually the first drug of choice. A recent Cochrane review[11] concluded that it is equally or more effective than IV diazepam and possibly produces less respiratory depression.[9] It also has a longer duration of action (12–24 hours) than diazepam (less than 1 hour).[4]

Midazolam is an effective quick-acting anticonvulsant which takes effect within minutes but has a shorter lasting effect than lorazepam. It can be administered via the buccal or the IV route. It has a depressant effect on respiration that occurs in only about 5 % of patients. Buccal midazolam has been shown to be more effective than rectal diazepam.[13] It is also easier to administer, more socially acceptable, and also preferred by parents.[9]

Seizures that have not responded to 2 doses of benzodiazepines are much less likely to respond to further doses.[7] There is also an increased risk of side effects with multiple doses, especially respiratory depression.[14,15]

Step 3

Phenytoin is the most commonly used second line antiepileptic drug in the UK. It has been shown to be effective in terminating seizures in 30–50 % of cases.[13,16] It can cause dysrhythmias and hypotension, therefore the child should be monitored closely. It has little depressant effect on respiration.[4]

Do not give a loading dose of phenytoin if the child is known to take oral phenytoin until the blood level of phenytoin is known. Then only give it if the phenytoin level is less than 5 micrograms/ml. In the case of children already receiving phenytoin as maintenance treatment for their epilepsy, phenobarbital (20 mg/kg IV over 5 minutes) should be used in place of phenytoin. Alternatives include IV sodium valproate or levetiracetam.[4]

Step 4

If the seizure continues 20 minutes after Step 3 preparation should be made for a rapid sequence induction of anaesthesia.

Answer

The Advanced Paediatric Life support algorithm should be followed with intravenous lorazepam as the first-line treatment if available.

Case progression

Her seizures terminated immediately after arriving in the ED. She did not require any further treatment. The duration of her seizure was less than 15 minutes in total.

✚ Clinical tip Administration of benzodiazepines

It is important to clarify if a benzodiazepine has been administered at home or en route to the hospital by the parents or by a pre-hospital care practitioner.

The patient may have already received 2 doses prior to arriving to the emergency department.

If so it is important to alter the entry point into the algorithm.

❢ Expert comment

The administration of antipyretics will not guarantee that a febrile convulsion cannot recur but may help the child feel better owing to fever reduction.

Practice internationally may vary[17] with certain differences in the management of the child with febrile convulsions varying according to location in the world and resource-poor or rich environments.

✚ Learning point Precipitating factors

- The height and duration of fever may be important
- Synthesis of immunoglobulin in the CSF of children with febrile convulsions has been demonstrated, suggesting that encephalitis may occur and not be recognized
- There may be an association with the HHV-6
- There is a risk of febrile seizures on the day of receipt of DPT vaccine and 8–14 days after MMR vaccine

Data from Verity CM. Febrile convulsions—a practical guide. Chapter 8. <http://www.epilepsysociety.org.uk/FileStorage/Professionalsarticles>.

Clinical examination reveals that she is maintaining her airway, her RR is 20 with saturations of 100 % on 15 litres, HR 145 cap refill < 2, and she responds to verbal stimuli. Her temperature is 38.2 °C. She has evidence of a runny nose, and mild erythema to the throat. She has no focal neurology but remains drowsy.

Intravenous access was obtained on arrival and a venous blood gas was also taken, the result is: pH 7.39 PCO2 5.6 PO2 6.0 HCO3 19 BE -5, lactate 4 glucose 7.4 Na 135 K 3.6 Ca 1.2. Bloods are taken for FBC, renal function, inflammatory markers, and culture. The child has very mild coryza but you are uncertain if this is enough of a focus to explain the fever and the seizure. You consider if this is a simple febrile convulsion or if a there is an underlying cerebral disorder you consider what further investigations are required.

You consider if this is a simple febrile convulsion and wonder if any further investigations or imaging are required.

✪ **Learning point** Classification of seizures

The commission on Epidemiology and Prognosis of the International League Against Epilepsy[18] defined febrile seizures / convulsion as: '[a]n epileptic seizure … occurring in childhood after age one month, associated with a febrile illness not caused by an infection of the CNS, without previous neonatal seizures or a previous unprovoked seizure, and not meeting criteria for other acute symptomatic seizures'.

Complex febrile seizures are defined by the presence of at least one of the following:[19]

- Duration longer than 15 minutes (9 % of children)
- Multiple seizures within a 24-hour period
- Focal features

Simple febrile seizures do not have any of these features and make up 75 % of the attacks.[19]

Febrile myoclonic seizures are similar to myoclonic jerks. They occur in febrile patients, and may develop into a febrile seizure.[20]

Febrile status epilepticus occurs when the duration of seizures are greater than 30 minutes. These occur in 5 % of patients and are more likely to have focal features.[21]

Multiple febrile seizures are more than 1 convulsion during an episode of fever.[1]

Recurrent febrile seizures are more than one episode of febrile seizures.[1]

The commission on Epidemiology and Prognosis of the International League Against Epilepsy[18].

Young age (less than 15 months) at onset and a family history of febrile seizures predict increased risk. Most recurrences occur within 3 years of the first seizure. A prolonged initial seizure does not substantially increase the risk of recurrent febrile seizures.[1]

Clinical question: Which children require acute neuroimaging?

The discussion of whether the child needs a CT head commonly occurs when children present with seizures and fever. The concern is usually that the child has an underlying neurological problem or cerebral pathology.

Underlying pathology should be suspected on the basis of the history and examination findings. It may then be appropriate to perform a scan to investigate this possibility further. This situation will only exist in a small number of children with febrile seizures.

✪ **Learning point** Neuroimaging in seizures

Acute neuroimaging should be performed if there is clinical suspicion of:

- Space-occupying lesion
- Intracranial haemorrhage
- Hydrocephalus
- Abscess
- Cerebral oedema
- History or risk of HIV

MRI should be considered in children with recurrent complex febrile seizures who have other neurological findings, including:[22]

- Abnormal head circumference,
- Significant developmental delay, and
- Persistent focal neurology in a child with normal CT.

✓ **Evidence base** Neuroimaging in febrile convulsions

Teng *et al.* (2006)[23] performed a retrospective case series review and looked at 71 children who presented with their first complex febrile seizures. 51 (72%) had a single complex seizure (20 focal, 22 multiple, and 9 prolonged), and 20 (28%) had multiple complex seizures. None of the 71 patients had intracranial pathological conditions that required emergency neurosurgical or medical intervention. The authors concluded that acute neuroimaging was not required for children with a first complex febrile seizure.

Answer

There is no evidence to suggest that neuroimaging should not be performed routinely in children with simple febrile seizures.

Neuroimaging should be considered on an individual basis if there is suspicion of underlying intracranial pathology.

Case progression

It is decided that the child does not require any brain imaging but concern exists regarding the focus of the fever. A chest X-ray and urine sample are requested whilst the blood tests are still being processed. You consider whether a lumbar puncture is required as part of the septic screen.

Clinical question: Which children requires a lumbar puncture?

Meningitis is rare in children presenting with seizures and fever in the developed world. Nevertheless, meningitis presents with seizures in about a quarter of children. It is therefore essential that associated central nervous system (CNS) infections with their consequent mortality and morbidity are not overlooked.[24]

> ⊘ **Evidence base** Lumbar puncture in febrile convulsions
>
> **N.B.** Studies completed in developing counties were excluded due to the higher incidence of CNS infections as a cause of their seizures.
>
> **Hom J, Medwid K (2011)**[25] performed an evidence-based review. They included 2 studies that looked at children aged 6–18 months who presented with simple febrile seizures. Of the 150 children who had a lumbar puncture (LP) no child was diagnosed with bacterial meningitis (95% confidence interval [CI] = 0.0–3.0%). One of the 40 children who had been pretreated with antibiotics or 2.5% (95% CI = 0.0–14.0%), had leukocytosis in the CSF. The authors conclude that the findings suggest that rate of acute bacterial meningitis in children who present with simple febrile seizure and had a lumbar puncture performed is very low.
>
> **Kimia A et al. (2010)**[26] performed a retrospective cohort review of 526 patients aged 6 months to 5 years who presented to a pediatric ED between 1995 and 2008 for their first complex febrile seizure. 90 patents (17%) had a previous history of simple febrile seizures. 340 patients (64%) had a LP. Three patients had acute bacterial meningitis (0.9% [95% CI: 0.2–2.8]). None of the patients for whom an LP was not attempted subsequently returned to the hospital with a diagnosis of ABM. The authors conclude that few patients who experienced a complex febrile seizure had ABM in the absence of other signs or symptoms.
>
> **Carroll W, Brookfield (2002)**[27] completed a systematic review. They reviewed 15 articles. The overall incidence of ABM was 0.8% (95% CI 0.73–0.88%). The authors conclude that bacterial meningitis in the absence of associated signs (irritability, lethargy, and/or bulging fontanelle) is extremely uncommon. The routine lumbar puncture following a febrile convulsion in infancy is unjustified and potentially hazardous in an infant without signs of meningitis. Observation and regular review by the nursing and medical staff in the first few hours after the convulsion, with an emphasis on examination for signs of meningitis, is more likely to detect children with bacterial meningitis.
>
> **Chin et al. (2008)**[28] performed a prospective cohort study over a 6-month period of 24 children that presented to a north London Hospital with convulsive status epilepticus (CSE) with fever. On presentation, 16 (67%) had parenteral antibiotics for ABM. Diagnostic cerebrospinal fluid (CSF) sampling was conducted in nine (30%). Four (17%, 95% CI 15–18%) children were confirmed to have ABM. None of these 4 children had signs of meningism. The authors therefore suggest that the most appropriate management for children with CSE with fever is to start parenteral antibiotics early, perform an LP when there are no contraindications, and then base duration and type of therapy on CSF findings. Early treatment of ABM may decrease morbidity and mortality.

Answer

Lumbar puncture should be performed if there is clinical suspicion of meningitis.

A higher index of suspicion of meningitis should be present if the child is less than 18 months and presents with a complex seizure. If there is any doubt, a senior clinician should be involved in the decision-making process.

Children that present with febrile status epilepticus should be treated with early parenteral antibiotics, followed by lumbar puncture when safe.

> ✪ **Learning point** National guidelines
>
> In 1991 the Royal College of Paediatricians and the British Paediatric Association Joint working group recommended a lumbar puncture if:[29]
>
> - a clinical diagnosis of meningitis or encephalitis is suspected
> - after a complex seizure
> - if the child is drowsy/irritable or systemically unwell
> - if the child is less than 18 months (probably) and almost certainly if the child is aged less than 12 months.
>
> (continued)

In February 2011 The American academy of pediatrics published an updated clinical practice guideline that recommended[30]:

- A lumbar puncture should be performed in any child who presents with a seizure and a fever and has meningeal signs and symptoms, or in any child whose history or examination suggests the presence of meningitis or intracranial infection. Evidence level: B (over- whelming evidence from observational studies).
- In any infant between 6 and 12 months of age who presents with a seizure and fever, a lumbar puncture is an option when the child is considered deficient in Haemophilus influenza type b (Hib) or Streptococcus pneumoniae immunisations (ie, has not received scheduled immunisations as recommended) or when immunisation status cannot be determined because of an increased risk of bacterial meningitis. Evidence level: D (expert opinion, case reports).
- Lumbar puncture is an option in the child who presents with a seizure and fever and is pretreated with antibiotics, because antibiotic treatment can mask the signs and symptoms of meningitis. Evidence level: D (reasoning from clinical experience, case series)

Data from Joint working group of the research unit of the Royal College of Physicians and the British Paediatric Association. Guidelines for the management of convulsions with fever. BMJ 1991; 303(6803):634–6, and Subcommittee on Febrile Seizures. Febrile seizures: Guideline for the neurodiagnostic evaluation of the child with a simple febrile seizure. Pediatrics 2011; 127(2):389–94.

Expert comment

The full NICE guidance on the management of bacterial meningitis and meningococcal septicaemia in children and people younger than 16[31] provides in-depth systematic analysis of the literature on the indication for lumbar puncture and treatment modalities of bacterial meningitis.

⊕ Clinical tip Contraindications to lumbar puncture

It is important to remember not perform a lumbar puncture if:[24]

- there are signs of raised intracranial pressure
- altered level of consciousness
- focal neurological signs
- cardio-respiratory compromise
- abnormal clotting
- infection in the area the needle will traverse.

If there is any doubt, treatment with antibiotics should not be delayed.

Case progression

After 1-hour's observation, she has improved significantly. She is playing games with her mother and father. On repeat examination her observations are within normal limits. She is apyrexial. She has a runny nose, a dry cough, and erythema to her pharynx. Otherwise clinical examination is normal. The blood tests reveal a CRP of 12 and a normal white cell count. The child is admitted to the ambulatory unit for a period of observation and to educate the parents, before safely discharging her home.

Observation and discharge advice

Not all children that present with febrile seizures require admission.
The following factors would favour admission after a first febrile convulsion:[32]

- Complex convulsion
- Child less than 18 months
- Early review by doctor at home not possible
- Home circumstances inadequate or unusual parental anxiety or parents' inability to cope

Most parents/carers are very distressed when they witness febrile seizures, and it should be a priority to inform them about the essentially benign nature of most febrile convulsions. Parents should be assured that most children who have febrile seizures of any type (simple or complex) are subsequently normal in intellect, neurological function, and behaviour. For most children the risk of developing epilepsy is similar to that of the general population, which is around 1 in 100.

Parents should be advised that antipyretic agents do not prevent febrile convulsions and should not be used specifically for this purpose,[33] but should be considered for comfort. Ideally written information should supplement the consultation.[1]

A Final Word from the Expert

Febrile convulsions are a common presentation of children aged under 5 years to EDs. A holistic approach, excluding other pathologies that may be associated with fever and seizure activity, is mandatory. The source of fever should be ascertained and the management of the age group under 5 years should also adhere to NICE guidance.[33]

The diagnosis of a febrile convulsion requires careful explanation to the child's parents/carers about the consequences with reassurance given when appropriate.

References

1. Verity CM. Febrile convulsions—a practical guide. Chapter 8. <http://www.epilepsysociety.org.uk/FileStorage/Professionalsarticles>
2. Verity CM, Golding J. Risk of epilepsy after febrile convulsions: a national cohort study. *BMJ* 1991; 303(6814):1373–6.
3. American Academy of Pediatrics, Committee on Quality Improvement, Subcommittee on Febrile Seizures. Practice parameter: long term treatment with simple febrile seizures. *Pediatrics* 1999; 103 (6 Pt 1):1307–9.
4. The Advanced Life Support Group. Advanced paediatric life support: the practical approach. 5th edition. Oxford: Blackwell Publishing, 2010.
5. Appleton R. Choonara I, Martland T, *et al*. The treatment of convulsive status epilepticus in children. The status epilepticus working party. *Arch Dis Child* 2000; 83(5):415–9.
6. Shinnar S. Who is at risk for prolonged seizures? *J Child Neurol* 2007; 22(5 Suppl): 14S–20S.
7. Chin RF, Neville BG, Peckham C, *et al*. Treatment of community-onset, childhood convulsive status epilepticus: a prospective, population-based study. *Lancet Neurol* 2008; 7(8):696–703.
8. Mazarati AM, Baldwin RA, Sankar R, *et al*. Time-dependent decrease in the effectiveness of antiepileptic drugs during the course of self-sustaining status epilepticus. *Brain Res* 1998; 814:179–85.
9. Yoong M, Chin RFM, Scott RC. Management of convulsive status epilepticus in children. *Arch Dis Child Educ Pract Ed* 2009;94:1–9.
10. Scott RC, Besag, FMC, Boyd SG, *et al*. Buccal Absorption of Midazolam: Pharmokinetics and EEG Pharmacodynamics. *Epilepsia* 1998; 39(3):290–4.
11. Appleton R, Macleod S, Martland T. Drug management for acute tonic–clonic convulsions including convulsive status epilepticus in children (Review). The Cochrane collaboration. Chichester: John Wiley and Sons, Ltd, 2010. <http://onlinelibrary.wiley.com/doi/10.1002/14651858.CD001905.pub2/full>
12. Appleton RE, Sweeney A, Choonara I, *et al*. Lorazepam versus diazepam in the acute treatment of epileptic seizures and status epilepticus. *Dev Med Child Neurol* 1995; 37(8): 682–8.

13. McIntyre J, Robertson S, Norris E, *et al*. Safety and efficacy of buccal midazolam versus rectal diazepam for emergency treatment of seizures in children: a randomised controlled trial. *Lancet* 2005; 366(9481):205–10.

14. Chin RF, Verhulst L, Neville BG, *et al*. Inappropriate emergency management of status epilepticus in children contributes to need for intensive care. *J Neurol Neurosurg Psychiatry* 2004; 75(11):1584–8.

15. Stewert WA, Harrison R, Dooley JM. Respiratory depression in the acute management of seizures. *Arch Dis Child* 2002; 87(3):225–6.

16. Brevoord JC, Joosten KF, Arts WF, *et al*. Status epilepticus: Clinical analysis of a treatment protocol based on midazolam and phenytoin. *J of Child Neurology* 2005 20(6): 476–81.

17. <http://www.who.int/mental_health/mhgap/evidence/epilepsy/q3/en/>

18. Commission on Epidemiology and Prognosis, International League against Epilepsy. Guidelines for epidiologic studies on epilepsy. *Epilepsia* 1993; 34(4):592–6.

19. Nelson K.B, Ellenberg JH. Predictors of epilepsy in children who have experienced febrile seizures. *N Engl J Med* 1976; 295(19):1029–33.

20. Narula S, Goraya JS. Febrile myoclonus. *Neurology* 2005; 64(1):169–70.

21. Berg AT, Shinnar S. Unprovoked seizures in children with febrile seizures: short term outcome. *Neurology* 1996; 47(2):562–8.

22. Waruiru C, Appleton R, Febrile seizures: an update. *Arch Dis Childhood* 2004; 89(8):751–6

23. Teng D, Dayan P, Tyler S, *et al*. Risk of intracranial pathologic conditions requiring emergency intervention after a first complex febrile seizure episode among children. *Pediatrics* 2006; 117(2):304–8.

24. Sadlier LG, Scheffer IE. Febrile seizures. *BMJ* 2007; 334:307–11.

25. Hom J, Medwid K. The low rate of bacterial meningitis in children, ages 6 to 18 months, with simple febrile seizures. *Acad Emerg Med* 2011; 18(11):1114–20.

26. Kimia A, Ben-Joseph EP, Rudloe T, *et al*. Yield of lumbar puncture among children who present with their first complex febrile seizure. *Pediatrics* 2010; 126(1):62–9.

27. Carroll W, Brookfield D. Lumbar puncture following febrile convulsion. *Arch Dis Child* 2002; 87(3):238–40.

28. Chin RFM, Neville BR, Scott RC. Meningitis is a common cause of convulsive status epilepticus with fever. *Arch Dis Child* 2005; 90(1):66–9.

29. Joint working group of the research unit of the Royal College of Physicians and the British Paediatric association. Guidelines for the management of convulsions with fever. *BMJ* 1991; 303(6803):634–6.

30. Subcommittee on Febrile Seizures. Febrile seizures: Guideline for the neurodiagnostic evaluation of the child with a simple febrile seizure. *Pediatrics* 2011; 127(2):389–94.

31. The management of bacterial meningitis and meningococcal septicaemia in children and young people younger than 16 years in primary and secondary care Clinical guidelines, CG102. June 2010. <http://www.guidance.nice.org.uk/CG102>

32. Vestergaard M, Pedersen MG, Ostergaard JR, *et al*. Death in children with febrile seizures: a population-based cohort study. *Lancet* 2008 (9637); 372:457–63.

33. National Institute for Health and Clinical Excellence. Feverish illness in children-assessment and initial management in children younger than 5 years, <http://www.nice.org.uk/nicemedia/live/11010/30525/30525.pdf>

18 Right lower quadrant abdominal pain in women: gynaecology or surgery?

Olumayowa Adenugba

Expert commentary Ed Glucksman and Duncan Bew

Case history

A 27-year-old woman presents to the ED with a 24-hour history of right lower quadrant abdominal pain. The pain was sudden in onset, not migratory, and has gradually worsened, associated with nausea and vomiting but no diarrhoea. She denies any fever, back pain, dysuria, or frequency of micturition. There is no vaginal discharge or bleeding and her last menstrual period was 2 weeks earlier.

There is no history of similar pain in the past. There is no history of previous abdominal surgery and she is otherwise fit and well. She is not on any medication, has no known allergies, and does not smoke. Her partner looked on the internet earlier and feels her symptoms suggest acute appendicitis and hence brought her to the ED.

On examination her oral temperature is 37.4 °C and her heart rate and blood pressure are normal. She exhibits tenderness in the right iliac fossa with a positive psoas sign. There is no rebound tenderness with both Rovsing's and obturator signs being negative. A urine pregnancy test is also negative.

See Box 18.1 for a clinical summary of abdominal pain.

Box 18.1 Clinical summary of abdominal pain

- Abdominal pain in a pre-menopausal woman can be one of the most difficult clinical scenarios in the ED.
- The goal of the emergency physician in this situation is to exclude acute causes of abdominal pain that could result in high morbidity and mortality such as ectopic pregnancy and acute appendicitis.
- The incidence of appendicitis is reported to be declining in western countries with a slightly higher incidence in men than women (male:female ratio of 1.4:1).[1]
- Historically clinical evaluation has been the mainstay of the diagnosis of acute appendicitis, despite advances with laboratory and radiological tests.
- The symptoms and signs elicited still remain a very important aspect of the assessment of these patients. When patients present with typical features, diagnosis is usually straightforward. However, this is the exception and not the rule, especially in pre-menopausal women.[1]
- Clinical features associated with a diagnosis of acute appendicitis include migratory abdominal pain, RLQ pain, nausea/vomiting, fever, anorexia, RLQ tenderness, abdominal rigidity, rebound tenderness, Rovsing's sign, obturator sign, and psoas sign.

⊕ **Clinical tip** Special signs in acute appendicitis

Psoas sign: Put the patient in the left lateral decubitus position and passively extend the right hip with both knees already in extension. The sign is positive when abdominal pain increases with this manoeuvre. This sign is reported to have a sensitivity of 13–42 % and specificity of 79–95 %.[1]

(continued)

> **Obturator sign**: This sign is considered positive if pain is increased when the examiner internally and externally rotates the right hip in flexion with the patient supine. This sign is reported to have a sensitivity of only 8% and specificity of 94%.[1]
> **Rovsing's sign**: This sign is considered positive when deep palpation of the left lower quadrant and then sudden release of this pressure elicits tenderness or referred rebound tenderness in the right lower quadrant. Although this sign is mentioned historically, its added value is questionable.[1]

Clinical question: In women with right lower quadrant (RLQ) abdominal pain, are there any clinical features or a constellation of features which specifically differentiates appendicitis from other pathology?

The reliability and positive predictive value of clinical features in pre-menopausal women is questionable due to the broader diagnostic considerations needed with this clinical presentation (see Table 18.1). It is no surprise that misdiagnosis is more

Table 18.1 Evidence for clinical features differentiating appendicitis from other pathology

Author, date, country	Design, subjects, and intervention.	Key results
Wagner et al. 1996[3] USA	Meta-analysis of 10 studies Over 4000 patients in 10 studies with RLQ abdominal pain Performance of various aspects of the history and clinical examination in the assessment of suspected acute appendicitis using 95% confidence intervals	The best-performing aspects of history and examination in suggesting acute appendicitis were RLQ pain (+LR=7.31 − 8.46), abdominal rigidity (+LR=2.96 − 4.78), and migration of pain from periumbilical region to RLQ (+LR=2.41− 4.21). Psoas sign had a +LR of 1.21− 4.67, fever had a +LR of 1.63-2.32, and anorexia +LR of 1.16 − 1.38 The best-performing features in excluding acute appendicitis were absence of RLQ pain (−LR=0−0.28) and presence of similar pain in the past (−LR=0.25 − 0.42)
Andersson 2004[4] Sweden	Meta-analysis of 24 studies 5833 patients with suspected acute appendicitis Meta-analysis of 24 studies Diagnostic value of elements of history, physical examination, and laboratory data (WCC, CRP) individually and in combination	The only useful elements suggestive of appendicitis were pain migration (+LR=2.06 [95% CI 1.63-2.60]), vomiting (+LR=1.63 [95% CI 1.45-1.84]), pain progression (+LR=1.39 [95% CI 1.29-1.50]), and aggravation of pain by cough (+LR=1.49 [95% CI 1.40-1.59]) Useful elements to exclude appendicitis were absence of aggravation by cough (−LR=0.38 [95% CI 0.32-0.46]), absence of pain progression (−LR=0.46 [95% CI 0.27-0.77]) absence of direct tenderness (−LR=0.25 [95% CI 0.12-0.53]), and absence of rebound tenderness (−LR=0.39 [95% CI 0.32-0.48]) White cell count (WCC) >10×10^9 +LR=2.47, −LR=0.26 and CRP >10 mg/l (+LR=1.97, −LR=0.32) were weak in ruling in a diagnosis of acute appendicitis while useful in ruling out the diagnosis A combination of abdominal guarding or rebound tenderness, WCC>10.0×10^9, and CRP >8 mg/l had a +LR of 23.32 (95% CI- 6.87-84.79) and −LR of 0.03 (95% CI- 0.0-0.14)

Data from various sources (see references)

frequent and negative appendicectomy rates are also higher in women.[1] A study carried out on patients with suspected acute appendicitis undergoing CT scan evaluation showed that of the alternative diagnoses made, ureteric/renal calculi accounted for 30 % of cases.[2] Other diagnoses made included gynaecologic disorders (25 %), ascending colon and sigmoid diverticulitis (24 %), small bowel disease (8 %), mesenteric adenitis (5 %), and neoplasm (3 %).[2]

Answer

There is no single symptom or sign that can be considered diagnostic in appendicitis. Right lower quadrant pain, rigidity, and migration of peri-umbilical pain to the right lower quadrant had high positive likelihood ratios.

Case progression

The patient has analgesia and undergoes laboratory tests. Her urinalysis has a trace of blood, CRP is 28, white cell count 9.7, and all other tests are within normal limits. She is referred to the surgical team for review. The surgical registrar is keen to discharge her home with analgesia with a suspected diagnosis of a ruptured ovarian cyst. The ED consultant advises otherwise.

Clinical question: What is the role of the C-reactive protein (CRP) and white cell count (WCC) in ruling in or excluding acute appendicitis in women with RLQ abdominal pain?

The use of clinical symptoms and signs to make a diagnosis of acute appendicitis has been noted to be especially difficult in women (see Table 18.2). Many studies have evaluated the use of simple laboratory tests to improve the diagnostic accuracy. The white cell count (WCC) and C-reactive protein (CRP) have been the focus of most of these studies.

Table 18.2 Evidence evaluating the role of CRP and WCC in appendicitis

Author, date, country	Design, subjects, and intervention	Key results
Sengupta 2009[5] UK	Prospective case series. 98 adult (75 % women) presenting with clinically suspected acute appendicitis. Correlation of operative records and pathological specimen reports with pre-operative WCC and CRP values	Both inflammatory markers elevated had a PPV of 56 % for acute appendicitis. Both inflammatory markers normal had an NPV of 100 % and sensitivity of 100 % Elevated WCC specificity was 63 % while for CRP was 75 %. Both markers elevated had specificity of 88 %
Khan 1999[6] UK	Retrospective study. 259 patients presenting with RLQ pain and operated on for suspected acute appendicitis. Pre-operative blood WCC and CRP correlated with three groups (normal appendix, inflamed appendix and perforated/ gangrenous appendix) based on histopathological reports	14.3 % negative appendicectomy rate. Sensitivity and specificity of WCC when elevated was 83 % and 62 % while for elevated CRP it was 75 % and 83.7 % respectively

(continued)

Expert comment

The fact that there are a number of potentially useful clinical and/or laboratory findings suggests that none is sufficiently diagnostic on its own. The 'psoas sign' is probably most useful in patients with a retro-caecal appendix. It is important to recognize the value of *serial* examinations to assess progression of symptoms and signs and the *early* involvement of a senior clinician.

Author, date, country	Design, subjects, and intervention	Key results
Gronroos 1999[7] Finland	Retrospective case series 200 fertile aged women with suspected appendicitis undergoing appendicectomy Correlation of raised and normal inflammatory markers (WCC and CRP) in patients with surgically confirmed acute appendicitis and those with negative appendicectomies	Mean leucocyte count and CRP for acute appendicitis (13.7×10^9/L, and 42 mg/L) significantly higher than in those with normal appendix (10.6×10^9 /L and 29 mg/L) $p < 0.001$ and $p < 0.05$ respectively. Normal WCC and CRP had 100% NPV 24% of normal appendices at appendicectomy had normal levels of both WCC and CRP pre-operatively
Vaughan-Shaw 2011[8] UK	Multicentre retrospective study 297 adult patients undergoing surgery for suspected acute appendicitis (50% women) Pre-operative inflammatory marker results (WCC, neutrophils, CRP) compared to histological report of resected appendix at surgery	Overall negative appendicectomy rate of 20.5%. Sensitivity of more than 1 inflammatory marker raised was 94% and 92% in both centres while specificity was 60% and 64% respectively

Data from various sources (see references)

Answer

A normal WCC and CRP have a high negative predictive value to rule out acute appendicitis; however, abnormal results have poor sensitivity and therefore should not be used to aid diagnosis.

---

① Expert comment

Individual inflammatory markers are not sufficiently discriminatory in isolation for diagnosing acute appendicitis, but when used in combination they are very sensitive. When both markers are negative acute appendicitis is very unlikely. If there is a rise in either one or both markers this is not specific for acute appendicitis and poorly reflects a pathological process causing an acute phase response of which appendicitis is only one of many causes. The Alvarado score tends to be used more in research than in clinical practice, but the 10 components included are important features to consider in the assessment of patients with possible acute appendicitis.

✪ Learning point The Alvarado score

Scoring systems have been derived to attempt to improve the diagnostic accuracy for acute appendicitis. The Alvarado score is one such scoring system that combines clinical and laboratory findings to assign a score from 0 to 10^9 (see Figure 18.1). Higher scores (≥ 7) are associated with a high likelihood of appendicitis and lower scores (< 5) imply that appendicitis is unlikely. Many studies have been performed to evaluate the sensitivity and specificity of this score in the general population with varying results.

All studies have been carried out in the general population with none specifically on women. A short-cut review concluded that the score should be used in the assessment of any patient with RLQ

(continued)

pain as it showed consistently high sensitivity and specificity.[10] In this review, a score <5 had 100% NPV and 100% sensitivity. The authors acknowledged the limited use of the score in women and recommend its use in conjunction with imaging in this group. Ohle et al.[11] performed a systematic review including 42 studies on the performance of the Alvarado score for predicting acute appendicitis. Overall a score of less than 5 was 99% sensitive and reliable to exclude acute appendicitis. A score of 7 or greater was poorly specific in ruling in disease with specificity of 81%. Sub-group analysis of women in this review showed that the score was very sensitive (99%) at cut-off score of <5 but poorly specific (73%) at a cut-off score of ≥7, thereby over-predicting the probability of appendicitis and leading to an unacceptably high negative appendicectomy rate. The authors advise caution on the use of this scoring system to clinically predict appendicitis in women. The accuracy of the Alvarado score is affected by gender. It is a useful risk stratification tool that can be applied to determine which women can be discharged with a safety net that reassessment may be required if symptoms deteriorate (score <5). Female patients with a score of ≥7 will benefit from admission and use of diagnostic imaging before proceeding to surgery.

Alvarado score	
Feature	**Score**
Migration of pain	1
Anorexia	1
Nausea	1
Tenderness in right lower quadrant	2
Rebound pain	1
Elevated temperature	1
Leucocytosis	2
Shift of white blood cell count to the left	1
Total	**10**

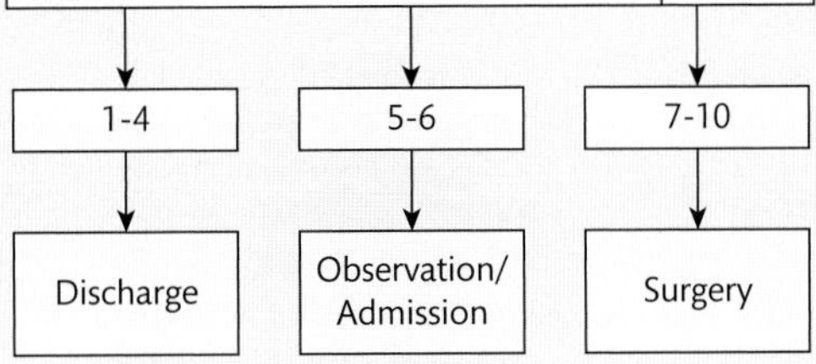

Figure 18.1 The Alvarado score[11]

Reproduced from Ohle R, O'Reilly F, O'Brien K, et al. The Alvarado score for predicting appendicitis: A systematic review. 2011. BMC Med 9:139. This is an Open Access article distributed under the terms of the Creative Commons Attribution License <http://creativecommons.org/licenses/by/2.0>, which permits unrestricted use, distribution, and reproduction in any medium, provided the original work is properly cited. Data from Alvarado A. A practical score for the early diagnosis of acute appendicitis. Ann Emerg Med. 1986: 15(5):557–64.

1-4 → Discharge

5-6 → Observation/Admission

7-10 → Surgery

Predicted number of patients with appendicitis:
- Alvarado score 1-4 -30%
- Alvarado score 5-6 -66%
- Alvarado score 7-10-93%

⚖ Expert comment

Appendicitis remains the commonest surgical emergency in pregnancy. There is the added challenge of delaying diagnosis and treatment to 'be sure' to avoid operating unnecessarily on a pregnant patient, and this delay contributes to complications not only at the time but the subsequent potential impact on fertility from perforation and peritonitis.

Sudden onset of non-migratory pain is more commonly associated with a cause of RLQ pain other than appendicitis.

Ask yourself, why this isn't appendicitis and why this isn't this an ectopic pregnancy?

It may help to identify symptoms or signs that positively suggest that another diagnosis is more likely perhaps analogous to risk assessments in patients with possible venous thromboembolism.

Case progression

The patient is admitted to a surgical ward for observation and further evaluation. The surgical registrar decides radiological imaging is warranted but is unsure whether an ultrasound scan (US) or a computed tomography scan (CT) is most appropriate.

Clinical question: Which imaging modality (ultrasonography or computed tomography) is most accurate in the diagnostic work-up of women with RLQ abdominal pain?

For the surgeon, a high negative appendicectomy rate (> 20 %) is unacceptable (see Table 18.3). In women with RLQ abdominal pain the negative appendicectomy rate is reported as high as 45–50 %.[3,7,8] Many patients get admitted for observation and re-examination with some eventually having surgery. It is generally recognized that

Table 18.3 Evidence evaluating the role of CT and ultrasound in the diagnosis of appendicitis

Author, date, country	Design, subjects, intervention, and outcome	Key results
Van Randen et al. 2008[13] Netherlands	Meta-analysis 6 studies with total of 671 adult patients comparing graded compression ultrasound with CT scan in same population with suspected acute appendicitis Estimates of mean sensitivity, specificity, negative and positive likelihood ratios (LR) for both tests.	Mean sensitivity for CT scans was 91 % (95 % CI- 84–95 %) compared to US with sensitivity of 78 % (95 % CI- 67–86 %) ($p<0.17$). Specificity of CT was 90 % (95 % CI- 85–94 %) compared to that of US which was 83 % (95 % CI 76–88 %) (($p<0.37$). The positive LR of CT was 9.29 (95 % CI 6.86–12.58) while that of US was 4.5 (95 % CI 3.03–6.68) ($p=0.011$), and negative LR of CT was 0.10 (95 % CI 0.06–0.17) compared to that of US of 0.27 (95 % CI 0.17–0.43) ($p=0.013$)
Hlibczuk et al. 2009[14]	Systematic review 7 studies with 1060 adult patients undergoing unenhanced CT for evaluation of suspected acute appendicitis Sensitivity and specificity of unenhanced CT scan use in suspected acute appendicitis	Pooled estimate sensitivity of 92.7 % (95 % CI: 89.5–95.0 %) and specificity of 96.1 % (95 % CI: 94.2–97.5 %)
Krajewski et al. 2011[15] Canada	Systematic review 28 studies including total of 9330 adult patients undergoing CT scan as part of their evaluation for suspected acute appendicitis Clinical outcomes such as negative appendicectomy rates, perforation rates and time to surgery	Overall negative appendicectomy rates were 8.7 % when CT used vs 16.7 % when using clinical evaluation alone. Appendiceal perforation rate was 23.4 % when CT used vs 16.7 % when clinical evaluation used alone. Mean time to surgery was 13.3 hours in the CT group vs 7.8 hours in the clinical evaluation group Subgroup analysis of the women showed a negative appendicectomy rate of 9.6 % in the CT group vs 27.3 % in the clinical evaluation only group ($p<0.001$)

(continued)

Author, date, country	Design, subjects, intervention, and outcome	Key results
Morse et al. 2007[16] USA	Retrospective chart review Reproductive-aged women undergoing appendicectomy Negative appendicectomy rates in groups undergoing preoperative CT scan and those that did not cost effectiveness analysis	Negative appendicectomy rates of 17% in group receiving pre-operative CT scans vs 42% in the group that did not CT scan saved average $1412 per patient
Wilson et al. 2001[17] USA	Prospective study 99 adult patients undergoing CT and US as part of evaluation for suspected acute appendicits Impact of CT and US and repeat clinical examination on clinical outcomes such as surgeon's decision making, negative appendicectomy rates, unnecessary admissions, and inappropriate discharges	A total of 34 patients had their initial management plan changed in the study. CT scan alone accounted for 53% of these changes compared to 0% by US alone. CT in combination with repeat examination changed the surgeon's decision making in 12% of these cases compared to 3% with US use instead Overall use of CT and repeat examination reduced negative appendicectomy rate from potential 25-11%. In women, the potential negative appendicectomy rate was reduced from 50-17%. 49% of patients initially designated for observation were re-designated from observation to either surgery or discharge with CT and repeat clinical examination accounting for 96% of these decisions

delay in diagnosis of appendicitis can result in perforation which leads to increased morbidity with prolonged hospital stay or mortality.

Imaging tests such as compression US and CT scans (with or without contrast) can be used to improve diagnostic accuracy with both easily accessible to clinicians.

The diagnostic accuracy of US has been reported to vary from 71–97 % while that of CT is reported as 93–98 %.[12] An appraisal of the literature revealed enormous heterogeneity in the population and methodology used in the studies, and none of the studies was carried out exclusively in women.

The American College of Emergency Physicians in its clinical policy on the evaluation and management of suspected appendicitis in the ED[18] acknowledges the superior diagnostic value of abdominal CT in the evaluation of adult patients. Ultrasonography is mentioned only with regards to the paediatric population due to the possible risk of an association with cancer from exposure to ionizing radiation.

Answer

In women with RLQ abdominal pain, equivocal clinical and laboratory findings are not uncommon. When this happens and radiological imaging is considered, CT scan is recommended as the imaging test of choice. It has a higher diagnostic accuracy than ultrasonography thereby expediting the surgeon's decision to operate or discharge, and reducing negative appendicectomy rates. The appropriate use of imaging, its benefits, risks, and cost-effectiveness, however, remains controversial (see Figure 18.2 and Figure 18.3).

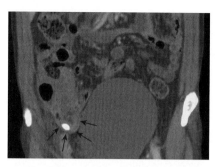

Figure 18.2 Non-enhanced coronal CT scan of a 34-year-old woman with RLQ pain showing a dilated appendix (arrows) with an appendicolith and peri-appendiceal stranding confirming acute appendicitis.

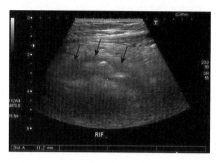

Figure 18.3 Compression ultrasound image of the RLQ in an 18-year-old woman showing a dilated non-compressible Hypo-echogenic tubular structure (arrows) measuring 11 mm in AP diameter with echogenic structures within suggestive of an inflamed appendix with appendicoliths.

❝ Expert comment

If imaging is required, a risk/benefit analysis and cost may influence discussions. The choice (ultrasound, CT, or MRI) will reflect local resources and expertise, but ultrasound is probably still the initial imaging of choice for women, including the pregnant patient, and is particularly useful if there is a faecolith or free fluid from a ruptured ovarian cyst.

If a faecolith is identified via imaging, it is imperative that it is found and retrieved at surgery (as there may have been a perforation).

Where the diagnosis is in doubt, laparoscopy is important as a diagnostic tool. Diagnostic laparoscopy is not explicitly discussed in this chapter but contributes significantly in many cases, especially where there is lingering doubt about the surgical vs gynaecological aetiology of the pain.

Diagnostic laparoscopy should be done jointly by surgery/gynaecology so that whatever pathology is found, the therapeutic intervention can proceed without delay.

✪ Learning point Appendicitis in pregnancy

- Acute RLQ abdominal pain in a pregnant woman poses a diagnostic challenge.
- The focus of the ED clinician is to exclude ectopic pregnancy and other diagnoses with high mortality/ morbidity.
- Acute appendicitis is the most common non-obstetric cause of abdominal pain with a reported incidence of 1 in 766 pregnancies.[19]
- In pregnant patients prompt and accurate diagnosis is particularly vital because of the high rate of fetal mortality associated with perforated appendicitis (up to 37%).[20,21]
- Appendicectomy carries a risk of pre-term contractions; therefore, unnecessary surgery (with negative appendicectomies) should be avoided in the pregnant patient.

The need for early accurate diagnosis is made particularly difficult with the non-specific clinical presentation, and impact of the anatomic and physiological alterations of pregnancy on the sensitivity and specificity of clinical findings and laboratory data. On a background of gastrointestinal discomforts that are associated with pregnancy, common presenting symptoms of acute appendicitis such as abdominal pain, nausea, and vomiting can be difficult to differentiate.[19] Furthermore, laboratory data such as elevated WCC are even less specific because of the physiological leucocytosis of pregnancy. As a result diagnostic imaging or laparoscopy is critical to the effective and efficient evaluation of the pregnant patient with abdominal pain. The selection of the imaging modality to be utilized is, however, the challenge.

Imaging in the pregnant patient

In the pregnant patient with suspected acute appendicitis, ultrasonography should be the imaging technique of first choice.[19,24] When ultrasound produces equivocal results, unenhanced MRI is the preferred imaging of choice. MRI is highly specific in the diagnosis of acute appendicitis and also very useful in eliciting alternative diagnoses.[22,23,25] The use of abdominal CT scan in pregnancy should be avoided whenever possible given the risks of ionizing radiation to the patient and the fetus.

A Final Word from the Expert

The clinical challenge remains as does the risk of delayed diagnosis verses unnecessary surgery in women without acute appendicitis. Earlier involvement of senior clinicians should help to highlight the value of clinical assessments and to limit requests for imaging.

It is important to emphasize the value of serial examinations to assess symptom/sign progression and recognize the contribution of diagnostic laparoscopy done jointly by the surgeon and the gynaecologist.

References

1. Cole MA, Maldonado N. Evidence-based management of suspected appendicitis in the emergency department. *Emerg Med Pract* 2011; 13 (10):1–29.
2. Lane MJ, Liu DM, Huynh MD, *et al.* Suspected acute appendicitis: non-enhanced helical CT in 300 consecutive patients. *Radiology* 1999; 213(2):341–6.
3. Wagner JM, McKinney WP, Carpenter JL. Does this patient have appendicitis? *JAMA* 1996; 276(19):1589–94.
4. Andersson RE. Meta-analysis of the clinical and laboratory diagnosis of appendicitis. *Br J Surg* 2004; 91(1):28–37.
5. Sengupta A, Bax G, Paterson-Brown S. White cell count and C-reactive protein measurement in patients with possible appendicitis. *Ann R Coll Surg Engl* 2009; 91(2):113–5.
6. Khan MN, Davie E, Irshad K. The role of white cell count and C-reactive protein in the diagnosis of acute appendicitis. *J Ayub Med Coll* 2004; 16(3):17–19.
7. Grönroos JM, Grönroos P. A fertile aged woman with right lower abdominal pain but unelevated leucocyte count and C-reactive protein. Acute appendicitis is very unlikely. *Langenbecks Arch Surg* 1999; 384(5):437–40.
8. Vaughan-Shaw PG, Rees JR, Bell E, *et al.* Normal inflammatory markers in appendicitis: evidence from two independent cohort studies. *JRSM Short Rep* 2011;2(5):43.
9. Alvarado A. A practical score for the early diagnosis of acute appendicitis. *Ann Emerg Med* 1986: 15(5):557–64.

10. Haldane C. The Alvarado scoring system is an accurate diagnostic tool for appendicitis. 2008. <http://www.bestbets.org/bets/bet.php?id=1671>

11. Ohle R, O'Reilly F, O'Brien K, *et al*. The Alvarado score for predicting appendicitis: A systematic review. *BMC Med* 2011; 9:139.

12. Rao PM, Boland GW. Imaging of acute right lower abdominal quadrant pain. *Clin Radiol* 1998; 53(9):639–49.

13. Van Randen A, Bipat S, Zwinderman AH, *et al*. Acute appendicitis: Meta-analysis of diagnostic performance of CT and graded compression US related to prevalence of disease. *Radiology* 2008; 249(1):97–106.

14. Hlibczuk V, Dattaro J, Jin Z, *et al*. Diagnostic Accuracy of Noncontrast Computed Tomography for Appendicitis in Adults: A Systematic Review. *Annal Emerg Med* 2009; 55(1):51–9.

15. Krajewski S, Brown J, Phang P, *et al*. Impact of computed tomography of the abdomen on clinical outcomes in patients with acute right lower quadrant pain: a meta-analysis. *Can J Surg* 2011; 54(1):43–53.

16. Morse BC, Roettger RH, Kalbaugh CA, *et al*. Abdominal CT scanning in reproductive age women with right lower quadrant abdominal pain: does its use reduce negative appendectomy rates and healthcare costs? *Am Surg* 2007; 73(6):580–4.

17. Wilson EB, Cole JC, Nipper ML, *et al*. Computed tomography and ultrasonography in the diagnosis of appendicitis: when are they indicated? *Arch Surg* 2001; 136(6):670–5.

18. Long SS, Long C, Lai H, *et al*. Imaging strategies for right lower quadrant pain in pregnancy. *Am J Roentgenol* 2011; 196(1):4–12.

19. Babaknia A, Parsa H, Woodruff JD. Appendicitis during pregnancy. *Obstet Gynecol* 1977; 50(1):40–4.

20. Mourad J, Elliott JP, Erickson L, *et al*. Appendicitis in pregnancy: new information that contradicts long-held clinical beliefs. *Am J Obstet Gynecol* 2000; 182(5):1027–9.

21. Rosen MP, Ding A, Blake MA, *et al*. Expert panel on gastrointestinal imaging. ACR appropriateness criteria right lower quadrant pain — suspected appendicitis. *J Am Coll Radiol;* 2011; 8 (11):749–55.

22. Israel GM, Malguria N, McCarthy S, *et al*. MRI vs ultrasound for suspected appendicitis during pregnancy. *J Magn Reson Imaging* 2008;28(2):428–33.

23. Cobben L, Groot I, Haans L, *et al*. MRI for clinically suspected appendicitis during pregnancy. *Am J Roentgenol* 2004; 183(3):671–5.

24. Lim HK, Bae SH, Seo GS. Diagnosis of acute appendicitis in pregnant women: value of sonography. *Am J Roentgenol* 1992; 159(3):539–42.

25. Oto A, Ernst RD, Shah R, *et al*. Right lower quadrant pain and suspected appendicitis in pregnant women: evaluation with MR imaging — initial experience. *Radiology* 2005; 234(2):445–51.

19 Dentofacial emergencies

Chet Trivedy

❻ Expert commentary Sunil Bhatia

Case history

A 16-year-boy presents to the ED after having sustained an injury whilst playing rugby at school. He was elbowed accidentally in the face during a scrum formation and sustained a facial injury. His front central incisors were avulsed and found in the grass. The school nurse placed them in milk within 15 minutes of the injury. He also has bruising and swelling over the left side of his maxilla and swelling below his left eye. He denies any loss of consciousness.

He is otherwise fit and well and has no relevant medical history apart from an innocent murmur as a baby, which he is not currently followed-up for.

His observations are as follows: HR 68, BP 118/82, 02 saturation 98 % on air, BM 5.8, GCS 15. The teeth are in a small cup of milk. His teacher reports to the triage nurse that the injury occurred 40 minutes ago.

See Box 19.1 for a clinical summary of dentofacial emergencies.

Box 19.1 Clinical summary of dentofacial emergencies

Dentofacial emergencies are a common presentation to the ED and it has been estimated that over 600 000 patients present to the ED with these types of emergencies in England and Wales every year, and this makes up 4 % of the ED workload.[1]

There is little consensus on what constitutes a 'maxillofacial emergency' there are few time-critical maxillofacial emergencies: major dental haemorrhages, fractures, or infections, which may compromise the airway require urgent referral. Displaced mandibular fractures are often admitted for surgical intervention whereas undisplaced fractures are often reviewed on an outpatient basis.

Complex lacerations of the facial structures requiring debridement and closure are often better managed by a maxillofacial specialist given the constraints of specialist equipment, assistance, and time within the ED.

Dental avulsion injuries should be classified as time-critical emergencies and any delays beyond 90 minutes in replanting a permanent tooth following a traumatic dental injury (TDI) will have a significant impact on the prognosis of tooth survival.[2,3]

The global prevalence of TDI in permanent teeth (adults and children combined) is between 4.7–44.2 %.[4] The UK prevalence rates in children aged 14–15 is in the region of 23.7–44.2 %.[5,6]

It is important to appreciate the difference between deciduous (baby) and permanent (adult) teeth. Deciduous teeth have a poor prognosis for replanting and as the roots of the deciduous teeth lie in close proximity to the developing permanent teeth, there is risk of further damage to the permanent teeth. Permanent teeth come through between 6 and 12 years of age.

---

❻ Expert comment

Some dentofacial emergencies such as avulsed teeth are time-critical emergencies and it is important that ED clinicians have a basic understanding and skills required to manage these emergencies. Studies have shown that ED clinicians have poor awareness as well as little or no formal training

(continued)

✚ Clinical tip Examination

As a part of the assessment it is important that the patient is examined to exclude a significant head or c-spine injury. Where the tooth/teeth are unaccounted for against a background of a period of a loss of consciousness; however, imaging of the chest may be warranted to look for inhaled teeth. A detailed assessment of the maxillofacial system should be performed (see Table 19.1).

in managing these types of emergencies.[7,8] This may lead to suboptimal care, which may result in significant morbidity, and life-long costs of dental treatment for the patient. Basic knowledge of dental anatomy, pathology in addition to practical skills such as replanting avulsed teeth, splinting teeth, dental blocks, and interpretation of facial X-rays are essential in improving the prognosis of these emergencies.

Table 19.1 Examination of the maxillofacial system

Key areas for examination in the maxillofacial system	Important abnormalities to detect
Scalp	Lacerations. Boggy haematoma
Forehead and supraorbital region	Bony tenderness. Step deformity. Paraesthesia
Ophthalmic examination including acuity and fundoscopy	Intraocular injury, diplopia, opthalmoplegia, restricted or painful eye movements, subconjunctival haemorrhage
Infraorbital margin	Bony tenderness. Step deformity. Paraesthesia
Nose	Deformity. Deviation. Septal haematoma, CSF rhinorrhoea
Ears	Haemotympanum, post-auricular bruising, CSF otorrhoea
Tempromandibular joints	Limited, painful, or asymmetrical mouth opening
Dental occlusion	Change in bite
Teeth	Displaced or fractured teeth
Soft tissue of oral cavity	Bruising under the tongue or soft palate

Clinical question: What is the best transport medium for an avulsed tooth?

The transportation and handling of an avulsed tooth is one of the key factors in determining the prognosis of the subsequent replantation. The cells of the periodontal ligament (PDL), which cover the root surface, play a central role in re-attaching the tooth within the socket and preventing ankylosis. Ensuring the viability of these cells is paramount and it is therefore essential that the tooth is rapidly transferred to a suitable transport medium which will maximize the survival of the cells of the PDL as early as possible; after 60 minutes of dry time, the PDL cells are likely to be non-viable. A variety of transport media have been suggested including saliva, tap water, saline, contact lens solution and milk. Specialist transport media such as Hanks balanced salt solution (HBSS), which contain nutrients, minerals as well a buffered isotonic environment have also been proposed.

✔ Evidence case Transport of an avulsed tooth

Doshi D, Hogg K (2009):[9] The authors carried out a BEST BET analysis, which examined 8 publications for evidence into which was the best transport medium. They concluded that for the emergency situation, milk or a special medium used for storage and transport of avulsed teeth was the best.

Gomes MC *et al.* (2009)[10]: The authors conducted a review of the literature and looked at several transport media including tap water, normal saline, saliva, milk, Gatorade, contact lens solutions, HBSS, Viaspan (used for transporting organs for transplantation), egg white, Propolis, and Emdogain. They concluded that HBSS was the best transport medium but as it is not readily available in the emergency setting, milk was preferred as it is more readily available and was preferred to saliva, tap water, or normal saline, which should be avoided

Huang SC, Remeikis NA, Daniels JC (1996):[11] PDL cells from extracted teeth were cultured in 5 transport solutions. Normal saline, HBSS, 2 types of commercially available contact lens solution,

(continued)

and milk at 4 °C and 20 °C. The study found normal saline was superior to the contact lens solutions at maintaining viability of the PDL cells. Milk at 20 °C degrees retained 24.4 % of the cells. HBSS was found to be the best transport medium, which resulted in 46.8 % cells remaining viable after 72 hours. They concluded that milk is a good short-term storage medium for maintaining viability of the PDL.

Courts FJ, Mueller WA, Tabeling HJ (1983):[12] The investigators looked at the effect of different storage media such as water, saliva, milk, and HBSS on the viability and proliferation of PDL cells obtained from extracted teeth. They found that HBSS followed by milk were superior transport media for supporting PDL cells in vitro.

> **❝ Expert comment**
>
> In the emergency pre-hospital environment where no special equipment is available, it would seem that milk is an appropriate transport medium to use whilst the patient is transferred to hospital. It may be appropriate that in such environments where the probability of dental avulsion is higher (e.g competitive combative sports), that a more specialist medium be available.

Answer

Although studies have demonstrated that HBSS is the ideal transport medium for avulsed teeth it is impractical to have this storage medium widely available in the emergency setting.

Case progression

The socket is inspected and there is clot visible so the socket is irrigated with saline, once clean there is no evidence of a socket fracture or gingival laceration. The teeth are removed from the milk and inspected by holding the crown. The teeth are both quite dirty from where they have been on the rugby pitch, therefore they are washed briefly (less that 10 seconds) under cold running water. Once clean, both teeth appear healthy. It is now 45 minutes since this incident and you consider what the next appropriate course of action is.

Clinical question: Should this tooth be replanted?

There are relatively few absolute contraindications for replanting an avulsed tooth in adults. Deciduous (baby) teeth should never be replaced.[3] Teeth that are fractured can still be replanted as long as the root is intact. If the tooth is split vertically along the long axis replantation is unlikely to be successful and the tooth should not be replanted. Time should not be seen as an absolute contraindication and teeth that have been out of the mouth for more than an hour should still be consider for replantation providing the patient understands the limited prognosis in terms of long-term survival.

The International Association of Dental Traumatology has developed a consensus statement regarding the management of avulsion of permanent teeth[13] (see Table 19.2).

Table 19.2 Treatment guidelines for the management of avulsed permanent teeth[13]

Classification of PDL	Treatment guidance
The PDL is likely viable: The tooth has been implanted immediately or a very short time after the incident.	• Leave the tooth in place • Clean the area with water spra/saline • Confirm position of tooth clinically and radiologically • Splint for 2 weeks • Systemic antibiotics and tetanus if required

(continued)

Classification of PDL	Treatment guidance
The PDL may be compromised: The tooth has been kept in a storage medium and the total dry time was less than 60 minutes	• Clean the root surface and apical foramen with a stream of saline and soak tooth in saline removing contamination and dead cells from the root surface • Irrigate and examine the socket • Replant the tooth with gentle digital pressure • As above
The PDL is probably non-viable: There is a total extra oral dry time of greater than 60 minutes regardless of whether the tooth was stored in a storage medium	• Remove attached non-viable tissue (best method not yet evident) • Consider root canal prior to replantation (discuss with maxillofacial team) • As above

13. Reproduced from Andersson L *et al*. International Association of Dental Traumatology guidelines for the management of traumatic dental injuries. 2. Avulsion of permanent teeth. *Dental Traumatology*. 2012; 28:88–96, John Wiley and Sons and International Association of Dental Traumatology and the Academy for Sports Dentistry

Careful consideration has to be given to situations where the risk of replantation potentially outweighs the benefits of putting a tooth back in the mouth (see Table 19.3). In these situations the treatment plan should be made after discussing the case with the specialist advice from the on call maxillofacial specialist. The Table 19.3 lists special circumstances which are NOT necessarily contraindications but require further consideration, and it is imperative the risks and benefits of the procedure be fully discussed with the patient.

Table 19.3 Considerations in replantation of teeth

Potential contraindications to replantation	Complication
Poorly controlled epileptics	• A seizure during the healing phase may result in the tooth becoming dislodged and inhaled • Ensure adequate splint
Severe learning difficulties	• Possible poor cooperation necessitating GA • Follow up treatment such as root canal treatment may be difficult.
Cardiac defects	• A dead tooth is a potential source of infection and may pose a risk to a prosthetic heart valve • Discuss antibiotic cover with cardiology
Immunosuppression	• Potential risk of infection • Discuss antibiotic cover with patient's specialist team
Compliance	• Heavily intoxicated or aggressive patients may not be candidates for replantation • May pose risk to healthcare professional
Poor dentition	• Replantation is less likely to be successful in those who have a very poor dentition and poor periodontal state • Ascertain how loose the tooth was before it was dislodged by a traumatic event

❻ Expert comment

The avulsed tooth should be replanted at the earliest opportunity. The tooth socket should also be irrigated and aspirated with gentle suction to remove debris or clots which may prevent the tooth being repositioned in the socket. Local anaesthetic can be administered as an infiltration block around the socket. The key to successful management is the early replantation of the tooth with minimal handling of the root followed by a period of immobilization that allows physiological movement for a maximum duration of 14 days. Restoration of the bite is a useful indicator that the tooth is in the correct position and it is important to check this with the patient prior to splinting.

The administration of local anaesthetic (LA) as in the form of dental blocks is a useful skill to have in the ED (see Figure 19.1). In this particular case, infiltration of lignocaine with adrenaline will provide sufficient anaesthesia to successfully replant the teeth. The technique involves the placement of the needle at the junction of the gingival (gum) margin and the mucosa of the lip as is demonstrated in Figure 19.1. Self-aspirating dental syringes are preferable as they are finer and longer than the conventional needles available in the ED. The self-aspirating syringes also reduce the risk of intravascular injection.

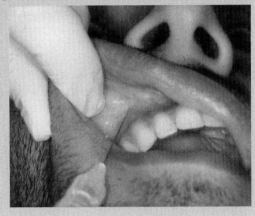

Figure 19.1 Image illustrating the position of the needle for infiltration of local anaesthetic in a dental block.

Reproduced with permission from the London Deanery.

Case progression

It is decided to replant the tooth. An infiltration block is performed and the teeth are replanted but do not feel stable.

Clinical question: What is the most appropriate type of splinting for this type of injury in the ED by emergency physicians?

Splinting (immobilization) of a replanted tooth following a TDI is crucial to the subsequent prognosis of survival. The ideal splint should allow physiological movement of the tooth and therefore be semi-rigid. It should also not encroach on the gingival margin and should allow for oral hygiene to be maintained. Metal wire splints, which are bonded onto the teeth with composite resin, have been used as the mainstay of splinting techniques.[14] This type of splint which some may see as the gold standard, may be totally impractical in the hands of an ED clinician who has no formal dental training, working single-handed in a busy ED. The splinting method employed with therefore depend upon the skills and materials available in the ED.

Trivedy et al. (2012):[15] there are no studies that have looked at the viability and efficacy of splinting avulsed teeth by ED clinicians in the ED setting. However, a recent study of 103 UK-based ED clinicians found that only 36.4% of the consultants (n=33), 18.4% of senior trainees (n=38), and 6.3% of junior trainees (n=32) had the confidence to replant and manage an isolated dental avulsion without supervision.

Answer

This study suggests that with the current knowledge and skills ED clinicians have in managing dentofacial emergencies, it is unlikely that ED clinicians will adopt the use of conventional splinting methods as standard practice in the ED. However, splinting methods which are more ED-friendly may be used as emergency splints when expert on-site support is not available.

A method of splinting which is quick, requires no specialist dental skills, involves the use of commercially available condensation cured-silicone impression material which is widely used by dentists to take dental impressions. The product usually comprises a 2-part putty and activation gel. These are mixed together by hand and then applied to teeth as a pliable mouthguard. This full coverage splint acts like a protective mouthguard and can be left in situ for a period of up to 24 hours. Although the splint is bulky and not aesthetic, it provides adequate protection for the replanted teeth and the surrounding soft tissues until a specialist sees the patient (see Figures 19.2, 19.3, 19.4).

Step 1: Silicone impression putty and activation gel are mixed together (Figure 19.2).

Step 2: The activated putty is made moulded in to the shape of the dental arch (Figure 19.3).

Step 3: The putty is applied to the teeth like a gum shield (Figure 19.4).

However, not all EDs may have this equipment, particularly if there is no dental service on site, and emergency physicians will require orientation in its use.

Another splinting method which has been suggested and utilizes equipment available in most EDs in the use of tissue adhesive and skin closure strips.[16] The method

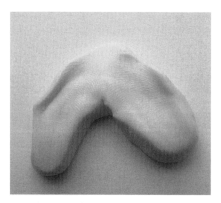

Figure 19.2 Mixing of putty and activation gel.

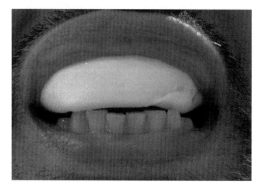

Figure 19.3 Moulding of putty.

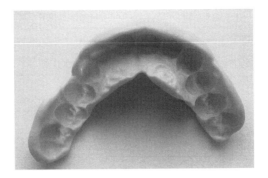

Figure 19.4 Application of putty.

described in these 2 case studies involved using the tissue adhesive to glue the replanted tooth to the neighbour tooth and also to glue skin adhesive strips across the relevant teeth. It was concluded that this method was suitable for short-term dental splinting.

> ❝ **Expert comment**
>
> The minimum requirements for any splinting method is that it should feasible to perform in a busy ED where there may not be access to specialist equipment or support. The splint should be seen as an emergency splint, which would protect the teeth for a short period of time until a specialist for definitive care could see the patient. With the advances in safe dental materials such as the silicone putty described earlier it is no longer acceptable to use items such as milk-bottle tops, lead foil, or paper clips within the ED setting. Maxillofacial teams should provide the materials as well training to their local ED to replant and splint avulsed teeth quickly and safely.

Case progression

The tooth is splinted in place and the rest of the facial skeleton is examined. Significant positive findings are swelling, bruising, and tenderness in the infraorbital region with possible altered sensation below the left eye; swelling and tenderness over the left maxilla; eye movements and acuity are normal. You consider if this patient requires any imaging.

> ✪ **Learning point** Imaging in facial trauma
>
> At present there are no guidelines on who should be imaged in facial trauma and there is work in progress to look at the clinical indicators for predicting facial trauma. Clinicians should correlate the clinical findings with the potential risks of ionizing radiation. The key outcome is not just the presence or absence of a fracture but also the significance of the findings on the subsequent management. Facial imaging should not be routinely be performed on every patient but when there is a high suspicion that the patient has symptoms such as:
>
> - A change in bite
> - Facial asymmetry
> - Neuropraxia
> - Eye signs
>
> Such findings may suggest surgical intervention is required. Although there is no evidence base to support this work is in progress to develop decision rules to support the use of these criteria. Once a decision to image is made it is essential to order the correct form of imaging (see Table 19.4).

Table 19.4 **Radiological examination of the face**

Imaging in facial trauma	Indication
Orthopantamogram	Dental root fracture or dentoalveolar fracture through the socket. View of the temporomandibular joint (TMJ) and the identification of condylar or coronoid fractures or fracture of the ramus/angle/body of the mandible
PA Mandible	Mandibular fractures
Occipitomental (OM) 15 and 30 degrees	Maxillary skeleton fractures, fractures of the orbital complex

> ❝ **Expert comment**
>
> Imaging in facial trauma is common practice and a controversial area in particular what types of imaging should be employed and when is the best time to request this imaging. Unnecessary imaging results in irradiating the brain and eyes (one facial X-ray is equivalent to 6–8 months of background radiation). Requesting the wrong type of facial view increases the likelihood of the fracture being missed, is not cost-effective, and may waste precious NHS resources. It increases the overall time the patient spends in the department and in inappropriate referrals to maxillofacial surgeons, and this may result in patients being bought back for review unnecessarily.

Case progression

In view of the infra-orbital numbness, facial views are requested. In view of the patient being in possession of 2 complete undamaged teeth an OPG is not requested. The following images are obtained (see Figures 19.5 and 19.6).

The facial views reveal opacification of the left maxillary antrum and a fracture of the left orbital floor. The case is discussed with the maxillofacial surgeons who are not on site and they agree to review the patient in clinical the following morning. The child is given systemic antibiotics for 7 days to minimize the effects of root resorption and pulpal necrosis[2] and a soft diet is advised.

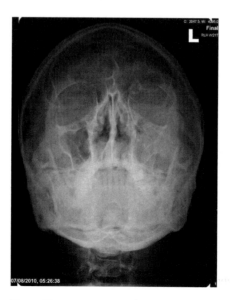

Figure 19.5 Facial X-ray OM (15 degrees).

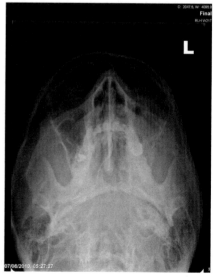

Figure 19.6 Facial X-ray OM (30 degrees).

A Final Word from the Expert

Patients with a traumatic dental injury where there is an avulsed tooth should be fast-tracked in the triage system as any delay will impair the prognosis. Patients should always be advised that there is a risk the tooth may not survive and that they will require close follow-up by a dentist, particularly if there has been a long delay in seeking medical attention and the tooth has not been stored in an appropriate medium. The consideration as to whether the patient requires X-ray imaging at present in governed by abnormalities found on clinical examination. It may be that with development of clinical decision rules for this group of patients we may be able to become more selective in who we X-ray.

References

1. Hutchinson IL, Magennis P, Shepperd JP, Brown AE. The BAOMS United Kingdom Survey of Facial Injuries Part 1: Aetiology and the association with alcohol consumption. *BJOMS* 1998; 36:3–13.
2. Hammarstrom L, Pierce A, Blomlof L, *et al.* Tooth avulsion and replantation: a review. *Endod Dent Traumatol* 1986; 2:1–9.
3. Flores MT, Malmgren B, Andersson L, *et al.* Guidelines for the management of traumatic dental injuries. III. Primary teeth. *Dent Traumatol* 2007; 23:196–202.
4. Glendor U. Epidemiology of traumatic dental injurie – a 12 year review of literature. *Dental Traumatology* 2008; 24:603–11.
5. Hamilton FA, Hill FJ, Holloway PJ. An investigation of dento-alveolar trauma and its treatment in an adolescent population. Part 1: The prevalence and incidence of injuries and the extent and adequacy of treatment received. *Br Dent J* 1997; 8:182.
6. Rodd HD, Chesham DJ. Sports-related oral injury and mouthguard use among Sheffield school children. *Community Dent Health* 1997; 14:25–30.
7. Patel KK, Driscoll P. Dental knowledge of accident and emergency senior house officers. *Emerg Med J* 2002; 19(6):539–41.
8. Trivedy, *et al.* The attitudes and awareness of emergency department (ED) physicians towards the management of common dentofacial emergencies. *Dent Traumatol* 2012; 28(2):121–6.
9. Doshi D, Hogg K. Best Evidence Topic reports. BET 3: Avulsed tooth brought in milk for replantation. *Emerg Med J* 2009; 26:736–7.
10. Baggio Gomes MC, *et al.* Study of storage media for avulsed teeth. *Brazilian Journal of Dental Traumatology* 2009; 1(2):69–76.
11. Huang SC, Remeikis NA, Daniel JC. Effects of long-term exposure of human periodontal ligament cells to milk and other solutions. *J Endod* 1996; 22(1):30–3.
12. Courts FJ, Mueller WA, Tabeling HJ. Milk as an interim storage medium for avulsed teeth. *Pediatr Dent* 1983; 5(3):183–6.
13. Andersson L, *et al.* International Association of Dental Traumatology guidelines for the management of traumatic dental injuries. 2. Avulsion of permanent teeth. *Dental Traumatology* 2012; 28:88–96.
14. Andreasen JO, Andreasen FM. *Textbook and color atlas of traumatic injuries to the teeth*, Third Edition. Copenhagen/St. Louis: Munksgaard/CV Mosby, 1994.
15. Trivedy C, Kodate N, Ross A, *et al.* The attitudes and awareness of emergency department (ED) physicians towards the management of common dentofacial emergencies. *Dent Traumatol* 2012; 28(2):121–6.
16. Cobb AR, Ahmad S, Kumar M. Use of n-butyl 2-cyanoacrylate tissue adhesive to splint traumatised teeth in the emergency department. *Br J Oral Maxillofac Surg* 2011; 49(6): 483–5.

Safeguarding: recognizing the abused child and acting on the evidence base

Jessica Spedding and Simon Walsh

Expert commentary Anna Riddell

Case history

You are asked to go and see a 6-month-old boy called Joseph. The nursing assessment states that he is unsettled and may have a leg injury following a fall from the bed the previous day. The nurse comes to speak to you because she is not happy with the mechanism which is being offered to explain the injury. Looking at the patient's records, you see that he has been to your department twice before. The nurse has contacted social services and the family are not known to them.

See Box 20.1 for a clinical summary of non-accidental injury.

Box 20.1 Clinical summary of non-accidental injury

Children account for a significant part of the workload for EDs; 25 % of patients attending EDs in the UK are children, comprising 3.5 million attendances per year (England).[1]

There were 50 573 children on child protection registers or the subject of child-protection plans in the UK as at 31 March 2012 (or 31 July 2012 in Scotland).[2]

According to the CEMACH review 'Why Children Die', over one-quarter of child deaths have 'avoidable' factors, due to 'neglectful' behaviour by adults.[3]

The NSPCC[4] carried out research which interviewed 1761 young adults aged 18–24 years, 2275 children aged 11–17 years, and 2160 parents of children aged under 11 this found that:

- 1 in 4 (25.3 %) of young adults had been severely maltreated during childhood.

- 1 in 6 (16.5 %) children aged 11–17 have experienced sexual abuse.

- 1 in 14 (6.9 %) have experienced physical violence at the hands of an adult.

- Neglect was the most prevalent type of maltreatment in the family for all age groups with 1 in 6 young adults experiencing some sort of neglect.

- I in 14 young adults (6 %) experienced emotional abuse in childhood.

⊕ Clinical tip Safeguarding checklists

It is important in all childhood injuries presenting to the ED that you look for any features that could point towards abuse or neglect. Many EDs have a safeguarding checklist printed onto the front of paediatric notes, such as the one in Table 20.1.

(continued)

Table 20.1 Safeguarding checklist

Safeguarding checklist	Please circle:	
Delay in presenting to A&E	Y	N
Mechanism inconsistent with injury sustained	Y	N
Relationship between child and parent inappropriate	Y	N
Recurrent attender to A&E with injuries	Y	N
Child has a Child Protection Plan/family has a social worker	Y	N
If you answered yes to any of the above discuss with senior or paediatric registrar		

Such lists act as an aide memoire to ensure that risk factors for abuse are considered in all children who present to the ED and not just those who are known to social services.

> **🎓 Expert comment**
>
> The consultation between the ED doctor and the child's parent is usually the first time the parent will have given a description of events. It is crucial you go into adequate detail in your history. Areas of particular importance are the developmental history of the child, particularly gross motor skills as it is important to ascertain what the child would be capable of doing him/herself, and the social history. It is important to document any additional siblings' names, dates of birth, and who they live with. If the family is known to social services, document social worker's name and contact details.
>
> You must examine the whole of the child undressed, not just the area of the reported injury. The use of body maps to document any marks on child's body is recommended and should be available in all EDs.

> **✖ Learning point** National guidance
>
> The National Institute for Health and Clinical Excellence (NICE) published the clinical guideline[5] 'When to suspect child maltreatment' in 2009, updated in 2013. This guideline summarises the 'alerting features that should prompt you to CONSIDER or SUSPECT child maltreatment' under the following headings:
>
> - physical features
> - sexual abuse
> - neglect
> - emotional functioning
> - clinical presentations
> - fabricated or induced illness
> - parent–child interactions

Case progression

The mother explains that her husband had been looking after the child and his two older siblings at home yesterday while she worked late. She says that her husband told her that Joseph had been placed on his parents' bed whilst his older brothers were playing in the room. The father had left the room and came back in and the baby was on the floor; he was not certain what had happened but thought the baby may have rolled off. There was a delay in presentation as the father had checked Joseph over and could find no injury but the parents became concerned when he was unsettled overnight and appeared reluctant to move his leg. Joseph has been to your ED twice before with injuries. He has no past medical history. When asked about motor milestones, she reports that he can roll over front to back and back to front, and is starting to sit unaided. The family of 5 live together and no-one else is involved in childcare.

> **✪ Learning point** Gross motor milestones
>
> **Table 20.2 Gross motor milestones**
>
> | Gross motor skill | Usually achieved by (months)[6] |
> |---|---|
> | Raises head when on stomach | 1 |
> | Supports head and upper body when on stomach | 3 |
> | Rolls over both ways (stomach to back, back to stomach) | 7 |
> | Gets on hands-and-knees position and crawls | 9 |
> | Cruises furniture | 11 |
> | Walks holding hands with an adult with one hand | 12 |
> | Walks independently | 15 |
> | Climbs up and downstairs | 24 |
>
> Data from www.emedicinehealth.com/infant_milestones

Making a judgement about whether abuse has occurred is difficult, but the judgement does not need to be made by one person in isolation. What is important is a thorough and accurate assessment, accompanied by detailed documentation which is then helpful to the senior paediatric staff who will make the safeguarding decisions. It is the accuracy of your clinical assessment and the recognition of sinister pointers in the assessment which will alert others to the fact there may be underlying abuse or neglect.

Case progression

There are some factors in the history which you find worrying; you are uncertain as to whether the child would be able to roll from the bed at this age if he was placed in its centre. You also wonder if it is reasonable for a parent to leave the child in a room unsupervised with younger children and whether this may constitute neglect. You question the mother further and she is not able to give you any further information as to how long the child was left unsupervised, but she becomes a little angry and suggests that her husband probably just 'popped out of the room' to get something for the baby. She agrees to call the father and ask him to attend the ED in order to provide a more detailed history. You carry out your own thorough examination of the child undressed to look for signs of injury and come across a number of bruises on his forehead, back, and shins.

> **❝ Expert comment**
>
> Be aware that pressing the parent for rapid answers by using a closed question approach may lead to dangerous misinterpretations. Document exact quotations of the description the parent gives. This should prevent any subsequent changes in the story from going unnoticed.
>
> Never make assumptions of parental guilt or innocence based on their appearance, perceived intelligence or socio-economic status, remain as objective as possible when assessing the likelihood of abuse and never collude with parents. Document what you have told the family about your concern, the action you will take, any aggression or violence towards you, other staff, or the child.

Clinical question: When assessing the bruises found on children is there any way of gauging whether they are accidental or inflicted?

> ✔ **Evidence base** Bruising in non-accidental injury
>
> **Maguire *et al.* (2008)[7]** performed a systematic review of studies from 1951–2004 to define patterns of bruising in non-abused or abused children <18 years of age. 23 studies identified: 7 looked at non-abusive bruising, 14 at abusive bruising, 2 at both.
>
> **Conclusions:**
>
> **Prevalence of bruising**
> <1% in non-independently mobile children
> 17% of infants starting to mobilze
> 53% of walkers
> The majority of school-age children
>
> **Patterns of bruising that are suggestive of physical abuse**
> Bruising in babies and children who are not independently mobile
> Bruises that are seen away from bony prominences
> Bruises to the face, back, abdomen, arms, buttocks, ears, and hands
> Multiple bruises in clusters
> Multiple bruises of uniform shape
> Bruises that carry the imprint of implement used or ligature

Answer

Bruising is common and its prevalence increases with age. A bruise must not be assessed in isolation but in the medical and social context in which it is seen. However, there are certain presentations which should alert the clinician to the possibility of physical abuse.

It has been reported that bruising is the most common manifestation of physical abuse in children.[8] De Silva and Oates[9] found 41 % of fatally injured children had multiple bruises on the trunk and limbs, whilst Pierce[5] found that 40 % of fatally or near-fatally abused children had presented on a prior occasion with highly suspicious bruising which was not acted on appropriately in order to protect the child. Explanations for bruises must be sought from parents and should not be ignored if found. The size and shape of any bruises should be clearly documented on a body map (see Figure 20.1 and Figure 20.2).

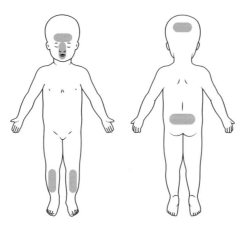

Figure 20.1 Patterns of accidental bruising.

Reproduced from Sabine Maguire and Mala Mann, 'Systemic reviews of bruising in relation to child abuse – what have we learnt: an overview of review updates', *Evidence-Based Child Health: A Cochrane Review Journal*, 8, 2, pp. 255–263, Copyright Wiley 2013, with permission

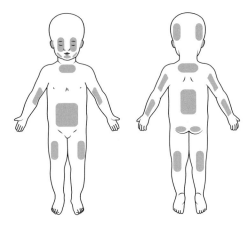

Figure 20.2 Patterns of abusive bruising.

Reproduced from Sabine Maguire and Mala Mann, 'Systemic reviews of bruising in relation to child abuse - what have we learnt: an overview of review updates', *Evidence-Based Child Health: A Cochrane Review Journal*, 8, 2, pp.255–263, Copyright Wiley 2013, with permission

---

ⓘ Expert comment

This evidence points to how important it is to look for bruising and to consider aetiology, particularly if the age of the child, or location of the bruise make an accidental cause unlikely. However, to-date, evidence suggests that even forensic clinicians cannot accurately date bruises based on their appearance and colour.[11]

Remember, bruising is often missed because the clinician does not think to look, as its importance as an abuse indicator is not recognized. However, it is often the only visible sign in cases of abuse. So although the patient may need no MEDICAL intervention because of bruising, they do need SOCIAL intervention to prevent further harm.

Case progression

On examination of the left leg there appears to be some warmth and swelling over the mid shaft of the tibia. It appears tender to touch. You provide the child with some analgesia and arrange for an X-ray to be taken of the lower leg. In view of the bruising and the possible leg injury, you begin to activate your local child protection procedures which in the first instance involves discussing the case with the safeguarding team and the paediatric registrar. They agree to attend to the department to assess the child.

The patient returns from X-ray and the X-ray reveals a spiral fracture of the mid shaft of the tibia. Whilst in a mobile child with a witnessed fall the film may suggest a toddler's fracture, you are concerned that in a non-mobile child it may suggest a twisting mechanism consistent with non-accidental injury.

Clinical questions: What is the likelihood that these bony injuries occurred as a result of an accident?

✓ Evidence base Fractures in non-accidental injury

Kemp *et al.* (2008)[12] performed a systematic review of studies published up until 2007 to establish features which differentiate fractures resulting from abuse from those sustained from other causes, in children <18 years of age.

32 studies were found:
- 26 cross sectional used for a meta-analysis
- (6 further studies with useful data not suitable for meta-analysis)

(continued)

Of these 26:
- 7 studies looked at the age distribution of fractures in abuse vs non abuse
- 13 studies looked a femoral fractures, 6 looked at humeral fractures, 7 looked at rib fractures
- 7 looked at skull fractures

Conclusions:

Multiple fractures are more common after physical abuse than after non-abusive traumatic injury

A child with rib fractures has a 7 in 10 chance of having been abused

Femoral fractures resulting from abuse are more commonly seen in children who are not yet walking

The probability that a femoral fracture was due to confirmed abuse was 0.28 (95% CI 0.32–0.54)

Mid-shaft fractures of the humerus are more common in abuse than in non-abuse, whereas supracondylar fractures are more likely to have non-abusive causes

The probability that a humeral fracture was due to abuse was 0.48 (95% CI 0.06–0.94)

An infant or toddler with a skull fracture has a 1 in 3 chance of having been abused

80% of fractures secondary to non-accidental injury (NAI) are in the under 18 month age group

One of the papers within this review article, by Carty and Pierce,[13] carried out retrospective analysis of 467 children suspected of being victims of abuse. They found no particular radiological features of long bone fractures to distinguish accidental from non-accidental injuries.

Answer

There is no pathognomonic features of a fracture which can distinguish accidental from non-accidental injury. During assessment the site, fracture type, and developmental stage of the child can help determine the likelihood of abuse.

Case progression

You inform the mother of the results of the X-ray and discuss the medical management. You also inform the mother that you are concerned about some of the bruises you have seen and for that reason will need to keep the child in hospital for further investigation. At that point the father attends the department. He smells strongly of alcohol and begins to shout at the mother, questioning why she brought the child to the hospital. He then leaves. You go back in to see the mother. She is very upset and discloses that she has been physically assaulted by her husband a number of times. However, she insists you do not disclose this to anyone else. She is not aware of him ever having hurt this child or their other two children.

There are a number of social determinants which put a child at risk of harm. Some of these risk factors will be sought on the standard social history; however, others are more difficult to query and may even evoke anger if parents are questioned and feel they are in some way being judged. If you are concerned a child is at risk it is important to information gather as much as you can about the family unit. This may involve contacting the GP, social services, or health visitor.

Clinical question: Can you share information about this case without Joseph's mother's permission?

Current legislation found in section 115 of the Crime and Disorder Act 1998[16] states it is permissible to pass information to another agency in situations where there is significant risk of harm to the woman, her children, or somebody else if information is not passed on.

Again, the Department of Health's handbook[13] offers guidance on this issue: 'There are limits to confidentiality. For example, if there is reason to suspect children are at risk, safeguarding and protection should always take precedence over confidentiality. The only acceptable reason for sharing information is to increase a woman's safety and that of her children. Even then, only share information that is relevant.'

Answer

If necessary, information can be shared between agencies if you believe a child is at risk. It would be considered best practice to obtain informed consent however unless you believe this may impinge on the child's immediate safety.

Case progression

It is decided to admit the child to the ward overnight and provision is made to bring the other children to the hospital. Social services are contacted and they agree to attend the department in order that a place of safety can be organized for the family whilst further information is obtained. The mother agrees to this plan.

As ED physicians, our role is to consider abuse, to look for it and to act on it, document appropriately, and escalate according to local policy. It is, however, important to have some understanding of what the next steps in the process are and what may happen to the child/family next. This is useful as you are able to advise families of the process (see Figure 20.3).

⊕ Clinical tip Child Protection Glossary

In serious case reviews relating to child protection, poor communication between agencies is a reason commonly cited as a contributory factor in cases in which child protection concerns have been missed or delayed.[17] It is essential therefore that we all use a common language when sharing information.

Child Abuse

Falls into four subsets:

Physical abuse: hitting, shaking, throwing, poisoning, burning or scalding, drowning, suffocating, or when a care-giver fabricates symptoms or deliberately induces illness in a child

Emotional abuse: persistent emotional mistreatment such as to cause severe and persistent adverse effects on the child's emotional development

Sexual abuse: forcing or enticing a child or young person to take part in sexual activities whether or not the child is aware of what is happening and including non-contact activities such as looking at pornography. All sexual contact between an adult and a child under 13 years is rape, and all sexual contact between an adult over 20 years of age and a girl under 16 years is rape

Neglect: persistent failure to meet a child's basic physical and or psychological needs, such as adequate food, clothing, housing, protection for harm, adequate supervision, and access to medical care. Neglect is also possible in pregnancy as a result of maternal substance abuse

Safeguarding

Protecting children from maltreatment, preventing impairment of children's health or development, ensuring children are growing up in circumstances consistent with the provision of safe and effective

(continued)

care. Undertaking the role so as to enable those children to have optimum life chances and to enter adulthood successfully.

Child in need

a. those children, identified by social services, whose vulnerability is such that they are unlikely to reach or maintain a satisfactory level of health or development or their health and development will be significantly impaired without the provision of services
b. those who are disabled

Child Protection Plan

A child with a Child Protection Plan is the replacement terminology for what was a child on the Child Protection Register (CPR). This is a child who after thorough social assessment (s47) has been deemed to be at continuing risk of significant harm

Each social care department holds details of all those children in the area who have been made subject to a Child Protection Plan for consistency

Emergency protection powers

There are a range of powers available to local authorities, the NSPCC and the police to take emergency action to safeguard children

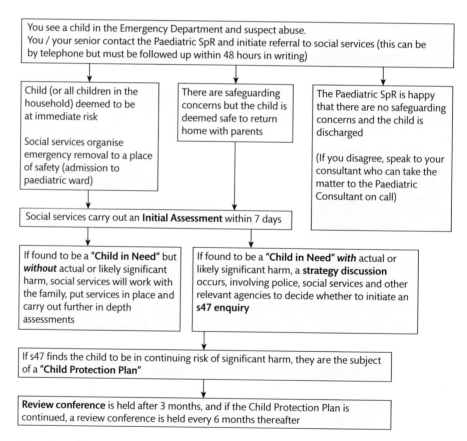

Figure 20.3 Flowchart: ED management in cases of suspected child abuse.

Data from 'What to do if you're worried a child is being abused', Crown Copyright 2006, Department of Education and Skills, https://www.gov.uk/government/publications/what-to-do-if-youre-worried-a-child-is-being-abused-summary

A Final Word from the Expert

Child protection in the ED can be a challenging and difficult area even for the most experienced of clinicians. It is important to ensure you are up-to-date with local and national safeguarding procedures and to ensure that every suspicion or concern is documented and discussed and information is shared with relevant agencies.

The Department of Child Health and Cardiff University together with the NSPCC have published a series of CORE INFO booklets based on the findings of the Welsh Child Protection Systematic Review Group in 2009, covering key clinical considerations in suspected child abuse. They are available at <http://www.core-info.cf.ac.uk> and include: Bruises on Children, Fractures in Children, Head Injuries in Children, Thermal Injuries on Children, and Oral Injuries & Bites on Children.

References

1. Services for children in Emergency Departments. April 2007. Report of the Intercollegiate committee for services for children in Emergency Departments.
2. NSPCC Child Protection Register statistics. April 2012. <http://www.nspcc.org.uk/Inform/research/statistics/child_protection_register_statistics_wda48723.html>
3. Pearson, G A (Ed) Why children die: a pilot study 2006;England (South west, North east and west midlands), Wales and northern Ireland: CEMACH.2008.
4. Radford L, Corral S, Bradley C, *et al. Child abuse and neglect in the UK today*. London: NSPCC, 2011. <https://www.nspcc.org.uk/Inform/research/statistics/prevalence_and_incidence_of_child_abuse_and_neglect_wda48740.html>
5. National Institute for Health and Care Excellence July 2009 (last modified: March 2013). When to suspect child maltreatment. CG89. London: National Institute for Health and Care Excellence. <http://publications.nice.org.uk/when-to-suspect-child-maltreatment-cg89>
6. <http://www.emedicinehealth.com/infant_milestones>
7. Maguire S, Mann MK, Sibert J, *et al.* Are there patterns of bruising which are diagnostic or suggestive of abuse? A systematic review. *Arch Dis Child* 2005;90:182–186.
8. Smith SM, Hanson R. 134 Battered children: a medical and psychological study. *BMJ* 1974; 3:666–70.
9. de Silva S, Oates K. Child homicide–the extreme of child abuse. *Med J Aust* 1993; 158:300–1.
10. Pierce MC, Kaczor K, Acker D, *et al.* Bruising missed as a prognostic indicator of future fatal and near-fatal physical child abuse. E-PAS2008:634469.46 Presentation at the Pediatric Academic Societies Meeting, Honolulu HI May 2008.
11. Visual assessment of the timing of bruising by forensic experts. *J Forensic Leg Med* 2010; 17I(3):143–9.
12. Kemp AM, Dunstan F, Harrison S, *et al.* Patterns of Skeletal Fractures in Child Abuse *BMJ* 2006; 337:a1518–25.
13. Carty H, Pierce A. Non-accidental injury: a retrospective analysis of a large cohort *Eur Radiol* 2002; 12:2919–25.
14. Responding to domestic abuse: A handbook for health professionals. 2005. <http://www.dh.gov.uk>
15. <http://www.patient.co.uk/doctor/Child-Abuse-Recognition-of-Injuries.htm>
16. 'Crime and Disorder Act 1998. <http://www.legislation.gov.uk>
17. 'What to do if you're worried a child is being abused' 2006 found at <https://www.gov.uk/government/publications/what-to-do-if-youre-worried-a-child-is-being-abused-summary>

21 Femoral nerve block for fractured neck of femur

Samy Sadek and Sam Thenabadu

ⓘ **Expert commentary** Michael Stone

Case history

An elderly woman of 85 years of age is brought to the ED after sustaining a fall. She has a background history of mild dementia, hypertension, and diabetes. Her social circumstances are that she lives in a residential home and mobilizes with a Zimmer frame. On examination she has an obviously shortened and rotated left hip but no other injuries. She is given simple analgesia in the form of intravenous paracetamol and undergoes a radiograph that confirms a fractured neck of femur.

Clinically she looks frail and unwell. Although drowsy and confused, she cries out in pain occasionally. A nurse asks you for some 'strong analgesia' for the patient, but you feel reluctant to give intravenous opioids. Her initial observations are heart rate 105 bpm, BP 100/60 mmHg, and saturations 92 % on room air.

You wonder if regional anaesthesia would be a better alternative to treat this patient's pain safely and effectively, and you have been trained to perform a femoral nerve block. A colleague is, however, dubious of the block's effect and tells you 'that they don't work for neck of femur fractures' and suggest you give small cautious doses of morphine instead.

See Box 21.1 for a clinical summary of fractured neck of femur.

Box 21.1 Clinical summary of fractured neck of femur

The average age of patients with a fractured neck of femur is over 80 years.[1] Those affected are often frail, vulnerable patients, many of whom have significant comorbidities, and reflecting this, the injury carries a mortality rate of 10 % at 1 month, and 30 % at one year.[1]

Managing pain is essential, not only for humanitarian reasons, but also it is likely to improve patients' outcome by reducing complications such as pressure necrosis, malnourishment, dehydration, and acute confusion.

A national clinical audit by the Care Quality Commission[2] found that in 2008 only 10 % of patients received adequate pain relief before arrival in the ED, 30 % within 30 minutes, and 52 % within 60 minutes of arrival. For those patients in whom a pain score was recorded, 32 % were judged to be in severe pain, and a further 37 % in moderate pain. The College of Emergency Medicine neck of femur audit in 2012 reiterated these statistics highlighting that in nearly three-quarters of UK EDs less than 50 % of patients received any analgesia or had radiographs performed to confirm the fracture in the first 60 minutes.[3]

ⓘ **Expert comment**

Traditionally, the pain of a hip fracture is treated with systemic analgesia, including non-steroidal anti-inflammatory drugs (NSAIDS) and strong opioids. Unfortunately, these medications have many

(continued)

side effects, to which elderly patients are more sensitive. Together with a high incidence of cognitive impairment, the assessment and management of the older adult's pain can be extremely challenging.

There are of course other options for managing this type of pain, not least regional anaesthesia, a practice that is gaining increasing credence in the ED. Peripheral nerve blocks are not without risks, but the incidence is low. These include nerve injury (permanent nerve dysfunction <1 per 10 000),[4–7] local infection (<2.5 per 1000),[7] and local anaesthetic toxicity (1 per 1000).[7,8]

The femoral nerve block (FNB) is a procedure that is taught within the CEM curriculum, and is technically one of the simplest regional anaesthetic techniques.

⊗ **Learning point** Anatomical landmarks

See Figure 21.1.

1. **Inguinal ligament:** Runs from anterior superior iliac spine (ASIS) to pubic tubercle.
2. **Inguinal crease.** Skin crease running parallel to the ligament, 1–2 cm below it. (At this level the femoral nerve is most superficial, wide, and consistent in its position).
3. **Femoral artery.** Crosses the inguinal ligament at its midpoint. Femoral nerve is **lateral** to the artery, femoral vein is medial to the artery. (Remember IVAN: Inner > Vein > Artery > Nerve)
4. **Femoral nerve.** Lies lateral to the artery, on the anterior surface of the psoas muscle, 3–5 cm below the skin and deep to 2 fascial planes.

Data from Moore KL, Agur AM. *Essential Clinical Anatomy*. USA. Baltimore: Williams & Wilkins. 1995.

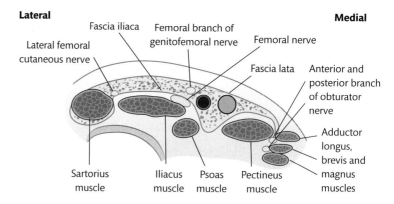

Figure 21.1 Anatomical landmarks—cross-section of the thigh.

Reproduced with permission from C Range and C Egeler, 'Fascia Iliaca Compartment Block: LANDMARK AND ULTRASOUND APPROACH ANAESTHESIA TUTORIAL OF THE WEEK 193', Copyright 2010, http://www.frca.co.uk/Documents/193%20Fascia%20Iliaca%20compartment%20block.pdf

The term '3-in-1' block is often used when high volumes of local anaesthetic (20 mls or greater) are injected whilst pressure is applied distal to the injection site. This theoretically encourages proximal spread of the local anaesthetic to block the femoral, lateral femoral, cutaneous and obturator nerves.

Numerous studies exist surrounding the use of the FNB for peri-operative pain control in femoral neck surgery, and its use by anaesthetists in this setting is now widely accepted. Consideration now is needed as to whether the same strategies can be used by the emergency physician at the first point of contact with a patient.

The FNB has long been recognized as an effective form of analgesia for femoral shaft fractures as the femur gains most of its nerve supply from the femoral nerve. Hilton's law[8] states that the nerve supplying a joint also supplies the muscles that move the joint, and by this theory the sensory nerve supply to the hip joint should come from the femoral, obturator, and sciatic nerves. It seems likely, referring to Hilton's law, that the pain from a femoral neck fracture would be reduced but not abolished by a femoral nerve block, the question being to what extent?

> **⊕ Clinical tip** Pain management
>
> The College of Emergency Medicine has set out guidance for the treatment of pain in the ED, with the crucial first step being to quantify the level with a pain score (see Figure 21.2). Frequently this can immediately limit the applicability to patients with a fractured neck of femur as they may often be cognitively impaired and elderly. Such patients are notoriously difficult to assess for their level of pain, and are particularly sensitive to the side effects of opioids, as well as the complications of poor pain control.
>
> Seeking out the correct class of analgesia, method, and frequency of delivery remains paramount. Finding a method that avoids side effects and does not require regular titration or patient feedback is therefore very desirable.

Algorithm for treatment of acute pain in the Emergency Department

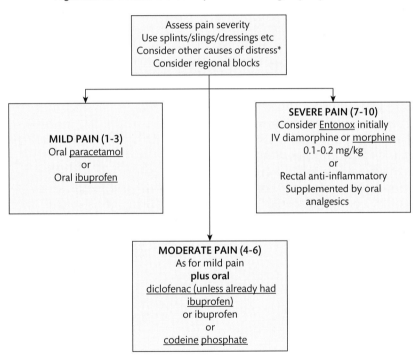

*Other causes of distress include: fear of the unfamiliar environment, needle phobia, fear of injury severity etc.

Figure 21.2 CEM algorithm for treatment of acute pain in the ED.
Reproduced with kind permission from the College of Emergency Medicine.

College of Emergency Medicine—neck of femur audits

The CEM clinical effectiveness committee has frequently highlighted the need to improve the management of patient's with neck of femur fractures. Since 2004, 6 national audit cycles have taken place examining key aspects of the management.

As discussed earlier, pain scores are advised in all patients with a recommendation of analgesia being delivered within 60 minutes; however, only 46 % of patients in the 2012 audit achieved this.[3] Reasons for failure focused upon difficulties in obtaining the prescription for opioids and the lack of manpower required to sign out controlled drugs safely. Timely radiographs and reassessment of pain were also key audit standards, however only 45 % of patients in 2012 were imaged within the expected 60 minutes, and a disappointing 35 % had a documented re-evaluation of pain.

These audit findings have led to the inclusion of new recommendations for early regional anaesthesia in the ED. Streamlining processes to initiate early regional anaesthesia could potentially obviate the need for opiate analgesia, make patients more compliant with transfer to X-ray departments and allow early transfer to the ward setting.

Clinical question: Is there a role for intravenous paracetamol in fractured neck of femurs?

In the elderly population, the pain ladder must be carefully utilized to avoid the side-effect protocols of stronger analgesia overriding the positive pain-relieving outcomes. The patient with a presumed neck of femur fracture may well be relatively comfortable when still on the ED trolley, but the need for quality radiographs may cause pain when the limb is positioned in the X-ray room. Effective and timely analgesia becomes a priority but reservations will occur due to concern over use of large quantities of opioids and potential hypotension and respiratory complications whilst out of the department.

Tsang *et al.* performed a prospective study of 72 patients comparing IV paracetamol use with IV morphine.[10] Encouraging findings in this trial demonstrated a non-significant 0.5-point scale difference in pain scores between the 2 groups ($p=0.173$), and an outcome recommendation that all patients with an NOF should be given IV paracetamol in the first instance to reduce the potential opiate requirement.

The 2011 NICE hip fracture guidelines reiterate the drive for considering early administration of paracetamol in the ED with regular doses 6 hourly (see Figure 21.3).

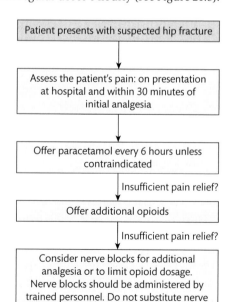

Figure 21.3 NICE Hip fracture guideline analgesia recommendation.

National Institute for Health and Care Excellence (2011) Reproduced from 'CG 124 Hip fracture: The management of hip fracture in adults'. London: NICE. Available from www.nice.org.uk/guidance/CG124. Reproduced with permission.

If pain relief appears insufficient, only then are opioids advised to be trialed. NSAIDS are not recommended on this guideline due to the increased risk of GI bleeds in the elderly.[11]

Answer

IV paracetamol should be initiated as soon as a neck of femur fracture is suspected and could reduce the need for larger doses of subsequent opiate analgesia.

Clinical question: Are femoral nerve blocks effective analgesia for patients with a fractured neck of femur and is this true for both intra and extra-capsular fractures?

> ⊘ **Evidence base** Femoral nerve block for fractured neck of femur
>
> In 1995, **Haddad** *et al.*[12] randomized 50 patients with extra-capsular femoral neck fractures to receive either femoral nerve block or no intervention. There were significantly fewer requests for analgesia (pethidine) in the FNB group. Mean pain scores were significantly reduced in the FNB group at 15 mins: 4.8 vs control 6.4 ($p < 0.05$) and 2 hours: 3.7 vs control 5.9 ($p < 0.01$).
>
> In 2003, **Fletcher** *et al.*[13] randomized 50 patients to receive either a '3-in-1' femoral nerve block or no intervention. The pain scores demonstrated that mean morphine dose required per hour and 'time to best response' were significantly lower in the FNB group.
>
> A Swedish study by **Kullenberg** *et al.*[14] in 2004 randomized 80 patients to receive either a femoral nerve block or systemic analgesia. The study found a significant reduction of mean VAS in both the nerve block and the control groups but there was no statistically significant difference between them. Overall, the FNB group required markedly less tramadol and ketobemidone (an opioid with similar strength to morphine), but no statistical values were given for this difference.
>
> A German study by **Gille** *et al.*[15] in 2006 randomized 100 patients to receive a femoral nerve block or IV metamizol (an NSAID) and PO tilidine (a weak opioid in the same WHO class as codeine and tramadol). The results showed the FNB group to have a greater reduction in mean pain score at 15 mins and 30 mins, both at rest and on movement.
>
> In 2006, a French study by **Murgue** *et al.*[16] randomized 45 patients with fractured neck of femur into three groups, comparing a femoral nerve block to either IV morphine or IV paracetamol + ketoprofen. There was a significant reduction in the mean pain score for the FNB group and, to a lesser degree, in the morphine group. There was a lower proportion of patients with a pain score >4 in the FNB group. There was no significant effect on pain scores in the paracetamol + ketoprofen group.
>
> A trial by **Graham** *et al.*[17] in 2008 randomized 40 patients with fractured neck of femur to receive either a femoral nerve block or IV morphine. Analysis showed a significant drop in pain scores at 30 mins for both groups, and this was greater in the FNB group. There were no statistically significant differences between the pain scores between the two groups at any other times up to 12 hours, and no significant difference in the amount of morphine given over 24 hours.
>
> **Parker** *et al.*[18] published a Cochrane systematic review in 2002, updated in 2009, to determine the effects of nerve blocks for pain relief after a hip fracture. The authors asked a broader question as they included all forms of regional anaesthesia and also included intra- and post-operative analgesia. The authors did, however, conclude that the use of nerve blocks pre- or peri-operatively reduced the degree of pain and the need for parenteral analgesia.

Answer

These studies were relatively small, excluded patients with cognitive impairment, and only one was truly double blinded. However, despite their flaws, all studies show a significant reduction in pain, although not always superior to IV opioids. The evidence suggests that routine use of FNB in patients with a femoral neck fracture is safe, and would reduce opiate consumption, though not necessarily replace it.

A femoral nerve block can be considered in all patients with a fractured neck of femur, particularly those with multiple comorbidities and greater susceptibility to the side effects of systemic opiates.

Case progression

You decide you will perform a nerve block to treat this patient's pain and reduce her need for morphine. Whilst planning and preparing for your nerve block you review the X-ray and your colleague who is standing next to you points out that this is an intra-capsular fracture, and he thinks that a femoral nerve blocks only work for extra-capsular fractures 'because of the nerve supply'.

> ✅ **Evidence base** FNB for intra- versus extra-capsular fractures
>
> In 1988, **Finlayson** *et al.* studied femoral nerve blocks for analgesia in femoral neck fractures in a case series of 36 patients.[19] It was noted that better analgesia was attained in those with extra-capsular compared to intra-capsular fractures. The authors therefore suggested that the more distal the fracture, the more likely it is to have a dominant femoral nerve supply. However, there have been no subsequent studies to confirm or refute this hypothesis. All but one[11] of the subsequent studies into the efficacy of femoral nerve blocks for fractured NOF have included both intra-and extra-capsular fractures, and all have shown an analgesic effect.

Answer

There is no strong evidence to suggest that femoral nerve blocks provide better analgesia in either type of fracture and the current body of evidence suggests that they are effective in all types.

Table 21.1 Comparison of femoral block techniques

Technique	Pros	Cons
Blind	Technically the simplest method	Likely to be less accurate and therefore have lower success rate and higher complication rate
	No specific equipment required	No feedback on symptoms of nerve injury in an obtunded or confused patient
Nerve stimulator	Improves accuracy	Stimulation of quadriceps muscle twitching by nerve stimulator may move the fracture and therefore cause pain—in practice this rarely causes pain unless there is a fracture extending into the femoral shaft, although the contractions may cause distress in confused patients
	No requirement for understanding of ultrasound, and technically simple to master with training	
	Gives clear visual confirmation that nerve is accurately located (muscle contractions)	
	Equipment less expensive than an ultrasound machine	Requires specific training

> ⭐ **Learning point** Ultrasound and nerve stimulator guidance
>
> The femoral nerve block was traditionally taught as a 'blind' technique guided by anatomical landmarks, however the use of a nerve stimulator or ultrasound guidance is now recommended by NICE and the Royal College of Anaesthetists as a means of improving efficacy and reducing the complication rate. There are pros and cons to all three methods (see Table 21.1).

(continued)

Technique	Pros	Cons
Ultrasound	Improves accuracy No movement of muscles or fracture.	Requires specific training—technically more difficult than a nerve stimulator and requires an understanding of ultrasound physics
		Ultrasound equipment is expensive and less portable

Case Progression

Whilst preparing your equipment and drugs in the resuscitation room, a senior anaesthetist that you have previously worked alongside takes an interest in what you are doing. She is pleased to hear that you are using regional anaesthesia for your patient and comments that there are many techniques for delivering this regional anaesthesia. She explains that she always gives a nerve block for these patients when they are in theatre, but prefers to use a fascia iliaca compartment block. She is enthusiastic to teach you and assures you that it is a simple procedure.

> ### ✚ Clinical tip Fascia iliaca block
>
> A (FICB) is an alternative method of blocking the femoral nerve. It involves instilling local anaesthetic into the fascial compartment that contains the femoral nerve. In addition, this compartment also contains the obturator nerve and lateral femoral cutaneous nerve of the thigh. The technique is usually performed 'blind', but more recently clinicians have begun to use ultrasound guidance. One method for performing a FICB is described here (See Figures 21.4 and 21.5):
>
> 1. Locate the site for injection—one-third of the way along the inguinal ligament from the ASIS at a point 2 cms below the ligament.
> 2. Inject a bleb of local aneasthetic subcutaneously at this point.
> 3. Make a 2 mm-long incision through the skin at this point.
> 4. Insert a blunt tipped needle through this incision and apply steady controlled pressure until a 'pop' is felt as the needle passes through the fascia lata.
> 5. Continue to advance the needle until a second 'pop' is felt as the needle passes through the fascia iliaca.
> 6. Aspirate to exclude intravascular injection and then instill 20 mls of local anaesthetic, there should be no resistance as you inject into the potential space.

> ### ⓕ Expert comment
>
> In experienced hands, the Fascia iliaca compartment block is a quick and simple technique. It relies heavily on tactile feedback that may be difficult to detect or even absent in some patient groups. If the initial skin incision is made too deep, the first 'pop' through the fascia lata may be lost and this may prove disorientating. The injection site is more lateral than that of the FNB and therefore the femoral nerve should be at less risk of damage. For the same reason there should also be less chance of vascular puncture. Some clinicians feel the FICB anaesthetizes the lateral femoral cutaneous nerve of the thigh more effectively and therefore lends itself to treating the pain of operative incision as well as the fracture itself.

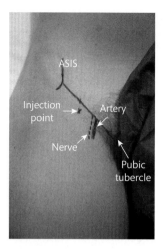

Figure 21.4 FICB anatomical landmarks on skin.

Reproduced with permission from C Range and C Egeler, 'Fascia Iliaca Compartment Block: LANDMARK AND ULTRASOUND APPROACH ANAESTHESIA TUTORIAL OF THE WEEK 193', Copyright 2010, http://www.frca.co.uk/Documents/193%20Fascia%20Iliaca%20 compartment%20block.pdf

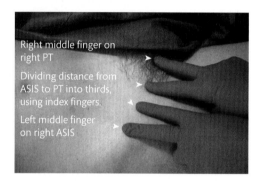

Figure 21.5 FICB injection site landmarks.

Reproduced with permission from C Range and C Egeler, 'Fascia Iliaca Compartment Block: LANDMARK AND ULTRASOUND APPROACH ANAESTHESIA TUTORIAL OF THE WEEK 193', Copyright 2010, http://www.frca. co.uk/Documents/193%20Fascia%20Iliaca%20 compartment%20block.pdf

Clinical question: Is a 'blind' fascia iliaca block equivalent to the femoral nerve block or pharmacological treatments?

✔ **Evidence base** FNB vs FICB

The Cochrane review by **Parker et al. (2002)**[18] attempted to make comparison between different blocks. They found the numbers insufficient to draw definite conclusions between the relative merits of each type of block.

Elkhodair (2007) performed a prospective cohort study on 137 patients utilizing a blind two-pop technique FICB.[20] This study revealed encouraging results and demonstrated a reduction of pain score of at least 3 points on a 10-point score in 77.4% of patients.

Foss et al. (2011)[21] randomized patients to receive either a fascia iliaca compartment block with 1% mepivacaine and epinephrine, or an IM injection of 0.1 mg/kg morphine. They found no statistically significant difference between the groups in pain at rest; however, there was significantly less pain on lifting the leg for those in the nerve block group ($p=0.04$). The total supplementary morphine use was less for the nerve block group ($p<0.01$).

Dickman et al. (2010)[22] published the results of a 3-armed randomized controlled pilot trial comparing IV morphine to ultrasound guided femoral nerve block and ultrasound guided fascia iliaca block. The authors found significantly lower pain scores in both nerve block groups compared to the

(continued)

morphine group, except at 8 hours, (which is consistent with the pharmacokinetics of bupivacaine). They also found a statistically significant difference between the 2 nerve block groups at 2 hours (p<0.05) and a trend at the other time points indicating that FICB may be superior to FNB.

A 2013 survey by **Mittal** *et al.* of UK femoral nerve block utilization revealed that of the 78% of departments surveyed, over half (55%) of the departments were regularly using nerve blocks, and a further 16% occasionally considering their use. In the peri- and post-operative phases of femoral nerve block use, anaesthetists are recommended by NICE to use either ultrasound or a nerve stimulator REF. The use of this ultrasound to guide these blocks only occurred in 10% of cases, and nerve stimulators rarely if ever used with again the blind two pop technique seem to be en vogue within the ED.

Answer

Currently there is not definitive evidence to recommend the FICB over the FNB, however, the decision should be made on the basis of the equipment, personnel, and expertise available.

See Box 21.2 for future advances in the field.

Box 21.2 Future advances

We are increasingly recognizing the avoidable element of the morbidity associated with hip fractures in the elderly. Protracted pain, immobility, and multi-system complications need not be tolerated as tradition dictates.

The hip fracture care of the future will include multidisciplinary review on admission in the ED, recognizing that this injury is not the remit of one specialty alone. Immediate input from the emergency medicine, orthogeriatric, and anaesthetic and acute pain teams will all play a role in the early control of pain, the optimization of comorbid state, and will prevent deterioration prior to surgery.

Early surgery, the same day as admission if physiological state allows, will also be key to reducing morbidity, mortality, and improving the patient's experience.

A Final Word from the Expert

Femoral nerve blocks and fascia iliaca compartment blocks appear to reduce pain significantly in elderly patients with hip. When balancing the risks of over-sedation, respiratory depression, and delirium it appears that regional anaesthetic techniques should be incorporated into the routine care of these patients.[23,24]

Ultrasound represents a widely available and familiar technology that can offer visual guidance for these peripheral nerve block procedures, and may provide a measure of additional safety and efficacy. More studies are needed to characterize the role of these techniques further in the care of the elderly patient with an acutely fractured neck of femur.

As part of this streamlined pathway we may see an increase in the provision of indwelling nerve block catheters with continuous local anaesthetic infusions, or patient-controlled pumps, allowing continuity of regional anaesthesia from the pre-op to post-op period and perhaps as a result, a greater opiate-sparing benefit.

The onus is on us to think laterally and consider carefully the impact of our interventions on this fragile patient population.

References

1. NHS Institute for Innovation and Improvement. Focus on: Fractured Neck of Femur. <http://www.institute.nhs.uk/>
2. The Care Quality Commission. CEM Clinical Audits: Fractured Neck Of Femur 2008. <http://www.collemergencymed.ac.uk>
3. CEM NOF Audit 2012 <http://www.collemergencymed.ac.uk/Shop-Floor/Clinical%20Audit/Previous%20Audits/>
4. Rastogi S, Turner J. Nerve damage associated with peripheral nerve block. In:Fischer B. (ed.) *Information for patients: Risks associated with your anaesthetic.* Revised Edition 2009. London: The Royal College of Anaesthetists; 2009. Section 12 pp. 1–4.
5. Nicholls B. Regional Anaesthesia. In: Allman KG, Wilson IH. (eds.) *Oxford Handbook of Anaesthesia.* New York, NY: Oxford University Press; 2004. p. 996.
6. Brull R, McCartney CJ, Chan VW, *et al.* Neurological complications after regional anaesthesia: contemporary estimates of risk. *Anesth Analg* 2007; 104(4):965–74.
7. Macintyre PE, Scott DA, Schug SA, *et al. Acute Pain Management: Scientific Evidence.* Third Edition. Melbourne AUS: Working Group of the Australian and New Zealand College of Anaesthetists and Faculty of Pain Medicine; 2010.
8. Barrington MJ, Watts SA, Gledhill SR, *et al.* Preliminary results of the Australasian Regional Anaesthesia Collaboration: a prospective audit of over 7000 peripheral nerve and plexus blocks for neurological and other complications. *Regional Anaesthesia and Pain Medicine* 2009; 34(6):534–41.
9. Moore KL, Agur AM. *Essential Clinical Anatomy.* USA. Baltimore: Williams & Wilkins. 1995.
10. Tsang K, Page J, Mackenney P. Can IV paracetamol reduce the opiate usage in fracture neck of femur patients? A district general hospital experience. *J Bone Joint Surg Br* 2011; 93-B(SUPP II):178–179
11. National Institute for Health and Care Excellence. *Hip Fracture. CG 124.* London: National Institute for Health and Care Excellence, 2011.
12. Haddad FS, Williams RL. Femoral nerve block in extracapsular femoral neck fractures. *J Bone Joint Surg* 1995; 77-B(6):922–3.
13. Fletcher AK, Rigby AS, Heyes FLP. Three-in-one femoral nerve block as analgesia for fractured neck of femur in the emergency department: A randomized, controlled trial. *Ann Emerg Med* 2003; 42(2):227–33.
14. Kullenberg B, Ysberg B, Heilman M, *et al.* Femoral nerve blockade as pain relief in hip fractures [Swedish]. *Lakartidningen* 2004; 101(24):2104–7.
15. Gille J, Gille M, Gahr R, *et al.* Acute pain management in proximal femoral fractures. Femoral nerve block (catheter technique) vs. systemic pain therapy using a clinical internal organisation model [German]. *Anaesthetist* 2006; 55(4):414–22.
16. Murgue D, Ehret B, Massacrier-Imbert S, *et al.* Equimolar nitrous oxide/oxygen combined with femoral nerve block for emergency analgesia of femoral neck fractures [French]. *Journal Europeen des Urgences* 2006; 19(1):9–14.
17. Graham CA, Baird K, McGuffie AC. A pilot randomised clinical trial of 3-in1 femoral nerve block and intravenous morphine as primary analgesia for patients presenting to the emergency department with fractured hip. *Hong Kong J Emerg Med* 2008; 15(4):205–11.
18. Parker MJ, Griffiths R, Appadu BN. Nerve blocks (subcostal, lateral cutaneous, femoral, triple, psoas) for hip fractures (Review). *Cochrane Database of Systematic Reviews.* 2002; Issue 2.
19. Finlayson BJ, Underhill TJ. Femoral nerve block for analgesia in fractures of the femoral neck. *Arch Emerg Med* 1988; 5:173–6.
20. Elkhodair S, Mortazavi J, Chester A, *et al.* Single fascia iliaca compartment block for pain relief in patients with fractured neck of femur in the emergency department: a pilot study. *Eur J Emerg Med* 2011 Dec; 18(6):340–3.

21. Foss NB, Kristensen BB, Bundgaard M, *et al.* Fascia iliaca compartment blockade for acute pain control in hip fracture patients: a randomized, placebo-controlled trial. *Anesthesiology* 2007; 106(4):773–8.

22. Dickman E, Haines L, Ayvazyan S, *et al.* Ultrasonography-guided nerve blockade for pain control in patients with hip fractures in the emergency department. *Ann Emerg Med* 2010; 56(3):s21–2.

23. Martin B, Ali B. Regional nerve block in fractured neck of femur. Towards evidence based emergency medicine: best BETs from the Manchester Royal Infirmary. *Emerg Med J* 2002; 19:144–5.

24. Hurley K. Do femoral nerve blocks improve acute pain control in adults with isolated hip fractures? *Can J Emerg Med Care* 2004; 6(6):441–3.

22 Sedation and restraint in the ED

Anna Johnson and Fleur Cantle

 Expert commentary Meng Aw-Yong

Case history

A 26-year-old man is brought to the ED at 10 p.m. by ambulance and police. He lives alone in a bed-sit and the emergency services were called by another resident who heard the man smashing things in his room. There is very little history available, but the other resident told the ambulance crew that he had not seen the patient around at all in the last few days.

The patient is being restrained by 4 police officers. He is highly agitated, aggressive, and shouting that he is in danger and being followed by MI5 and must leave as he is in fear of his life.

See Box 22.1 for a clinical summary of the disturbed patient.

Box 22.1 Clinical summary of the disturbed patient

The management of the disturbed patient presents a number of challenges to the ED physician. The patient can be difficult to assess and pose risk of harm to other patients and members of staff.

Disturbed patients present a diagnostic and management challenge as agitation, aggression, and psychotic symptoms can result from a psychiatric diagnosis or arise secondary to an underlying medical disorder (see Table 22.1). However, such conditions may coexist and disturbed behaviour may be exacerbated by a toxic component of overdose or withdrawal from prescription or illicit medications and alcohol.

Unfortunately it is difficult to distinguish between primary and secondary psychoses on the basis of psychopathology alone[1] as there are often few pathognomonic signs which are diagnostic of either aetiology.

A 2008 survey of over 3500 Emergency Department Doctors across 69 Emergency Departments in the United States found that 3461 physical on staff had occurred over a 5 year period.[2] No such large-scale survey has been conducted in the UK, however a retrospective study in Queens Medical Centre in Nottingham reported a total of 218 incidents of aggression and violence towards staff over a 1-year period.[3]

Table 22.1 Differential diagnosis of agitation in the ED

Infection/sepsis	Any infection can cause agitation and confusion, however infections which affect the brain often present bizarrely with neuropsychiatric type symptoms
Encephalitis	
Meningitis	
Urinary tract in fections	Travel history and immune status may help direct the physician to less-common infections.
Cerebral malaria	
Neurosyphillis	Abnormalities in baseline observations may aid the diagnosis
Respiratory tract	

(continued)

❻ Expert comment

It is important to utilize all available information regarding the patient from potential sources such as police, ambulance personnel, family, friends, and your trust's IT healthcare record system to prevent a potentially serious misdiagnosis.

Endocrine disorders Thyroid disease (hyper[5] or hypothyroid[6]) Cushing's disease or ectopic Cushing's syndrome.[7] Electrolyte disturbance: low sodium, potassium, calcium Hypoglycaemia/hyperglycaemia	Thyroid or adrenal disease may present with psychosis. The clinical examination may reveal other features of these disorders
Metabolic disorders Acute intermittent porphyria	May present with psychosis and abdominal complaints, e.g. abdominal pain and constipation
Autoimmune Systemic lupus erythematosus	Psychosis and seizures have long been recognized diagnostic criteria[8] secondary to brain involvement but also due to steroid treatment[9]
Neurological disorders Seizure disorders Space-occupying lesions CVA/subdural Dementia	Neuropsychiatric symptoms are more common in pathology involving the temporal lobe Psychosis can occur at the ictal, postictal or interictal phase of a seizure disorder. May present with very abrupt onset of symptoms May present with behavioural change and other neurological symptoms Rare but can be seen as a result of stroke related seizure activity
Trauma Head injury	Head injury related psychosis typically develops insidiously many years after injury.[10] Risk factors for developing psychosis following head injury being duration of loss of consciousness and family history of pschosis[11]
Toxins Illicit drug use: Cannabis Anabolic steroids Alcohol/drug toxicity/withdrawal Prescription medications: Steroids Anticholinergics, e.g. atropine Serotonin syndrome Liver cirrhosis	The causal link between substance abuse and psychosis can be difficult to prove as there are often many social, physical, and pharmacological influences in psychiatric pathology
Nutritional deficiencies B12 (Wernicke's) Folate	Often seen in the ED associated with chronic alcohol use

Case progression

The police tell you he's 'on a 136' but they are not certain if he has taken something. They brought him to the ED as he is not under arrest and they were concerned for his welfare. The ED charge nurse says the patient is far too violent to be assessed and the ED is not a designated place of safety. He thinks that the police should either have taken him to the local mental health unit or arrested him. The local mental health unit has a 136 assessment suite, but will not accept him, as they believe he is under the influence of drugs or alcohol.

He looks flushed and sweaty. The paramedic managed to take a pulse and says the patient is tachycardic.

Section 136

Section 136 (s136) is the most controversial section of the Mental Health Act (1983).[12] It allows a police officer to remove an individual from a public place to a 'place of safety' if that individual appears to be suffering from a mental illness. An s136 is valid for 72 hours whereupon a mental health assessment must be completed and cannot be renewed.[1]

Deprivation of liberty and removal from a public place, often to a police cell, on the 'appearance' of mental illness as observed by a police officer (without medical evidence or training) has led to criticisms of the ethical ambiguity of the section.[13]

✪ Learning point Place of safety

Much confusion exists surrounding the definition of 'place of safety'. A place of safety as defined by the Act[12] refers to:

'Residential accommodation provided by the local services authority, a hospital as defined by the Act, a police station, a mental health nursing home or residential nursing home for mentally disordered persons, or any other suitable place the occupier of which is willing to temporarily receive the individual'.

Whilst a designated place of safety should generally be a psychiatric facility, in real terms, due to the lack of availability of such facilities it is often a police cell or the ED.

In the Royal College of Psychiatrists College Report: Standards on the use of section 136 of the Mental Health Act 1983 (England and Wales) (2011)[14] it states:

'Police stations should only be used as the place of safety on an exceptional basis...

Emergency departments should be used as places of safety for those who need urgent physical health assessment and management'.

Case progression

You tell the charge nurse that you're not happy to send him away without further assessment because you are concerned there might be an underlying medical cause for his behaviour. The patient is becoming increasingly disruptive and the officers are struggling to contain him.

The charge nurse has managed to take some initial observations: pulse 140 bpm, temperature 37.8 °C, and oxygen saturations 100 %.

You realize that you urgently need to calm the patient and may need to sedate him to prevent him hurting himself and to make a full assessment to exclude serious illness.

➕ Clinical tip De-escalation techniques

The NICE Guideline on Violence[16] advises that de-escalation techniques should be tried before sedation and makes the following recommendations

- In a potentially violent or disturbed situation, 1 staff member should assume control.
- That person should then:
  - Manage the immediate environment—move to a safe space, remove unnecessary staff and other service users, give clear, concise instructions
  - Attempting to establish facts and encourage reasoning—try to establish a rapport, offer realistic options and avoid threats, use open questions to elicit the cause of the patient's aggression or anger, show concern and empathy, avoid being patronizing or dismissive of the patient's concerns.
  - Avoid provocation and use non-threatening non-verbal communication—remain calm, controlled and confident, allow personal space, adopt non-threatening posture.

Case progression

You ask the officers to move the patient to a quiet cubicle. De-escalation techniques are used to try and calm him and engage with him, but he becomes more agitated. You now have serious concerns for his safety and well-being. From what you have seen and heard so far, you are of the opinion that he lacks capacity and decide to act in his best interest and chemically sedate him. You require assistance to perform the sedation procedure and security are reluctant to assist and look to the police for help.

> **Ø Expert comment**
>
> The responsibility of restraint in a hospital is often delegated to security staff. It is best practice that the security staff have obtained a Security Industry Authority licence which covers aspect such as conflict management and physical intervention skills.[17] Training must be taken to ensure that restraint is undertaken to avoid injuries or death. Deaths related to restraint are highly topical, particularly where police have been involved,[18] with postural asphyxia, cocaine-related factors, serotonin, neuroleptic malignant syndromes as causative factors.
>
> The police are becoming reluctant to get involved in restraint of patients in hospital, especially with those with mental health issues due to recent high-publicity cases. Any death involving police officers will result in a referral to the coroner and the Independent Police Complaints Commission (IPCC), suspension from public contact for the officers involved and will cost around £1 million. Thus there is a growing trend to involve healthcare professionals.

Clinical question: Can a patient held under section 136 be physically restrained in the ED and who should restrain them?

- Patients can be physically restrained in the ED.
- The level of force applied must be justifiable, appropriate, reasonable, and proportionate to a specific situation, and should be applied for the minimum possible amount of time.[16]
- It is the responsibility of the healthcare staff to restrain the person where necessary but they may ask the police to assist in an emergency (e.g. while waiting for adequate staff trained in physical intervention to arrive). The staffing of a place of safety ought, therefore, to include the possibility of a maintained police presence to assist in the management of threatened or actual violence.[14]
- The police should not leave the unit until it is agreed with the senior nurse that it is safe for both the individual and staff for them to do so.[14]

A place of safety should include sufficient staff trained in physical intervention and readily available in an emergency situation. In reality, many ED do not have staff trained in physical intervention.

> **Ø Expert comment**
>
> The Mental Capacity Act 2005 (MCA)[19] is applicable to England and Wales, for those aged 18 and over, allows a patient to be restrained under section 6 of the Act. The MCA permits the use of force or threatening to use force to secure compliance with treatment, which will prevent a patient who lacks capacity coming to harm. Restraint is only permitted if the person using it reasonably believes
>
> (continued)

it is necessary to prevent harm to the incapacitated person, it is in their best interest, and provided the restraint used is proportionate to the likelihood and seriousness of the harm (always use the least-restrictive option).

Section 5 of the Mental Capacity Act provides protection for carers, healthcare, and social care staff against civil and criminal liability for certain acts done in connection with the care or treatment of a person. However, there is a new offence of ill treatment or neglect of a person who lacks capacity punishable with imprisonment for up to 5 years. Section 5.4 allows a nurse to lawfully prevent a patient from leaving hospital, and section 5.2 allows a clinician with authority to detain a patient for up to 72 hours.

Case progression

On the basis of the difficulties you are experiencing containing the patient and the ongoing suspicion relating to an underlying medical explanation for his behaviour, you decide that it is necessary to chemically sedate him. You are concerned that the patient will not comply with oral medication (see Table 22.2).

Table 22.2 Agents used for control of behavioural disturbance in the ED

Drug	Dose	Time to max plasma concentration	Approximate plasma half-life
Haloperidol injection* Can precipitate Long QT Baseline ECG required Not licenced for behavioural disturbance in dementia	2–10 mg	15–60 mins	10–36 hrs
Haloperidol tablet	0.5–5 mg	2–6 hrs	1–36 hrs
Lorazepam injection*	1–2 mg	60–90 mins	12–16 hrs
Lorazepam tablets	1–4 mg	2 hrs	12 hrs
Olanzapine injection* Caution in Ischaemic heart disease	5–10 mg	15–45 mins	32–50 hrs
Olanzapine tablets	5–10 mg	5–8 hrs	32–50 hrs

* administered intra-muscularly

Clinical Question: Haloperidol, lorazepam and olanzapine are all used in rapid tranquilisation, but which drug is most effective and safest?

The safety and efficacy of drugs used for rapid tranquilization was considered in a systematic review of randomized controlled trials of adults in the inpatient psychiatric setting.[20] Despite small sample sizes and variable outcome measures, some useful findings were reported. No significant difference was found between lorazepam and haloperidol, however the risk of dystonic reactions with haloperidol was reported. A comparison and olanzapine and haloperidol reported no difference in efficacy but olanzapine was felt to have a better safety profile.

> ❂ **Learning point** The NICE Guideline
>
> The NICE Guideline on Violence (2005)[16] provides guidance on all aspects of managing disturbed and violent behaviour in psychiatric inpatient settings and emergency settings.
>
> The NICE Guideline makes the following recommendations:
>
> - Where possible, oral medication should be offered before parenteral medication is used. When oral medication is refused or not appropriate, the intramuscular route should be used. Intravenous medication is not recommended for rapid tranquillization in the emergency setting.
> - 'The aim of rapid tranquillisation is to achieve a state of calm sufficient to minimise the risk posed to the service user and to others.' The aim is not to induce sleep and the patient should be able to communicate verbally at all times.
> - Clinicians should be aware of the potential complications and side effects of rapid tranquillization. Resuscitation equipment should be immediately available. If using haloperidol, an antimuscarinic agent such as procyclidine should be immediately available to treat dystonic reactions.
> - After rapid tranquillization, pulse, blood pressure, and oxygen saturations should be monitored and recorded regularly along with respiratory rate, temperature, and hydration.
> - In the ED setting:
>   - 'If rapid tranquillisation is considered necessary, prior to formal diagnosis and where there is any uncertainty about medical history... lorazepam should be considered as the first-line drug of choice. Where there is a confirmed history of previous significant anti-psychotic exposure, and response, haloperidol in combination with lorazepam is sometimes used.'

> ❝ **Expert comment**
>
> Patients should be given the option of taking an oral medication benzodiazepines are generally the medication of first choice, particularly in cases of known intoxication. If the patient has a known psychiatric disorder, consider using top-up doses of their regular medication. Rarely, administration of a benzodiazepine can result in paradoxical reactions with increasing agitation and anxiety as opposed to its normal sedating effect. This is more commonly seen in patients with developmental delay and/or a history of aggressive behaviour.

Case progression

You explain to the officers that you do not have staff trained in physical restraint in the ED and they agree to stay until the patient can be safely transferred to the psychiatric unit, or until suitable staff are available.

You move the patient to the resuscitation room and offer him oral lorazepam. He refuses and so you administer an intra-muscular injection of 2 mg lorazepam while the police officers continue to restrain him. As the patient begins to calm, the nurse applies cardiac and oxygen saturation monitoring. Thirty minutes after the injection the patient is calmer, but still able to talk to you and you are able to take a history and examine him.

An hour later the patient remains calmer and cooperative, although still anxious and saying that he is in danger from 'them' and that 'they' are trying to get inside his head. His observations are now all within normal limits, including his pulse, blood pressure, oxygen saturations, and temperature. He is not complaining of any physical symptoms and on direct questioning, denies headache or other pain. Physical examination was normal as were FBC, U&E, CRP, ECG, and urine dipstick.

The police have managed to contact the patient's mother who says that he has mental health problems and sometime 'kicks of'" like this and has not been taking his olanzapine for several weeks, but is unable to tell you any more than that. The police remain with the patient and are completing the s136 form. They have alerted to psychiatric unit who are happy for the patient to be transferred there once he is 'medically cleared'.

Clinical question: What is necessary when a patient is required to be 'medically cleared'?

It is a common request by psychiatric services that a patient receive some sort of medical work-up and assessment prior to review by the liaison team. This is important as the behavioural symptoms exhibited can be caused by an underlying medical cause and especially important in patients with ongoing mental health problems who are known to the mental health services as it is in this group that a coexisting medical issue may be missed. Once the decision has been made to transfer a patient to a psychiatric facility, the possibility of further medical work-up may not be easily available and hence this may be the most appropriate time to perform this assessment.

The literature suggests that there is great variation in what degree of workup is performed on this group of patients. A retrospective audit[21] of 17 defined variables agreed as commonly accepted components of the clinical examination in adult patients presenting to the ED with a disposition diagnosis of schizophrenia revealed marked inconsistencies in which components of the examination were performed at presentation. 51.9 % of patients had a complete set of vital signs recorded, 12.4 % had a cranial nerve examination documented, 53.5 % had a respiratory examination, and 51.5 % had a cardiovascular system documented. It was found that a patient was more likely to be completely examined if seen by a trainee emergency physician rather than a senior clinician.

It has been found that when investigations are performed they provide limited extra information.[22] In a prospective study of 375 patients with a primary psychiatric complaint and a pre-existing psychiatric disorder, 128 patients had abnormal laboratory results of which 72 had positive urine drug screens which were managed by observation and hydration. Of the 56 remaining patients with abnormal results 42 displayed abnormalities which was corroborated by the history and hence the abnormal test added no further information.

In a retrospective chart review[23] of the laboratory results of 502 consecutive adult patients admitted to inpatient psychiatric services, only 1 patient was found to have a result which may have altered disposition if it had been known about in the ED. The most common abnormalities in the study group were urine drug screen (221/502), hyperglycaemia (139/502), and anaemia (136/502).

This suggests that routine blood tests add little to the standard medical history and examination in patients with known mental health problems. A more extensive work-up may be required for those with a first presentation of psychiatric symptomatology.[24] In this study, 63/100 consecutive patients presenting with new psychiatric symptoms had organic aetiology.

It is very difficult to generalize and the degree of work-up to medically clear a patient is case-specific. As a general rule asymptomatic patients require a medical history, observations, and examination and symptomatic patients need investigations tailored to their presentation. Adults presenting for the first time with psychiatric symptoms may require a more extensive investigation including neuro-imaging and lumbar puncture.

Case progression

You refer the patient to the duty psychiatrist, reassuring him that the patient is medically cleared and inform him of the times and doses of medication given and the need for ongoing observation. The police officers accompany the patient to the s136 suite for assessment, thanking you as they leave.

A Final Word from the Expert

As physical restraint and sedation deprives the patient of autonomy, it should only be contemplated as a last resort. When physical restraint is required a coordinated team approach is essential, with roles clearly defined and swift action taken. Individual trusts should develop guidelines for pathways for managing violent patients (e.g. the Royal Children's Hospital Melbourne code grey protocol). This is a team-based approach with 5 staff members—supervising team leader, security holding arms (×2), and staff members holding upper and lower limbs (×2). Any protocol should include planning of the physical environment such as secure containing areas for managing violent patients, training in crisis prevention to anticipate and identify early irritable behaviour.

References

1. Freudenreich O. Differential diagnosis of psychotic symptoms: Medical 'mimics'. *Psychiatr Times* December 2010; 27(12):56–61.
2. Kasangra SM, Rao SR, Sullivan AF, *et al.* A survey of workplace violence across 65 U.S Emergency Departments. *Acad Emerg Med* 2008; 15:1268.
3. James A, Madeley R, Dove A. Violence and aggression in the emergency Department. *Emerg Med J* 2006 Jun; 23(6):431–4.
4. A Safer Place to Work: Protecting NHS Hospital and Ambulance Staff from Violence and Aggression, NAO, March 2003. <http://www.nao.org.uk/report/a-safer-place-to-work-protecting-nhs-hospital-and-ambulance-staff-from-violence-and-aggression/>
5. Brownlie BE, Rae AM, Walshe JW, *et al.* Psychoses associated with thyrotoxicosis – 'thyrotoxic psychoses'. A report of 18 cases with statistical analysis of incidence. *Eur J Endocrinol* 2000 May; 142(5):438–44.
6. Heinrish TW, Grahm G. Hypothyroidism presenting as psychosis:myxedema madness revisited. *Prim Care companion J Clin Psychiatry* 2003 (Dec); 5(6):260–6.
7. Bilgin YM, Van der Wiel HE, Fischer HR, *et al.* Treatment of severe psychosis due to ectopic Cushing's syndrome. *J Endocrinol Invest* 2007 Oct; 30(9):776–9.
8. American College of Rheumatology. The American College of Rheumatology nomenclature and case definitions for neuropsychiatric lupus syndromes. *Arthrtis Rheum* 1999 Apr; 42(4):599–608.
9. Appenzeller S, Cendes F, Costallat LT. Acute psychosis in systemic lupus erythematosus. Rheumatol Int. 2008 Jan; 28(3):237–243.

10. Fujii D, Ahmd I. Characteristics of psychotic disorder due to traumatic brain injury: an analysis of case studies in the literature. *J Neuropsychiatry Clin Neurosci* (2002) Spring; 14:130–40.

11. Sachdev P, Smith JS, Cathcart S. Schizophrenia like psychosis following traumatic brain injury: an analysis of case studies in the literature. *Psychol Med* 2001 Feb; 31(2):231–9.

12. Mental Health Act 1983. <http://www.legislation.gov.uk/ukpga/1983/20/section/136>

13. Jones SL, Mason T. Quality of treatment following police detention of mentally disordered offenders. *J Psychiatr Ment Health Nurs* 2002 (Feb); 9(1):73–80.

14. Royal College of Psychiatrists College Report CR 149. Standards on the use of section 136 of the Mental Health Act 1983 (England and Wales), 2011. <http://www.rcpsych.ac.uk/default.aspx?page=9768>

15. A criminal use of police cells? The use of police custody as a place of safety for people with mental health needs. HMIC, 2013. <http://www.hmic.gov.uk/media/a-criminal-use-of-police-cells-20130620.pdf>

16. National Institute for Health and Care Excellence. Violence. The short-term management of disturbed/violent behaviour in in-patient psychiatric settings and emergency departments. CG25. London: National Institute for Health and Care Excellence, 2005.

17. <http://www.sia.homeoffice.gov.uk/Pages/training.aspx>

18. <http://www.ipcc.gov.uk/en/Pages/deathscustodystudy.aspx>

19. Mental Capacity Act (2205). <http://www.legislation.gov.uk/ukpga/2005/9/contents>

20. Pratt JP, Chandler-Oatts J, Nelstrop L, *et al*. Establishing gold standard approaches to rapid tranquilisation: A review and discussion of the evidence of the safety and efficacy of medications currently used. *J of Psychiatr Intensive Care* (2008); 4:43–57.

21. Szpakowicz, M, Herd, A. 'Medically Cleared': How well are patients with psychiatric presentations examined by emergency physicians? *J Emerg Med* 2008; 35(4):369–72.

22. Amin M, Wang J. Routine laboratory testing to evaluate for medical illness in psychiatric patients in the Emergency Department is largely unrevealing. *West J Emerg Med* 2009 May; 10(2):97–100.

23. Janiak BD, Atteberry S. Medical clearance of the psychiatric patient in the emergency department. *J Emerg Med* 2012 Nov; 43(5):866–70.

24. Hennenman, PL, Mendoza, R, Lewis, RJ. Prospective evaluation of emergency department medical clearance. *Ann Emerg Med* 1994; 24(4):672–7.

25. Royal Childrens Hospital Melbourne code grey protocol for person restraint. <http://www.rch.org.au/clinicalguide/guideline_index/Emergency_Restraint_and_Sedation_Code_Grey/>

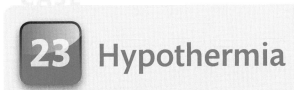

23 Hypothermia

Sarah Finlay and Sam Thenabadu

Expert commentary André Vercueil

Case history

An unkempt middle-aged man approximately in his mid-40s is brought by the paramedics to your resuscitation room on a cold and frosty December night. The paramedics report that they were called by a passer-by who noticed the man lying on an icy pavement and had feared that he was 'dead'. The ED nurse in charge immediately recognizes the patient as a regular attender with a long history of alcohol excess and of no fixed abode.

On arrival he is dressed in multiple layers of cold, wet, and dirty clothing. He smells mildly of alcohol and has signs of vomit on his attire. A search of his pockets reveals an empty can of strong-strength lager but no evidence of illicit drugs.

Immediate examination reveals that he has a patent airway with no obvious head or neck injury. Respiratory examination is grossly normal although saturations cannot be demonstrated due to his cold peripheries but of concern to the team is a cardiovascular examination showing a heart rate of 38 beats per minute and a BP of 82/40mmHg. His GCS is only a maximum of 10 (E-2, V-3, M-5) with sluggish but reactive pupils. A rapid secondary survey shows no signs of trauma. He feels very cold but the paramedics were unable to record a body temperature at scene with their portable thermometer and initial attempts in the ED fail to pick up a temperature.

See Box 23.1 for a clinical summary of hypothermia.

Box 23.1 Clinical summary of hypothermia

Hypothermia is defined as a core body temperature of less than 35 °C. It is categorized as mild (32–35 °C), moderate (30–32 °C) and severe (less than 30 °C).

Primary hypothermia is due to environmental exposure. Secondary hypothermia is due to a medical pathology lowering the body's temperature set point. In moderate to severe hypothermia, normal physiological thermogenesis progressively fails and cerebral and cardiac dysfunction ensues.

The mainstay of treatment is re-warming. Remember the old adage when treating the hypothermic patient in cardiac arrest: 'You're not dead until you're warm and dead'.

Therapeutic hypothermia now plays a role in intra-surgical procedures as well as in the care of the post-resuscitation patient.

The Swiss staging system[1] is frequently utilized in wilderness and rescue medicine. It is used at the scene (most often post avalanche-related accidents although applicable to any hypothermic patient) to describe the clinical state of the patient:

1. Patient is shivering but conscious
2. Patient has impaired consciousness and is no longer shivering

3. Patient is unconscious
4. Patient is not breathing
5. Patient has died due to irreversible hypothermia

✪ Learning point Temperature measurement in the hypothermic patient

To measure temperature in the hypothermic patient accurately, a low-reading thermometer is required.

Various methods of testing temperature are available in most EDs:

- Tympanic: this is readily available, but may be inaccurate when the ambient temperature is low or there is no flow in the carotid artery (as in the case of cardiac arrest).[2] These readings do not provide a good seal to the external acoustic meatus, and may in fact give falsely low readings.
- Axillary, rectal, and bladder temperature probes–more accurate than tympanic readings.
- Oesophageal: the temperature of the heart is closely correlated with the temperature in the lower third of the oesophagus.[2]

---

❻ Expert comment

The advantage of the Swiss staging system is that it does not require specialist low-reading thermometers, and it allows rapid triage of the patient.

Stage 1 patients can successfully be managed with simple interventions (warm environment, warm sweet drinks, and active movement).

Stage 2 patients require transfer to hospital for close monitoring for arrhythmia, but can be re-warmed using minimally invasive means (warm environment; chemical, electrical, or forced-air heating packs or blankets; warm parenteral fluids).

Stage 3 patients require treatment as for stage 2, but also require securing of the airway, and consideration of transfer to a specialist centre for CPB (cardiopulmonary bypass) or ECMO (extra-corporeal membrane oxygenation) for patients with cardiovascular instability.

Stage 4 patients require treatment as for stages 2 and 3, but with the addition of ongoing CPR and up to 3 doses of epinephrine and defibrillation. Active re-warming with CPB or ECMO is recommended, although alternative methods of internal re-warming should be instituted if this is not available. If successful, transfer to an intensive therapy unit (ITU) for ongoing management of organ failure if indicated.

Diagnosis

To diagnose hypothermia, an accurate body temperature measurement is required, thus the use of the correct equipment is paramount. It is important to remember that hypothermia may develop even in temperate climates, particularly in vulnerable groups such as the immobile and those at the extremes of age, as well as in patients exposed to wet or windy conditions.

It is also crucial not to miss other factors that may have contributed to the patient's clinical condition. In many cases such as in this scenario, the patient may have been drinking alcohol, ingested illicit drugs, taken a deliberate drug overdose, be hypoglycaemic, or had an acute myocardial or neurological event which has caused him to collapse on the pavement in cold weather; the possibilities are endless. In addition, the patient may be a victim of trauma, and precautions (e.g. c-spine control) should be taken if this is suspected. The patient should have necessary investigations to rule out any factors contributing to his hypothermia before being diagnosed with hypothermia alone.

Case progression

A temperature reading from a specific 'low-reading' tympanic temperature probe now shows his temperature to be only 28 °C.

A portable chest X-ray is ordered and the team debate whether a CT head is required now or after a period of resuscitation as no overt head injury can be seen. The ED team are also concerned that the rhythm strip on the resuscitation monitor appears to be irregular with ectopic beats and have performed a 12-lead ECG (see Figure 23.1).

Deep accidental hypothermia
QRS: 160ms, QT: 750ms

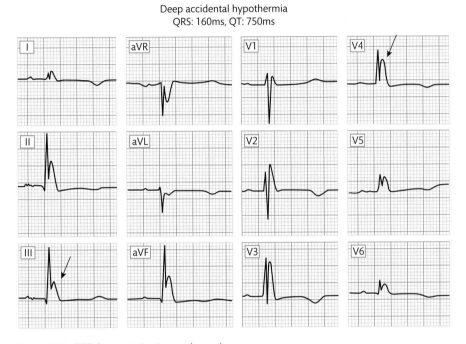

Figure 23.1 ECG demonstrating J waves (arrows).

Reproduced from AJ Camm *et al.*, *The ESC Textbook of Cardiovascular Medicine*, 2009, Figure 2.57, page 68, by permission of Oxford University Press on behalf of the European Society of Cardiology.

⊗ **Learning point** ECG changes in hypothermia

Multiple ECG changes are possible with the hypothermic patient.[3] The classic textbook finding of the 'Osborn' or J wave is, however, not always seen and a spectrum of ECG changes must be considered such as those listed here. Re-warming arrhythmias are also common.

- Sinus bradycardia
- Slow AF
- Prolonged QRS complex
- J waves (illustration) because of delayed cardiac repolarisation
- ST segment changes akin to ischaemia or infarction
- The hypothermic heart's function becomes progressively impaired with time and temperature fall, and the changes above can deteriorate in to VF then asystole

Data from Mattu A , Brady WJ, Perron AD. Electrocardiographic Manifestations of Hypothermia *Am J Emerg Med.* 2002; 20:314–326.

ⓕ Expert comment

Heat is lost through convection, evaporation, transduction, and conduction. Your aim is to minimize the possibility of further heat loss through these mechanisms, and warm the patient. First, remember to remove wet clothing and dry the patient if necessary. The ambient temperature should ideally be warm, with drafts minimized.

Re-warming can then commence, which may be active or passive.

Passive re-warming is suitable for cases of mild hypothermia. Warmed blankets are placed around the patient's head and body.

Active re-warming is more appropriate for cases of moderate or severe hypothermia.

Options include forced-air re-warming (by use of a Bair hugger), warmed IV fluids, warmed humidified air (via endotracheal tube if patient intubated), and infusion of warmed fluid into body cavities (peritoneum, pleural space, or bladder). Extracorporeal warming is also effective.[4]

Your junior doctors are aware that careful re-warming is necessary; having never seen a patient with a temperature this low they are now concerned whether active or passive re-warming is required and are unsure in which clinical setting this should occur in.

Clinical question: What are the most effective re-warming strategies in the hypothermic patient in the ED?

✓ Summary of evidence

Van de Ploeg et al. (2010) conducted a retrospective review of re-warming techniques used in 84 patients admitted to the ED with a core body temperature of less than 35 °C.[5] A variety of re-warming methods were used, and a variety of re-warming speeds. Whilst the power of the study was poor as numbers were low, no real difference was seen in outcome depending on the method used. The authors comment that controversy surrounding the best re-warming method remains, and note that controlled clinical trials looking into this are limited.

Danzi et al. (1989) performed a multivariate analysis of existing clinical data looking at different re-warming techniques but showed no significant difference in outcome dependent on the methods used.[6]

Extracorporeal blood re-warming in the form of CPB is now often cited as the ideal method of re-warming. **Walpoth et al. (1997)**[7] carried out a retrospective case series of 234 patients admitted with hypothermia, of whom 46 patients had a core temperature of less than 28 °C and circulatory arrest. In 32 of these 46, re-warming with cardiopulmonary bypass was attempted. 15 of these survived long term with no long-term disability attributable to hypothermia, leading the authors to conclude that this was indeed an effective re-warming strategy.

In 2010, a retrospective series by **Suominen et al. (2010)** of 9 drowned hypothermic paediatric patients admitted with severe hypothermia, all were re-warmed successfully with CPB; however, long-term outcome was not as favourable, with only one long-term survivor who sustained neurological deficit. Numbers were small and this was a drowned population, therefore less applicable.[8]

Coskun et al. (2010) demonstrated slightly better results in a case series of 13 children with core temperatures between 20 °C and 29 °C. When warmed by ECC, 11 regained spontaneous circulation and 5 survived to discharge, 2 of whom sustained no neurological complication.[9] Further case studies include a patient with a core body temperature of 13.7 °C was successfully resuscitated in this way,[10] as was an avalanche victim who was in cardiopulmonary arrest having been completely buried 3.0 m deep in snow for 100 minutes.[11]

(continued)

The recently developed 'Bernese Hypothermia Algorithm' draws in experience of treating avalanche victims and evidence in favour of early ECC. This suggests that patients with severe hypothermia should be taken to the operating theatre early, bypassing the ED, so ECC can be commenced as soon as possible.[12] A large retrospective study from Japan showed that in cases of stage 3 and 4 hypothermia, patients randomized to ECMO re-warming in the ED did significantly better than those re-warmed using conventional heating blanket and invasive warming measures (warmed IV fluids, warmed bladder, and gastric cavity irrigation). Re-warming was more rapid, with significantly fewer malignant arrhythmias, and also significantly improved Glasgow Outcome Scores (GOS) and survival benefit. A possible explanation for this may be the ongoing circulatory and respiratory support that can be provided using ECMO.[13]

Haemodialysis has also been used successfully as a re-warming technique[14] with a case of CVVH (continuous veno-venous filtration) being used to successfully warm a patient who was in cardiac arrest for 5 hours.[15] Warm pleurodesis has been successfully used,[16] as has thoracotomy for thoracic lavage.[17] This may be of use if ECW is unavailable. A case series by Plaiser (2010) of 14 patients who had thoracic lavage reinforced this message by showing a mean re-warming rate of 2.95 °C per hour and survival in 10, 8 of whom had normal neurology.[18]

Despite the variable success of these invasive measures, the benefit of non-invasive techniques should also not be underestimated. This is illustrated by Fisher (2011) with a case of a 2-year-old boy with a temperature of less than 20 °C who was successfully resuscitated using external techniques alone.[19]

Answer

Extracorporeal warming has shown to be effective in profound hypothermia. Non-invasive techniques have also, however, demonstrated good results and resource limitations should dictate that these basic methods should always be instigated in the first instance.

Case progression

As you are preparing to warm the patient, he becomes completely unresponsive and the alarms sound demonstrating that he has gone into VF. His core temperature reading still remains at 28 °C and you commence advanced life support.

✔ Evidence base Temperature cut-off levels and treatments

Animal studies in the most lead the way in our understanding of drugs in cardiac arrest. Studies looking at pigs noted the inefficacy of vasopressors in hypothermic cardiac arrest[21,22]—hence the guideline to administer drugs only at a core body temperature of greater than 30 °C. Another study looked at pigs in hypothermic cardiac arrest to note the automaticity of their heart at various temperatures.[23] At temperatures below 30 °C, the hearts were highly arrhythmogenic. In light of these findings, a temperature of 30 °C or above to start regular defibrillation has been recommended.

⊕ Clinical tip Changes to the ALS algorithm in hypothermia

Hypothermia remains a crucial 'H' of the Hs & Ts to exclude in cardiac arrest.

According to the new Resuscitation guidelines, in hypothermic cardiac arrest:[20]

- Only administer drugs once the core temperature has reached 30 °C. Then give them at double intervals (i.e. every 4 cycles, not every 2 cycles) until the temperature reaches 35 °C. Then proceed as normal.
- Below 30 °C, if the patient is in a shockable rhythm, only attempt defibrillation 3 times. If that is ineffective, delay further attempts until the core temperature is above 30 °C.

Data from Resuscitation Council UK. Advanced Life Support. 2011.

Case progression

Resuscitation has been continuing now for nearly 20 minutes. Your junior doctor astutely notes that the patient's pupils are fixed and dilated (without any atropine having been administered) and wonders why you are continuing despite this, as all previous cardiac arrests he has been involved in have stopped at approximately this duration. You wonder about prognostic indicators in cardiac arrest. You have heard the saying 'not dead until warm and dead' and wonder how long you should continue to attempt resuscitation.

> **❻ Expert comment**
>
> In the severely hypothermic patient, fixed dilated pupils may be seen and in this context are NOT an indication of brainstem death—hypothermia precludes the diagnosis of brainstem death.
>
> There is a risk that patients are wrongly diagnosed as dead when they are hypothermic. A case of a man whose temperature has been described 26.6 °C, who had falsely been diagnosed as dead on scene by fire services, but subsequently managed according to ALS principles with defibrillation for VF arrest. There was a delay to hospital and treatment of 4 hours; however, the patient survived to discharge with only mild neurological sequelae.[23]

Clinical question: In the patient with cardio-respiratory arrest secondary to hypothermia, how long should resuscitation continue?

The question of how long to continue any cardiac arrest is an important one, but especially challenging in the hypothermic cardiac arrest. As one of the 8 ALS 'reversible causes', logic would imply that until the temperature rose above 35 °C and thus hypothermia was excluded as the precipitant for cardiac arrest, full resuscitation should be performed. ALS quotes 'no-one is dead unless warm and dead', and suggests that senior doctors and clinical judgement should be used to decide when in fact to cease resuscitation.[19]

> **✔ Evidence base**   Timescales for continuing resuscitative efforts
>
> State of Alaska guidelines[25] state: '[a]ssume that the hypothermic patient can be resuscitated even if they appear to be beyond help because of skin colour, pupil dilation, and depressed vital signs. Patients suffering from severe hypothermia have been resuscitated. It is also wise to be cautious about what is said during the resuscitation. Seemingly unconscious patients frequently remember what was said and done.'
>
> Hypothermia has the effect of slowing metabolism, increasing the time for which the brain can tolerate ischaemia, and reducing oxygen consumption.[7]
>
> A case report of a patient in Spain who survived after 3 hours of CPR with external re-warming including warm IV fluids and gastric lavage, but no ECC, suggests that even in situations where only simpler methods of re-warming are available, survival after prolonged CPR is possible.[26]
>
> A case reports survival after 4 hours of CPR with extracorporeal warming.[27] Another case reports survival after 385 minutes of resuscitation.[28] A patient with a temperature of 22.0 °C survived after 90 minutes of CPR using a Lukas device.[29] One extreme case reports survival and good neurological recovery despite an initial temperature of 13.730 °C and 9 hours of CPR.[10]

Answer

There is increasing evidence that patients can have good neurological outcomes following even prolonged periods of resuscitation while re-warming. This is less likely if hypothermia was preceded by a hypoxic event, or if there is severe associated trauma or underlying comorbidity.

Case progression

You remind your junior doctors that hypothermia can cause dilated pupils, and that prolonged resuscitation may be necessary. Your team continues CPR.

You are presented with a blood gas result: it shows a pH of 7.01 and a profound metabolic acidosis of HCO3 8 mmol/L and base deficit of −19 mmol/L. You are aware that warming the patient whilst doing CPR will take time and resources and you wonder whether that low pH can be taken as a prognostic indicator that resuscitation will be unsuccessful.

Clinical question: What prognostic indicators can be used to guide decisions regarding resuscitation in hypothermic cardiac arrest?

> ✓ **Evidence base** Prognostic indicators in cardiac arrest
>
> **Hauty et al. (1987)** published a case series looking at victims of the May 1986 Mt Hood climbing disaster[30] (climbers from a school expedition were trapped by a blizzard, 9 died). Results from 10 severely hypothermic patients (of which there were 2 survivors) are presented. Indicators of a poor prognosis included factors from the history, including comorbidities, duration of exposure, initial low core temperature, abnormal heart rate and rhythm, altered mental status, and low pO_2. Laboratory markers of poor prognosis included severe hyperkalaemia and raised serum ammonium (indicating cell death), and high fibrinogen (suggesting intravascular thrombosis).
>
> **Silfvast et al. (2003)** conducted a 10-year retrospective chart review of 75 patients, 23 of whom were in cardiac arrest, which showed that of the 23 in cardiac arrest, the survival of 22 could be predicted based on a high serum potassium and pCO_2.[31] Other poor prognostic indicators were a low pH and increasing age. The authors summarize that more work needs to be done on the possibility of K and pH being used as prognostic indicators in hypothermic arrest.
>
> **Mair et al. (1994)** conducted a retrospective study of 22 patients with severe hypothermia to determine whether outcome in severe hypothermia could be predicted from serum investigations on admission.[32] Their data suggest that patients with a potassium of greater the 9 mmol/L, a pH of less than 6.5 or an activated clotting time of greater than 400 seconds were useful in predicting death in avalanche victims (where death was likely to precede cooling), but for situations where cooling is likely to precede death (e.g. cold-water submersion or prolonged exposure to cold), these were only of limited prognostic value. Their conclusions were that 'a decision to continue or terminate resuscitation cannot be based on laboratory parameters'.
>
> **Wolleneck et al.'s (2002)** description of a cohort study of 12 paediatric patients also emphasised this point:[33] the lowest recorded pH in a survivor was 6.29 and the lowest base excess −36.5. This study also concluded that initial serum potassium could also not be used as an indicator of prognosis.

Answer

No single parameter or constellation of features can be considered prognostic in outcome from a hypothermic arrest and as such each resuscitation attempt must be dealt with on its individual merits. A recent review of the evidence suggests that a Potassium level >12 mmol per litre may represent a cut-off above which CPR is considered futile, and discussion with the CPB or ECMO team when the level is between 10–12 mmol per litre.[34]

Case progression

Your team agrees that a pH of 7.01 should not be used as an indicator of poor prognosis and thus continues with CPR and active re-warming. The patient continues to be in VF and, as per ALS guidance, receives 3 shocks below the temperature of 30 °C, then shocks every 2 minutes and drugs every 8 minutes (as his core temperature is between 30 °C and 35 °C). He has return of spontaneous circulation after 50 minutes of resuscitation, with a core temperature of 33.5 °C. Post-resuscitation care ensues and despite the long period of resuscitation his blood pressure and heart rate are relatively stable at 90 systolic and 50 beats per minute in sinus rhythm and as such he is transferred to the ICU.

See Box 23.2 for future advances in the field.

Box 23.2 Future advances

It remains unclear which method of ECR is the most appropriate, and prospective studies randomizing patients with cardiac arrest to either CPB or ECMO are required. The increasing availability and safety of ECMO, as well as the possibility of medium to long-term support of ongoing organ failure following successful resuscitation, means that these trials are unlikely to be performed. Also uncertain is the optimal treatment modality for patients with stage 3 hypothermia, who have not yet suffered cardiac arrest—prospective studies comparing minimally invasive active re-warming with ECMO may help to answer this question. Information can also be gathered from Hypothermia Registries, and may help to inform future treatment strategies.

A Final Word from the Expert

The development and increasing availability of re-warming techniques continue to improve the outcome of patients admitted to the ED with hypothermia. A greater understanding of the most appropriate approach to re-warming, based on the clinical situation, means that cardiovascularly stable patients may be successfully treated with a combination of external and minimally invasive internal re-warming. Should the patient be cardiovascularly unstable, or have suffered cardiac arrest secondary to hypothermia, consideration should be given to transferring the patient to a specialist centre for CPB or ECMO. Prolonged CPR is indicated in such cases, and even if ECR is not available, minimally invasive active re-warming may result in a good clinical outcome. Therapeutic nihilism should be avoided, though if hypothermia was preceded by a hypoxic event, the outcome may be more guarded.

References

1. Davis PR, Byers M. Accidental Hypothermia. *J R Army Med Corps* 2006; (152):223–33.
2. Deakin CD, Nolan JP, Soar J, *et al.* European Resuscitation Council Guidelines for Resuscitation, Section 4. *Resuscitation* 2010; 10(81):1305–52.

3. Mattu A, Brady WJ, Perron AD. Electrocardiographic Manifestations of Hypothermia *Am J Emerg Med* 2002; 20:314–26.

4. Epstein E, Kiran A. Accidental Hypothermia. *BMJ* 2006; 332(7543):706–9.

5. Van der Ploeg G-J, Goslings JC, Walpoth BH, *et al.* Accidental hypothermia: Rewarming treatments, complications and outcomes from one university medical centre. *Resuscitation* 2010 Nov; 81(11):1550–5.

6. Danzl DF, Hedges JR, Pozos RS. Hypothermia outcome score: development and implications. *Crit Care Med* 1989 Mar; 17(13):227–31.

7. Walpoth BH, Walpoth-Aslan BN, Mattle HP, *et al.* Outcome of Survivors of Accidental Deep Hypothermia and Circulatory Arrest Treated with Extracorporeal Blood Warming. *N Engl J Med* 1997 Nov 20;337(21):1500–5.

8. Suominen PK, Vallila NH, Hartikainen LM, *et al.* Outcome of drowned hypothermic children with cardiac arrest treated with cardiopulmonary bypass. *Acta Anaesth Scand* 2010; 54(10):1276–81.

9. Coskun KO, Popov AF, Schmitto JD, *et al.* Extracorporeal Circulation for Rewarming in Drowning and Near-Drowning Pediatric Patients. *Artificial Organs* 2010; 34(11):1026–30.

10. Gilbert M, Busund R, Skagseth A, *et al.* Resuscitation from accidental hypothermia of 13.7 degrees C with circulatory arrest. *Lancet* 2000 29 Jan; (355):375–6.

11. Oberhammer R, Beikircher W, Ârmann C, *et al.* Full recovery of an avalanche victim with profound hypothermia and prolonged cardiac arrest treated by extracorporeal rewarming. *Resuscitation* 2008; 76(3):474–80.

12. Brodmann Maeder M, Martin D, Balthasar E, *et al.* The Bernese Hypothermia Algorithm: A consensus paper on in-hospital decision-making and treatment of patients in hypothermic cardiac arrest at an alpine level 1 trauma centre. *Injury* 2011; 42(5):539–43.

13. Morita S, Inokuchi S, Yamagiwa T, *et al.* Efficacy of portable and percutaneous cardiopulmonary bypass rewarming versus that of conventional internal rewarming for patients with accidental deep hypothermia. *Crit Care Med* 2011; 39(5):1064–8.

14. Sultan N, Theakston KD, Butler R, *et al.* Treatment of severe accidental hypothermia with intermittent hemodialysis. *CJEM* 2009 Mar; 11(2):174–7.

15. Alfonzo A, Lomas A, Drummond I, *et al.* Survival after 5-h resuscitation attempt for hypothermic cardiac arrest using CVVH for extracorporeal rewarming. *Nephrology Dialysis Transplantation* 2009; 24(3):1054–6.

16. Hall KN, Syverud SA. Closed thoracic cavity lavage in the treatment of severe hypothermia in human beings. *Ann Emerg Med* 1990; 19(2):204–6.

17. Tamminen O, Tiukka T. Thoracic cavity lavage in the resuscitation of the severely hypothermic patient. *Duodecim* 1990; 106(17):1224–7.

18. Plaisier BR. Thoracic lavage in accidental hypothermia with cardiac arrest--report of a case and review of the literature. *Resuscitation* 2005 Jul; 66(1):99–104.

19. Fisher JD, Schaefer C, Reeves JJ. Successful Resuscitation From Cardiopulmonary Arrest Due to Profound Hypothermia Using Noninvasive Techniques. *Pediatr Emerg Care* 2011; 27(3):215–7.

20. Resuscitation Council UK. Advanced Life Support. 2011.

21. Krismer AC, Lindner KH, Kornberger R, *et al.* Cardiopulmonary Resuscitation During Severe Hypothermia in Pigs: Does Epinephrine or Vasopressin Increase Coronary Perfusion Pressure? *Anesth Analg* 2000 Jan 1;90(1):69.

22. Kornberger E, Lindner KH, Mayr VD, *et al.* Effects of epinephrine in a pig model of hypothermic cardiac arrest and closed-chest cardiopulmonary resuscitation combined with active rewarming. *Resuscitation* 2001 Sep; 50(3):301–8.

23. Ujhelyi MR, Sims JJ, Dubin SA, *et al.* Defibrillation energy requirements and electrical heterogeneity during total body hypothermia. *Crit Care Med* 2001; 29(5):1006–11.

24. Lee CH, Van Gelder C, Burns K, *et al.* Advanced Cardiac Life Support and Defibrillation in Severe Hypothermic Cardiac Arrest. *Prehosp Emerg Care* 2009 Jan 1;13(1):85–9.

25. State of Alaska Cold Injuries Guidelines, Alaska Multi-level. 2003 Version. <http://www.chems.alaska.gov>

26. Kot P, Botella J. Cardiac arrest due to accidental hypothermia and prolonged cardiopulmonary resuscitation. *Medicina Intensiva* 2010; 34:567–70.

27. Masaki F, Isao T, Seiji H, *et al.* Revival From Deep Hypothermia After 4 Hours of Cardiac Arrest Without the Use of Extracorporeal Circulation. *J Trauma Acute Care Surg* 2009; 67(5):E173–6.

28. Hagiwara S, Yamada T, Furukawa K, *et al.* Survival after 385min of cardiopulmonary resuscitation with extracorporeal membrane oxygenation and rewarming with haemodialysis for hypothermic cardiac arrest. *Resuscitation* 2011; 82[6]:790–1.

29. HolmstrÂm P, Boyd J, Sorsa M, *et al.* A case of hypothermic cardiac arrest treated with an external chest compression device (LUCAS) during transport to re-warming. *Resuscitation* 2005; 67[1]:139–41.

30. Hauty MG, Esrig BC, Hill JG, *et al.* Prognostic factors in severe accidental hypothermia: experience from the Mt. Hood tragedy. *J Trauma* 1987 Oct; 27(10):1107–12.

31. Silfvast T, Pettiloñ V. Outcome from severe accidental hypothermia in Southern FinlandGÇöa 10-year review. *Resuscitation* 2003; 59[3]:285–90.

32. Mair P, Kornberger E, Furtwaengler W, *et al.* Prognostic markers in patients with severe accidental hypothermia and cardiocirculatory arrest. *Resuscitation* 1994 Jan; 27(1):47–54.

33. Wollenek G, Honarwar N, Golej J, *et al.* Cold water submersion and cardiac arrest in treatment of severe hypothermia with cardiopulmonary bypass. *Resuscitation* 2002; 52[3]:255–63.

34. Brown DJ, Brugger H, Boyd J, *et al.* Accidental Hypothermia. *N Engl J Med* 2012 Nov 15; 367(20):1930–8.

24 'Cocaine chest pain'

Gavin Wilson

ⓘ **Expert commentary** Geoff Hinchley

Case history

A 22-year-old Caucasian male presents to the ED at 6 a.m. on a Sunday morning having been brought in by ambulance from a nightclub. He complains of a 1-hour history of central chest pain that radiates to his left arm. The pain is severe and the patient complains of shortness of breath as well as appearing sweaty and mildly agitated. You note that he has widely dilated pupils.

He has no significant medical history to note, although he does admit to smoking 15 cigarettes per day. There is no familial history of cardiac disease and he is not taking any prescribed medications.

On further questioning, he admits to recreational cocaine use at weekends and occasional cannabis use during the week. He prefers to take cocaine intranasally and he states that he had taken '2 or 3 lines' in the hour preceding the onset of chest pain. He denies taking any other illicit drugs and cannot reliably recall how much alcohol he has had to drink.

On arrival, he is hypertensive with a blood pressure of 205/115 mmHg and tachycardic at a rate of 110/min. He is saturating 100 % on air and has a respiratory rate of 22/min. An initial ECG demonstrates a sinus tachycardia with non-specific ST changes (see Figure 24.1).

See Box 24.1 for a clinical summary of cocaine-induced chest pain.

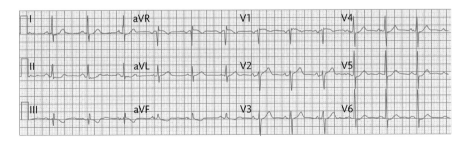

Figure 24.1 ECG with ST depression.

Reproduced from R Rajendram *et al.*, *Oxford Case Histories in Cardiology*, 2011, Figure 7.1, page 47, with permission from Oxford University Press.

Box 24.1 Clinical summary of cocaine-induced chest pain

- Cocaine is now one of the most abused drugs in western countries. Cocaine hydrochloride is a white powder that is highly water-soluble and is readily absorbed across mucous membranes. It is often taken via the intranasal route, although it may be injected intravenously.

- The free-base form, which includes the variant 'crack' cocaine, is typically smoked as it becomes volatile at considerably lower temperatures and is resistant to heat degradation.[1]
- Cocaine has similar stimulant effects to amphetamines and acts to increase the levels of adrenaline, noradrenaline, dopamine, and serotonin. As a result, it produces a sympathomimetic toxidrome in overdose but serotonin syndrome may also occur.
- The toxic dose of cocaine will depend on a number of factors including individual tolerance, route of administration, purity, and the presence of other drugs.[1] As an approximate estimate, a 'line of cocaine' contains 20–30 mg. Ingestion of 1 g or more is potentially lethal.[2–4]
- An abnormal ECG has been reported in 56–84% of patients with cocaine-associated chest pain.
- Evaluation of cocaine chest pain is similar to classic ACS, however treatment options will differ.

⊕ Clinical tip ECG changes associated with cocaine use

Acute cocaine ingestion[1,3,5]

- Sinus tachycardia, supraventricular tachycardia, ventricular tachycardia, and ventricular fibrillation
- ECG changes consistent with either myocardial ischaemia or infarction
- Prolongation of PR, QRS, and QTc intervals
- Brugada-type pattern may also occur

ECG change associated with chronic cocaine ingestion:[6] Prolongation of QTc interval which tends to reduce after a period of abstinence.

⏶ Expert comment

Emergency department staff should understand the legal framework governing the possession of, and potential to supply illegal drugs.

Where a patient is found to be in possession of an illegal drug, he or she should be advised that possession is unlawful and asked to hand it over voluntarily to a member of clinical staff, who should then contact the police? When the patient is unconscious, any suspicious or illegal substance should be removed and this should be recorded in the patient's notes.

Any illegal drugs should be placed in a sealed container that must be placed immediately in the Controlled Drug cupboard until a hospital pharmacist can safely collect it, and this should be witnessed and documented. The pharmacy department will then liaise with the local police, who will determine whether the drug should be destroyed or transferred to police care. The movement of the drugs must be clearly documented to ensure that the chain of evidence can be maintained. Medical staff in England, are also expected to notify cases of drug misuse that generates a treatment demand, to the National Drug Treatment Monitoring System (NDTMS) whose contact details can be found in the British National Formulary.

Clinical question: In patients presenting with cocaine induced chest pain, is GTN or a benzodiazepine more effective in relieving the symptoms of chest pain?

Unlike patients presenting with acute coronary syndrome, benzodiazepines in addition to nitrates are recommended as first-line agents in managing chest pain following cocaine use.[7] Benzodiazepines are thought to work by reducing the sympathetic response to cocaine and hence indirectly reduce myocardial oxygen demand.[7–13] Additionally, benzodiazepines may cause coronary vasodilation by the selective potentiation of A2A-adenosine receptors.[15] While there are a number of animal studies to support benzodiazepine use,[11–14] prospective control trials in humans have been more limited.

The evidence that nitrates improve coronary artery spasm in cocaine-induced chest pain in human subjects is attributed to a single cardiac catheterization study in patients pre-medicated with 5–10mg oral diazepam.[16] In this study, Brogan *et al.* randomized 23 patients who were undergoing cardiac catheterization for the evaluation of chest pain to receive either intranasal saline placebo (control group containing 8 patients) or 2mg/kg of intranasal cocaine administered in a 10 % solution (15 patients). Nine patients from the intervention group and 6 patients from the control group subsequently received sublingual glyceryl trinitrate (GTN). The study, although small, demonstrated that GTN was effective in relieving cocaine induced coronary artery vasoconstriction. Interestingly, the magnitude of cocaine induced vasoconstriction was greatest in segments of artery affected by atherosclerotic disease, an effect which has been demonstrated in other studies.[17] Relief of cocaine-induced chest pain in the clinical setting has been shown in only two randomised control trials,[9,10] and a single case series which demonstrated a beneficial effect in 49 % of patients given GTN (95 % CI, 38–60 %).[18] See Table 24.1.

> **Evidence base** Benzodiazepines versus nitrates
>
> Two papers were found to be relevant in addressing the question and these are outlined in Table 24.1. No further control trials or meta-analyses have been conducted since this initial review.

Table 24.1 Summary of evidence: benzodiazepines versus nitrates

Author, date, and country	Patient group	Study type	Outcomes	Key results	Weaknesses
Baumann B *et al.* (2000)[9]	40 patients, aged between 18–60 years, attending the ED with cocaine-induced chest pain All patients had taken cocaine within 24 hours (median 5 hr 37 mins) and had a history suggestive of IHD 3 Groups: diazepam alone (n = 12), GTN alone (n = 15), diazepam and GTN (n = 13)	Randomized, double-blind, placebo control trial	Pain score, chest pain severity, haemodynamic and cardiovascular performance	No difference in chest pain reduction, haemodynamic or cardiovascular performance when either agent was used alone or in combination Ischaemic ECG changes seen in 63 %, AMI in 7.5 % of patients No difference in final cardiological diagnosis in each group	Use of a convenience sample, failure to reach the minimum numbers in each group (n = 14) to achieve a power of 0.8
Honderick T *et al.* (2003)[10]	27 patients, aged between 18–45 years, attending the ED with chest pain and cocaine use over the preceding 72 hours. 2 Groups: GTN alone (n = 15) and GTN with lorazepam (n = 12) Recruitment stopped early due to significant statistical difference being seen in interim analysis	Randomised single blind placebo control trial	Pain score, chest pain severity	Mean chest pain scores were significantly lower in the group given both GTN and lorazepam [Chest pain at 5 minutes: difference in means = 1.24, 95 % CI 0.8–3.29, p = 0.02. Chest pain at 10 minutes: difference in means = 3.10, 95 % CI 1.22–4.98, p = 0.005]	Use of convenience sample, single blinded nature of the study introducing possible investigator bias, lack of lorazepam only arm, small sample size, patients with high-risk cardiovascular disease were excluded

Data from various sources (see references)

Expert comment

UK NPIS Toxbase advice is that cocaine causes coronary artery vasospasm and can precipitate infarction in some patients. If chest pain is not relieved with diazepam, aspirin, and nitrates, and there are ECG changes suggestive of myocardial infarction, conventional management should be followed to add in clopidogrel and low molecular weight heparin and to act according to local protocols for thrombolysis / primary angioplasty. Troponin I is a better marker of myocardial damage than other cardiac enzymes in cocaine-related myocardial infarction.

Answer

Both GTN and benzodiazepines appear to be equally effective when administered either alone or in combination. Given the evidence in animal models, benzodiazepines should be considered as the initial agent of choice if agitation or other sympathetic symptoms are present.

> **Learning point** Initial ED treatment strategies
>
> Coronary artery spasm and coronary artery thrombosis can result in myocardial infarction in the absence of coronary artery disease. As previously seen, cocaine-induced coronary spasm can be more severe in those segments of the coronary artery affected by atherosclerosis.
>
> Chest pain persisting after benzodiazepines and sublingual GTN should be treated with an intravenous infusion GTN in the first instance. Calcium channel antagonists such as verapamil should be considered as second line treatment if there is no evidence of myocardial infarction.[7]
>
> Aspirin should be given to all patients with cocaine-induced chest pain. At present, the American Heart Association (AHA)[7] recommends the early use of clopridogrel and a low molecular weight heparin in all high-risk patients (patients presenting with unstable angina, those patients diagnosed with acute ST elevation myocardial infarction, and those that are subsequently diagnosed with non-ST elevation myocardial infarction).

Case progression

Intravenous access is obtained and bloods are taken for urea, electrolytes, creatinine, liver function tests, troponin, and a clotting screen. The patient is initially given sublingual GTN with minimal effect, immediately followed by 300 mg aspirin orally and a total of 5 mg diazepam intravenously. The chest pain subsides after the benzodiazepines and sublingual GTN and the patient is considerably less agitated, but the does remains hypertensive with a blood pressure of 180/108 mmHg.

A repeat ECG demonstrates minimal ST segment depression in the infero-lateral leads. A chest radiograph is also performed which is essentially normal with no evidence of a pneumothorax.

In view of the ongoing hypertension and previous improvement in his clinical condition with nitrates, you commence a GTN infusion starting initially at 2 mg/hour. You consult with a senior colleague who suggests giving a calcium channel antagonist if the hypertension is not controlled with the GTN infusion. During the discussion, you consider whether β-blockers would be helpful in this situation given the new ECG changes.

> **Learning point** Pharmacokinetics of Cocaine.
>
> The half-life of cocaine is approximately 60–90 minutes. Cocaine is rapidly metabolized by hepatic esterases and plasma pseudocholinesterase. In the presence of alcohol, cocaine is trans-esterified to cocaethylene. This metabolite has similar pharmacological effects to cocaine itself and is generally more toxic with a longer half-life of 2.5 hours.[2]
>
> Cocaine and its derivatives are excreted in the urine within 100 minutes of its use. Urinary drug screen testing remains the quickest and most reliable way to test for recent cocaine use. Cocaine is usually detectable in the urine unchanged a few hours after the last dose, but the metabolites may be present up to 48 hours later.[8]

Clinical question: Is there a role for β-blockers in the acute management of cocaine-induced chest pain?

To evaluate this particular clinical question, it is necessary to consider the effects of β-blockers in two inter-related clinical circumstances; (1) in the setting of cocaine induced coronary artery vasoconstriction, and (2) cocaine induced systemic hypertension and tachycardia.

Part one: In the setting of cocaine induced coronary artery vasoconstriction.

The role of β-blockers in the management of cocaine-induced chest pain is controversial. β-blockers have been shown to decrease both mortality and morbidity in patients presenting with myocardial ischaemia and ST elevation myocardial infarction (STEMI).[19,20] Due to the potentiation of both α and β receptors by cocaine, it has been hypothesized that β-blockers should not be used acutely in patients with ST elevation (cocaine) myocardial infarction as this can potentially worsen coronary artery spasm. As a result, the latest AHA guidelines published in 2008 continue to stress that β-blockers should not be used in the acute management of cocaine-associated chest pain, unstable angina or myocardial infarction.[7] This recommendation is largely based on 2 studies produced in the early 1990s, 1 of which was performed on a cohort of canine subjects.[21]

Given the body of evidence (see Table 24.2) supporting the benefits of early β-blockade in patients presenting with acute coronary syndrome, is there any evidence to support a similar benefit in patients presenting with cocaine-induced chest pain?

Answer

Acute β-blocker use may actually reduce the incidence of myocardial infarction and may not be as harmful as initially feared. On current evidence, propranolol should be avoided acutely, but drugs like labetalol and carvedilol with both α and β adrenergic blocking activity may have a role although this needs to be evaluated further.

Part two: Cocaine induced systemic hypertension.

The use of β-blockers following recent cocaine use has also been cited to worsen systemic hypertension and tachycardia.[7,26,27] A retrospective case series of just 7 patients by Sand *et al.* in 1991 recommended that the routine use of esmolol be discontinued in patients presenting with cocaine-associated cardiotoxicity.[27] The main reason cited in the paper was a lack of consistent haemodynamic benefit despite the small sample size. As we have already seen in the previous section, there is some evidence emerging to indicate that β-blockers in the context of cocaine-induced coronary spasm may not be as harmful as previously thought and may actually be beneficial. In light of this, do β-blockers actually worsen systemic parameters when administered to patients with cocaine intoxication? See Table 24.3.

Table 24.2 Summary of evidence: β-blockers and cocaine induced coronary vasoconstriction

Author, date, and country	Patient group	Study type	Outcomes	Key results	Weaknesses
Boehrer JD et al. (1993)[22]	15 patients undergoing cardiac catheterization for the evaluation of chest pain. All patients were given intranasal cocaine, 2 mg/kg, and randomized to receive either intravenous saline ($n=6$) or intravenous labetalol 0.25 mg/kg ($n=9$) 15 minutes later	Randomized, single-blind, placebo control trial	Heart rate, MAP and coronary arterial area (measured by computer-assisted quantitative angiography)	Labetalol reduced MAP (from 117 ± 14 mm Hg after cocaine administration to 110 ± 11 mm Hg after labetalol, $p < 0.05$) There was no difference in the coronary artery cross-sectional area in either group after labetalol administration	Fixed dose of intranasal cocaine used; higher doses or other routes of administration not evaluated; small sample size used; randomization process not mentioned
Datillo PB et al. (2008)[23]	Cohort of 348 patients presenting with chest pain and positive urine test for cocaine. β-blockers were administered in 60 patients over the course of their admission (18 patients received β-blockers acutely in the ED)	Retrospective cohort study	Incidence of AMI, in-hospital mortality	The incidence of MI after administration of a β-blocker was significantly lower (6.1% versus 26.0%, difference in proportions 19.9%, 95% CI = 10.3–30.0%). Multivariate analysis demonstrated a reduced risk of myocardial infarction in patients treated with a β-blocker (odds ratio 0.06, 95% CI = 0.01–0.61)	Retrospective analysis (open to possible selection and investigator bias). Other possible confounders were accounted for in the statistical analysis
Lange RA et al. (1990)[24]	30 patients undergoing cardiac catheterization for the evaluation of chest pain. All patients were randomized to receive either intranasal saline ($n=15$) or 2 mg/kg intranasal cocaine ($n=15$). Patients from each group were then randomised to receive either 2 mg intracoronary propranolol or a saline push over 2 minutes	Randomized, double-blind, placebo control trial	Change in coronary blood flow and coronary vascular resistance	An additional decrease in coronary sinus blood flow seen in patients given both cocaine and propranolol (100 ± 14 ml/min, $p < 0.05$) and an increased coronary vascular resistance (1.20 ± 0.12 mm Hg/ml/min, $p < 0.05$)	Small sample size in each group
Rangel C et al. (2010)[25]	331 consecutive patients presenting with chest pain and positive urine toxicology test for cocaine. 46% received a β-blocker in the emergency department during their management (metoprolol was administered in 85% of cases)	Retrospective cohort study	Incidence of mortality, peak troponin level in first 24 hours, arrhythmias requiring defibrillation	No significant differences in either baseline ECG findings or subsequent ECG changes between those that received a β-blocker and those that did not. The proportions of positive troponins diagnostic for MI did not differ between the groups	History of cocaine use within 48 hours of presentation, wide variation of other drugs given which are potentially cardioprotective

Data from various sources (see references)

Table 24.3 Summary of evidence: β-blockers and cocaine-induced systemic hypertension and tachycardia

Author, date, and country	Patient group	Study type	Outcomes	Key results	Weaknesses
Hoskins MH et al. (2010)[28]	90 patients presenting to an emergency department with ACS and a positive urine drug screen for cocaine. Patients were randomized into 2 groups: oral labetalol (200 mg bd) plus standard ACS therapy (n=60) or oral diltiazem (240 mg daily) plus standard ACS therapy (n=30)	Prospective, single-blinded, randomised control trial	Blood pressure and heart rate at baseline and at 48 hours, cardiac enzymes	Both groups demonstrated a significant and equivalent decrease in both blood pressure and heart rate at 48 hours compared to baseline measurements Labetalol systolic blood pressure (1) baseline: 146.3±10.2 mmHg, (2) 48 hours: 133±7.2 mmHg, difference $p < 0.05$, diastolic blood pressure (1) baseline: 92.4±7.5 mmHg, (2) 48 hours: 79.4±7.0 mmHg, difference $p < 0.05$ There were no adverse events in the group receiving labetalol	Method of randomization suboptimal
Rangel C et al. (2010)[25]	331 consecutive patients presenting with chest pain and positive urine toxicology test for cocaine 46% received a β-blocker in the emergency department during their management. Overall, 65% received a β-blocker at some point during their hospitalization (metoprolol was administered in 85% of cases)	Retrospective cohort study Median follow-up 972 days	Incidence of mortality	After adjusting for potential confounders, patients that had received a β-blocker in the emergency department had a significantly lower blood pressure (mean reduction −8 mm Hg, IQR=−21–3 mm Hg, p=0.03). Patients discharged on a β-blocker had a significant reduction in cardiovascular death (hazard ratio 0.29, 95% CI=0.09–0.98, p=0.047)	History of cocaine use within 48 hours of presentation, wide variation of other drugs given which are potentially cardioprotective

Data from various sources (see references)

Answer

Selective β-blockers are associated with improved blood pressure control and may be associated with a reduced risk of cardiovascular death. It is reasonable to consider administering short-acting drugs with combined α- and β-blocking properties to patients following cocaine use that remain tachycardic and hypertensive following treatment with nitrates and benzodiazepines.

✪ Learning point Treatment of cocaine induced cardiac arrhythmias

Sinus tachycardia: parenteral diazepam

Supraventricular tachycardia: best treated with diazepam in the first instance. Intravenous verapamil (5–10 mg over 2–3 minutes) or adenosine (6–12 mg IV) can be used in those patients that are refractory to benzodiazepines, but these along with DC cardioversion my not be as effective as titrated doses of benzodiazepines. The United Kingdom National Poisons Information Service does not recommend the use of verapamil in the presence of pulmonary oedema or acute myocardial infarction.

Ventricular tachycardia: (See Figure 24.2) initially treat with intravenous 50–100 mmol sodium bicarbonate. If VT remains refractory to sodium bicarbonate and defibrillation, treat with intravenous lignocaine 1.5 mg/kg followed by an infusion of 2 mg min -1. Amiodarone is not as effective as it is a class 3 Vaughan William anti-arrhythmic.

Note: QRS widening can occur in acute cocaine toxicity due to the effect of cocaine on cardiac sodium channels. As a result, a broad complex tachycardia similar to that seen with a tricyclic antidepressant overdose may occur. Initial management is the same in both conditions: treat early by correcting the underlying metabolic acidosis with intravenous sodium bicarbonate and administer fluids.

Data from Nancy G, Murphy MD, Benowitz MD. Cocaine. In: Olson KR (Ed). *Poisoning and drug overdose*, Fifth Edition. San Francisco, CA: McGraw Hill, 2007, pp 170–3; Murray L, Cadogan M, Daly F, *et al.* Chapter 3.30: Cocaine. In: *Toxicology Handbook*, Second Edition. Sydney: Churchill Livingstone, 2011; Amin M, Gabelman G, Karpel J, Buttrick P. Acute myocardial infarction and chest pain syndromes after cocaine use. *Am J Cardiol* 1990; 66:1434–7.

Case progression

The hypertension is controlled with a GTN infusion and no further pharmacological intervention is required. The infusion rate of the GTN is reduced over the next 2 hours and repeat serial ECGs are performed which demonstrate normalization of

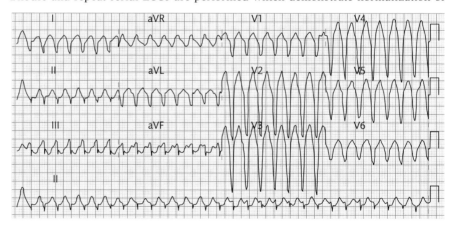

Figure 24.2 ECG of VT.

Reproduced from SG Myerson *et al., Emergencies in Cardiology, Second Edition*, 2010, Figure 21.35, page 421, with permission from Oxford University Press.

the ST segments. The patient does not complain of any further episodes of chest pain but a referral is made to the medical team for observations and ongoing management.

Clinical question: Do all patients attending with resolved cocaine-induced chest pain following treatment with benzodiazepines and nitrates require acute admission?

Dilemmas occur for the treating physician when the initial treatment in the ED of cocaine chest pain is effective and pain is abated and the ECG changes resolve. If vasospasm is the underlying mechanism and the initial drug therapies have worked, is there really a necessity to admit these patients and subject them to the same period of observation and follow up tests that would be performed in classic ACS? See Table 24.4.

Table 24.4 Admission versus discharge decision making

Author, date, and country	Patient group	Study type	Outcomes	Key results	Weaknesses
Amin, M et al. (1990)[31]	70 patients admitted with cocaine-induced chest pain	Retrospective cohort	Incidence of AMI	31% (n = 22)	Small sample, result skewed as AMI rates determined in admitted patients only. Average time from cocaine use to onset of chest pain reported as 18 hours
Feldman JA et al. (2000)[32]	Multicentre trial, 293 patients with cocaine-associated chest pain (subsection of ACI-TIPI trial)	Prospective cohort	Incidence of AMI Incidence of ACS	0.7% (95% CI 0.08–2.4%) 1.4% (95% CI 0.37–3.5%)	Wide variation of AMI incidence between study institutions
Hollander JE et al. (1994)[33]	Multicentre (COCHPA) trial: 246 patients presenting with chest pain following cocaine use	Prospective cohort	Incidence of AMI	5.7% (95% CI 2.7–8.7%)	Possible selection bias by recruiting investigators, inclusion criteria included use of cocaine in the week prior to presentation
Mittleman MA et al. (1999)[34]	Determinants of Myocardial Infarction Onset Study: 3946 patients with AMI interviewed within an average of 4 days of onset	Case cross over study	Cocaine use associated with 1% of cohort (n = 38). 9 patients reported cocaine use in 60 minutes prior to onset of AMI	Highest risk of AMI within 60 minutes of cocaine use (RR 23.7, 95% CI = 8.5–66.3)	Data relating to cocaine use based on self-reporting, absolute risk of AMI cannot be calculated

(continued)

Author, date, and country	Patient group	Study type	Outcomes	Key results	Weaknesses
Qureshi, AI *et al.* (2001)[35]	Survey of 10 085 Americans, aged between 18–45 years as part of the third National Health and Nutrition examination Survey	Retrospective cohort	Likelihood of non-fatal MI associated with frequent cocaine use	Persons who used cocaine regularly had a significantly higher likelihood of non-fatal MI than non-users (OR 6.9, 95% CI 1.3–58). Population-attributable risk% of frequent cocaine use for non-fatal MI estimated as 25%	Data relies on self-reporting of cocaine use and of self-reported physician diagnoses. Unable to calculate the likelihood of fatal AMI
Weber JE *et al.* (2000)[36]	250 patients presenting to ED with cocaine-associated chest pain	Retrospective cohort	Incidence of AMI	6% (95% CI 4.1–8.9%)	Patients over 50 years of age did not have routine urological testing for cocaine potentially missing a small, but important cohort of patients

Data from various sources (see references)

Answer

The incidence of acute myocardial infarction in cocaine associated chest pain may be as high as 6% and one paper has suggested that the risk is greatest within 60 minutes of cocaine use. Not surprisingly, patients that present with cocaine-induced chest pain are just as likely to continue taking the drug after hospital evaluation and are more likely to have multivessel disease.[37] As a result, it is advisable to exclude acute myocardial infarction using current ACS rule-out protocols in this cohort of patients.

A Final Word from the Expert

Whilst many of these are recreational drug users that tend to be young and otherwise physically fit, this is by no means guaranteed. Ike Turner, for example, is said to have died from acute cocaine toxicity at the age of 76.

As noted, the pathophysiological basis of cocaine-induced chest pain and myocardial infarction is primarily one of coronary vasospasm leading to reduced coronary blood flow and subsequent ischaemia. This is unlike the majority of myocardial infarctions, where atheroma leads to coronary occlusion, and it consequently requires a different treatment strategy, aimed at reducing coronary vascular spasm by reducing the sympathomimetic effects of cocaine and consequently increasing coronary blood flow.

As currently the chest pain stratification systems including the TIMI, GRACE, and HEART classifications relate primarily to atheroma-induced chest pain, they are not particularly helpful in risk stratification for cocaine-induced chest pain.

In UK practice, in the absence of a validated risk-scoring strategy for patients with cocaine-induced chest pain, they are likely to require hospital admission to demonstrate haemodynamic recovery and to exclude significant cardiac necrosis.

At present the use of serial cardiac biomarkers in these patients, such as troponin, determines the length of inpatient stay and need for further investigation and intervention. The use of new high-sensitivity troponin assays and developments in observational medicine within the ED setting may, however, result in changes to this practice for some low-risk groups. Further work would be required first, to create a validated risk-assessment methodology for this group of patients.

References

1. Nancy G, Murphy MD, Benowitz MD. Cocaine. In: Olson KR (Ed). *Poisoning and drug overdose*, Fifth Edition. San Francisco, CA: McGraw Hill, 2007, pp 170–3.
2. Farre M, de la Torre R, Gonzalez ML, *et al.* Cocaine and alcohol interactions in humans, neuroendocine effects and cocaethylene metabolism. *J Pharmacol Exp Ther* 1997; 283:164–7.
3. Henning RJ, Wilson LD, Glauser JM. Cocaine plus ethanol is more cardiotoxic than cocaine or ethanol alone. *Crit Care Med* 1994; 22:1896–1906.
4. Murray L, Cadogan M, Daly F, *et al.* Chapter 3.30: Cocaine. In: *Toxicology Handbook*, Second Edition. Sydney: Churchill Livingstone, 2011.
5. Beckman KJ, Parker RB, Hariman RJ, *et al.* Haemodynamic and electrophysiological actions of cocaine. Effects of sodium bicarbonate as an antidote in dogs. *Circulation* 1991; 83:1799–1807.
6. Levin KH, Copersino ML, Epstein D, *et al.* Longitudinal ECG changes in cocaine users during extended abstinence. *Drug Alcohol depend* 2008; 95:160—3.
7. McCord J, Jneid H, Hollander JE, *et al.* Management of Cocaine-Associated Chest Pain and Myocardial Infarction: American Heart Association Acute Cardiac Care Committee of the Council on Clinical Cardiology. *Circulation* 2008; 117:1897–907.
8. Bhangoo P, Parfitt A, Wu T. Cocaine–induced myocardial ischaemia: nitrates versus benzodiazepines. *Emerg Med J* 2006; 23:568–9.
9. Baumann BM, Perrone J, Hornig SE, *et al.* Randomized, double-blind, placebo-controlled trial of diazepam, nitroglycerin, or both for treatment of patients with potential cocaine-associated acute coronary syndromes. *Acad Emerg Med* 2000; 7:878–85.
10. Honderick T, Williams D, Seaberg D, *et al.* A prospective, randomized,controlled trial of benzodiazepines and nitroglycerine or nitroglycerinealone in the treatment of cocaine-associated acute coronary syndromes. *Am J Emerg Med* 2003; 21:39–42.
11. Catravas JD, Waters IW. Acute cocaine intoxication in the conscious dog: studies on the mechanism of lethality. *J Pharm Exp Ther* 1981; 217:350–6.
12. Guinn MM, Bedford JA, Wilson MC. Antagonism of intravenous cocaine lethality in non-human primates. *Clin Toxicol* 1980; 16:499–508.
13. Spivey WH, Schoffstall JM, Kirkpatrick R, *et al.* Comparison of labetalol, diazepam and haloperidol for the treatment of cocaine toxicity in a swine model. *Ann Emerg Med* 1990; 19:467–8.
14. Derlet RW, Albertson TE. Anticonvulsant modification of cocaine induced toxicity in the rat. *Neuropharmacology* 1990; 29:255–9.

15. Seubert CN, Morey TE, Martynyuk AE, *et al.* Midazolam selectively potentiates the A2A but not the A1-receptor-mediated effects of adenosine. *Anesthesiology* 2000; 92:567–77.

16. Brogan WC 3rd, Lange RA, Kim AS, *et al.* Alleviation of cocaine-induced coronary vasoconstriction by nitroglycerin. *J Am Coll Cardiol* 1991; 18:581–6.

17. Flores ED, Lange RA, Cigarrosa RG, *et al.* Effect of cocaine on coronary artery dimensions in atherosclerotic coronary artery disease: enhanced vasoconstriction by beta-adrenergic blockade. *Ann Int Med* 1990; 112:897–903.

18. Hollander JE, Hoffman RS, Gennis P, *et al.* Nitroglycerin in the treatment of cocaine associated chest pain– clinical safety and efficacy. *J Toxicol Clin Toxicol* 1994; 32:243–56.

19. Randomised trial of intravenous atenolol among 16,027 cases of suspected acute myocardial infarction: ISIS-1. First International Study of Infarct Survival Collaborative Group. *Lancet* 1986; 2:57–66.

20. Anderson JL, Adams CD, Antman EM, *et al.* ACC/AHA 2007 guidelines for the management of patients with unstable angina/non-ST elevation myocardial infarction. A report of the American College of Cardiology/American Heart Association task force on practice guidelines. *J Am Coll Cardiol* 2007; 50(7):e1–e157.

21. Shannon RP, Stambler BS, Komamura K, *et al.* Cholinergic modulation of the coronary vasoconstriction induced by cocaine in conscious dogs. *Circulation* 1993; 87(3):939–49.

22. Boehrer JD, Moliterno DJ, Willard JE, *et al.* Influence of Labetalol on Cocaine-Induced Coronary Vasoconstriction in Humans. *Am J Med* 1993; 94:608–10.

23. Dattilo PB, Hallpern SM, Fearon K, *et al.* β-Blockers are associated with reduced risk of myocardial infarction after cocaine use. *Ann Emerg Med* 2008; 51(2):117–25.

24. Lange RA, Cigarroa RG, Flores ED, *et al.* Potentiation of Cocaine-Induced Coronary Vasoconstriction by Beta-Adrenergic Blockade. *Annals Internal Med* 1990; 112:897–903.

25. Rangel C, Shu RG, Lazar LD, *et al.* β-Blockers for Chest Pain Associated with Recent Cocaine Use. *Arch Intern Med* 2010; 170(10):874–9.

26. Ramoska E, Sacchetti AD. Propanalol-induced hypertension in treatment of cocaine intoxication. *Ann Emerg Med*, 1985; 14(11):1112–1113

27. Sand IC, Brody SL, Wrenn KD, *et al.* Experience with esmolol for the treatment of cocaine-associated cardiovascular complications. *Am J Emerg Med* 1991; 9(2):163–5.

28. Hoskins MH, Leleiko RM, Ramos JJ, *et al.* Effects of labetalol on haemodynamic parameters and soluble biomarkers of inflammation in Acute Coronary Syndrome in patients with active cocaine use. *J Cardiovasc Pharmacol Ther* 2010; 15(1):47–52.

29. UK NPIS Toxbase: < http://www.toxbase.org/Poisons-Index-A-Z/C-Products/Cocaine/>

30. Amin M, Gabelman G, Karpel J, Buttrick P. Acute myocardial infarction and chest pain syndromes after cocaine use. *Am J Cardiol* 1990; 66:1434–7.

31. Feldman JA, Fish SS, Beshansky JR, *et al.* Acute cardiac ischemia in patients with cocaine-associated complaints: results of a multicentre trial. *Ann Emerg Med* 2000; 36:469–76.

32. Hollander JE, Hoffman RS, Gennis P, *et al.* Prospective multicentre evaluation of cocaine-associated chest pain. *Acad Emerg Med* 1994; 1:330–9.

33. Mittleman MA, Mintzer D, Maclure M, *et al.* Triggering of myocardial infarction by cocaine. *Circulation* 1999; 99:2737–41.

34. Qureshi AI, Suri FK, Guterman LR, *et al.* Cocaine use and the likelihood of nonfatal myocardial infarction and stroke. Data from the third national health and nutrition examination survey. *Circulation* 2001; 103:502–6.

35. Weber JE, Chudnofsky CR, Boczar M, *et al.* Cocaine-associated chest pain: how common is myocardial infarction? *Acad Emerg Med* 2000; 7:873–7.

36. Carillo X, Curos A, Muga R, *et al.* Acute coronary syndrome and cocaine use: 8-year prevalence and in-hospital outcomes. *European Heart J* 2011; 32:1244–50.

37. Weber JE, Shofer FS, Larkin GL, *et al.* Validation of a brief observation period for patients with cocaine associated chest pain. *N Eng J Med* 2003; 348:510–17.

38. Ambre J. The Urinary Excretion of Cocaine and Metabolites in Humans: A Kinetic Analysis of Published Data. *J Analytical Toxicology* 1985; 9:241–5.

39. Keller T, Zeller T, Ojeda F, *et al.* Serial changes in highly sensitive Troponin I assay and early detection of myocardial infarction. *JAMA* 2011; 306(24):2684–93.

25 Croup

Sam Thenabadu

ⓘ Expert commentary Sara Hanna

Case history

A 3-year-old boy attends the paediatric ED at 3 a.m. with a 4-hour history of a worsening barking cough and a mild coryza over the last 24 hours. His parents have been woken up by a 'seal-like' cough and have been concerned that although he 'sounds terrible', he still looks relatively well. They searched on the Internet and found advice to use steam to alleviate the cough; however, this hasn't worked and so they have brought him into the ED, fearful that the cough may be a sign of worsening illness.

He has no medical history of note, is not on any medications, and is fully immunized. He has two older siblings who are both well currently.

His observations on arrival are as follows: HR 145 bpm CRT<2 secs, O_2 sats 99 %, RR 24, and Temp 37.4°C

See Box 25.1 for a clinical summary of croup.

Box 25.1 Clinical summary of croup

- Classically 'laryngotracheitis'—inflammation of the larynx and trachea (less often involving the bronchi)
- Subglottic narrowing is the principle site of airway obstruction and the cause of stridor
- Parainfluenza II remains the predominant causative organism, although other virus including influenza, respiratory syncytial virus, measles, and herpes can cause a similar clinical picture
- Most commonly ages 6 months to 3 years and presentation outside of this age range should prompt consideration of another diagnosis
- Seasonal preponderance—autumn and winter
- 85 % are classified as mild with only 1 % being deemed severe
- Mortality rate low but deaths still reported, infants most at risk
- Symptoms usually resolve within 48–72 hours

Data from Cherry JD. Clinical practice: Croup *NEJM* 2008; 24:358(4):384–91.

ⓘ Expert comment

Croup is one of the 3 most common respiratory conditions seen in the paediatric ED and can pose quite a challenge to the untrained eye. A huge spectrum of croup is seen in the paediatric ED as the cough often concerns the parents. Typically this cough is exacerbated at night when children lie flat and are in drier room environments, meaning this presentation is one seen in the middle of the night when there is often less support for junior doctors.

It is important to realize that the bark itself is not an indicator of severity. More worrying is the presence of stridor, a harsh, high-pitched inspiratory noise, indicative of airway narrowing. This is worse when the child is excited or distressed. Again, the loudness of the stridor is not a marker of severity and other crucial parameters must be assessed quickly to determine if this is mild, moderate, or severe croup.

> ⭐ **Learning point** Stridor in children
>
> Stridor is a symptom caused by airway narrowing just above, within, or just below the larynx. Not all stridor is croup, and it is important for the clinician to have a list of differential diagnoses for both acute and chronic presentations in mind, when faced with such a case (see Table 25.1). An accompanying expiratory sound is a 'red flag' as this suggests either extreme airway narrowing or a diagnosis other than croup (obstruction within the chest, e.g. vascular ring). A history of previous stridor or 'noisy breathing' might suggest an underlying structural abnormality (e.g. acquired subglottic stenosis from previous intubation). Chronic airway obstruction may be tolerated well by the child and their family until a respiratory viral infection causes increased narrowing and sudden extreme symptoms.
>
> **Table 25.1 Causes of stridor**
>
> | Acute cause of stridor | Discriminating feature |
> | --- | --- |
> | Croup | Preceding coryza, barking cough, and often a well-looking child otherwise |
> | Inhaled foreign body | A rapid deterioration in breathing from a previous normal condition |
> | Bacterial tracheitis | A septic and unwell child who needs urgent attention |
> | Epiglottitis | High fever, severe signs of difficulty in breathing with soft stridor and drooling |
> | Anaphylaxis | Sudden onset often with other signs such as tongue and lip swelling, wheeze, rash, tachycardia, and hypotension |

Clinical question: Should we be recommending steam therapy for croup?

Parents have frequently used steam inhalation from boiled kettles, as well as purchased home-humidifier machines to treat a range of respiratory illnesses from bronchiolitis to croup. Is this advice still appropriate and based on any firm evidence? In the mid-1980s a theory existed that the moist air would reduce laryngeal inflammation and decrease the viscosity of secretions.[2,3] This has now been superseded by concerns that children may get more agitated by the steam and paradoxically worsen their breathing pattern. Greally (1990) highlighted 3 worse cases still where children were scalded or burnt from the hot steam, thus opinion now varies although many parents will recount successful experiences with the trial of steam.

> 🕐 **Evidence base** Humidity in croup?
>
> **Moore et al. (2006)**[4] conducted a systematic review and meta-analysis of 3 papers to assess the efficacy of humidified air in the treatment of croup. Three studies in the ED[5,6,7] were analysed with data cumulated for 135 patients with croup. The combined results from 20–60 minutes of the studies demonstrated an insignificant reduction of the croup score by –0.14 (95% CI=–0.75–0.47).
>
> **Scolnik D et al. (2007)**[8] hypothesized that a particular particle size of aerosolized air may improve croup symptoms. They conducted a randomized, single-blinded convenience sampling trial comparing placebo with blow-by technique vs 40% vs 100% humidified air. No significant reduction in croup score was found and humidity was not recommended in mild or moderate croup.

Answer

No evidence for the use of mist therapy or humidifiers either pre-hospital or in a hospital setting and should not be recommended at discharge.

Case progression

On reviewing the child, the doctor finds a happy child playing in the waiting room. He is chatty and interacts well with both you and his parents. Examination of the patient reveals a normal cardiovascular examination, with only mild recessions visible on the respiratory examination but nothing focal to auscultate. An ENT examination reveals mildly inflamed tonsils but no visible exudates, and no other positive findings. There are a few non-tender lymph nodes in the submandibular region only. Neurological examination is grossly normal and there is no evidence of rashes. Currently this child appears haemodynamically stable and does not require any urgent investigations. There are no indications at this point to place an IV cannula or obtain bloods, and similarly a chest X-ray is not needed as the child's saturations are normal.

> ✚ **Clinical tip** Indications for chest X-ray imaging in children
>
> There is often mixed opinion as to when a chest X-ray should be performed in the paediatric population. A good starting point is the NICE Feverish child guidelines which suggest that any child under 3 months with respiratory signs and symptoms should undergo a radiograph, whilst children over 3 months should undertake imaging if any 'red' features are present.
>
> The BTS/SIGN asthma guidelines suggest a chest X-ray should be performed if there is life-threatening asthma or if there is subcutaneous emphysema, persisting unilateral signs suggesting pneumothorax or lobar collapse.
>
> A chest X-ray should not be performed in a child with a clinical diagnosis of croup.[12] A requirement of oxygen to maintain normal saturations is a sign of severe airway obstruction and the priority is to reverse the swelling urgently or secure the airway. If the stridor is thought to be due to another mechanism such as inhalation of a foreign body, then a chest X-ray may be helpful. However, a normal radiograph does not exclude the diagnosis.
>
> Textbooks will describe the 'steeple sign' of a narrow airway visible on an AP soft-tissue neck film. There is no clinical indication for this imaging and may in fact jeopardize a potential obstruction airway.
>
> Other reasonable indications for a chest X-ray would include:
>
> - Suspected chest trauma—pneumothorax, haemothorax, and flail segment
> - Suspected NAI as part of a skeletal survey

Case progression

The history of a barking cough and examination signs are compatible with a self-limiting episode of croup. Stratification of the child is now required to gauge the severity of the croup episode and thus the treatment is required. You have performed a croup score on the child using the Westley Croup Score[9]. This child would only score 1 and would be classified as mild.

> ★ **Learning point** Croup scoring systems
>
> The Westley croup score is one of only 2 validated scoring systems in croup. It was devised in 1978 and is the most commonly used tool. It has been used in its original form or with minor modifications in the majority of croup trials, as on analysis the inter-rated reliability weighted kappa for the total croup score was 0.90.[10]
>
> The Westley score allows the clinician to grade the severity of the episode as:
>
> Mild   <4
> Moderate   4–7
> Severe   ->7
>
> The only other validated system created by Bjornson (2004)[11] as a 3-point telephone outpatient score (TOP) for following up patients in the community by asking parents about the presence of stridor and a barking cough. This score has not been taken up and used by any other large studies to-date.

Case progression

The family are concerned that it may get worse and are requesting a prescription for antibiotics and steroids as they have read about these treatments.

Clinical question: Are steroids required in cases of mild croup?

Mild croup poses significant debates—should dexamethasone be used in all cases of croup or is it unnecessary in the mildest of cases? With estimates that 85 % of cases presenting in the UK are mild, are steroids always needed?[10] Variation in practice does occur and URTIs are most often treated symptomatically with antipyretics and good oral hydration. This strategy is often mirrored in milder cases of croup but is there actually an evidence base to use steroids?

❝ Expert comment

Since the introduction of steroids, the number of children requiring airway intervention has reduced. However, re-emergence of symptoms after steroids have worn off should prompt re-evaluation both of the diagnosis and severity of the episode. Croup lasts for 2–3 days and therefore treatment should not be required beyond this timescale, especially due to the half-life of dexamethasone being 36–54 hours.

> ✓ **Evidence base** Treatment dilemmas in mild croup
>
> **Russell et al. (2011)**[11] performed a Cochrane review of glucocorticoid use in croup. 38 studies were included ($n=4299$) and glucocorticoids were associated with an improved Westley score at 6 hours with a mean difference of –1.2 (95 % confidence interval (CI) –1.6 to –0.8) and at 12 hours –1.9 (95 % CI –2.4 to –1.3).
>
> Additionally fewer return visits occurred in treated participants (risk ratio (RR) 0.5; 95 % CI 0.3–0.7) and length of time spent in hospital (mean difference 12 hours, 5–19 hours) was significantly decreased glucocorticoids.
>
> **Bjornson et al. (2004)**[12] conducted a double-blind RCT comparing dexamethasone 0.60 mg/kg vs placebo in mild croup. The primary outcome analysed was whether the patient required further review by a healthcare practitioner within 7 days. Return to medical care in the dexamethasone group was lower than the placebo group (7.3 % vs 15.3 %, $p=0.001$). This produced an odds ratio (OR) of 2.4 and an NNT to prevent one return of 13 (95 % CI 8–13). The authors conclude there is a small consistent but important clinical and socio-economic benefits, advocating use of steroids in all patients.

Answer

Steroids should be prescribed in all cases of croup indiscriminately of severity.

Clinical question: Is oral dexamethasone superior to nebulised budesonide in treating croup?

Having seen the evidence that all severities of croup should be treated with steroids, you wonder why some centres are using nebulizers and others insist on oral steroids. You have seen problems with both routes with children refusing to tolerate and cooperate with the nebulizer administration but also children readily vomiting the oral solution. Is there a superior drug and route?

> ✅ **Evidence base** Which steroid and which route?
>
> **Klassen T et al. (1997)**[14] performed a randomised controlled trial comparing oral dexamethasone and nebulized budesonide comparing reduction in croup scores. The mean change in the croup score was 2.3 (95% CI −2.6 to −2.0) in the budesonide group versus −2.4 (95% CI −2.6 to −2.2) in the dexamathasone group. The authors suggested that although there was no clinical difference, dexamethasone was better tolerated by children as well as being a cheaper alternative.
>
> **Geelhoed et al. (1995)**[15] conducted a randomized controlled trial examining the duration of time to reduce a croup score to <1 in hospital for children treated with oral dexamethasone versus nebulized budesonide. Median time to a croup score of < or = 1 was shorter for children treated with dexamethasone (2 hr) or budesonide (3 hr) compared to those who received placebo (8 hr) (p<0.01). Croup scores for both steroid groups were significantly lower than the placebo group by 1 hour and remained so subsequently. The croup scores did not differ significantly in the 2 steroid-treated groups. The authors conclude that oral dexamethasone and budesonide are both effective in reducing symptoms and duration of hospitalization in children with croup.

Answer

Oral dexamethasone and nebulized budesonide have no significant difference in efficacy on croup score reduction if tolerated by the child.

Case progression

The child is observed in the ED for a further 2 hours and another score performed which is now zero along with normal observations and repeat clinical examination.[8] You decide to send the patient home with printed advice sheets on croup and explain that as the aetiology is viral, no antibiotics are required.[9,10] You do emphasize, though, that the child should be encouraged to take oral fluids and antipyretics regularly for the next 48 hours. You ask the parent to attend the GP in 72 hours for review but advise that if the child deteriorates acutely to return urgently to the ED.[10]

> 🎙 **Expert comment**
>
> The quality of the re-evaluation before discharge from the emergency department and the advice given to the parents is key to ensuring safety for these children. TTO doses of dexamethasone are NOT recommended as the child should now be fine so if symptoms progress—the child develops stridor, difficulty breathing, refuses food or drink—they should be brought immediately back to the department. The child should be better by 3 days so review by the GP would seem unnecessary; however, good safety netting is always important.

✪ Learning point Advances in croup treatments

Further research is ongoing into the optimum dose of oral dexamethasone as a wide range of doses are used from 0.15–0.60 mg/kg. Several studies have examined whether smaller doses could be used especially in milder croup, as a dose of 0.60 mg/kg is equal to 6 mg/kg of prednisolone.[15,16,17] Opinion thus far is that an equivalent reduction in croup scores is seen; however, more robust trial data is required.

➕ Clinical tip Severe croup

Severe croup is a daunting clinical presentation, but the ED management is a 'less-is-more' approach as detailed following. The use of nebulized adrenaline as a holding measure until senior anaesthetic and ENT support are available to consider emergent intubation is the key principle, with clinicians well indoctrinated in the 'hands-off' strategy, to prevent a further precipitous deterioration. The adrenaline will reduce swelling acutely and can lead to a remarkable improvement in the child's condition. Thereafter ongoing observation and repeated review by an experienced clinician are mandatory because the effects can be short lived. Adrenaline can and should be repeated if the severity of symptoms recurs but only with a view to re-evaluating need for airway intervention.

- Westley score >7: requiring oxygen to maintain saturations, altered mental state, severe retractions
- Move to resuscitation room immediately—keep child in parents arms
- Cannulation is NOT recommended until specialist team assembled[11]
- Nebulised adrenaline 0.5 ml/kg of 1:1000 up to 5 ml—mask may be held under child's mouth rather than secured on
- Urgent anaesthetic review by senior anaesthetist

A Final Word from the Expert

Croup is a presentation that will commonly be seen in the paediatric ED but paradoxically continues to be managed differently across the UK and Europe with no national or internationally verified guidelines being in existence as yet.

The evidence demonstrates that steroids are of clinical use in all severities of croup, and that oral dexamethasone is equal to and perhaps superior to the alternate treatment of choice nebulized budesonide. On the milder spectrum there is now no evidence to support the use of antibiotics, salbutamol inhaler use, or humidified air, and these treatments should be discouraged.

The child with severe croup is significantly ill and requires a multidisciplinary team approach to optimize management. The key to management is to anticipate problems and mobilize key senior clinicians as soon as possible. Red flags include current severity of symptoms, poor response to adrenaline or repeated requirement, previous airway symptoms, and young age. Early involvement should be sought from senior members of the ED, anaesthetics, paediatrics, and ENT teams with conversations with paediatric retrieval teams also often providing a font of advice and reassurance that help is en route. Remember that it is a distressing event for the parent to witness, and as with all emergencies, a designated nurse or doctor should support the parents, as they are likely to remain at the bedside right until or even sometimes during intubation.

References

1. Cherry JD. Clinical practice: Croup *NEJM* 2008; 24:358(4):384–91.
2. Henry R. Moist air in the treatment of Laryngotracheitis. *Arch Dis Child* 1983; 63:1305–8.
3. Ophir D, Elad Y. The effects of steam inhalation on nasal patency and nasal symptoms with patients with the common cold. *Am J Otolaryngol* 1987; 8:149–53.
4. Moore M, Little P. Humidified Air inhalation for croup: a systematic review and meta analysis. *Family Practice* 2007; 24:295–301.

5. Bourchier D, Dawson KP, Fergusson DM. humidification in viral croup: a controlled trial *Aust Paediatric J* 1984; 20:289–91.

6. Neto G, Kentab O, Klassen TP, *et al.* A randomised controlled trial of mist in the acute treatment of moderate crop *Acad Emerg Med* 2002; 9:873–9.

7. Jamshidi P. The effect of humidified air in mild to moderate croup: evaluation using crop scores and respiratory induction plethysmography. *Acad Emerg Med* 2001; 8:417.

8. Scolnik D, Coates AL, Stephens D, *et al.* Controlled delivery of high versus low humidity versus mist therapy for croup in emergency departments. A randomised controlled trial. *JAMA* 2006; 295:1274–80.

9. Westley C, Cotton EK, brooks JG. Nebulized racemic epinephrine by IPPB for the treatment of croup: a double-blind study. *Am J Dis Child.* 1978 May; 132(5):484–7.

10. Klassen TP. The croup score as an evaluative instrument in clinical trials. *Arch Pediatr Adolesc Med* 1995; 149:60–1.

11. Bjornson CL, Klassen TP, Williamson J, *et al.* A randomised trial of a single dose of oral dexamethasone for mild croup. *NEJM* 2004; 351:1306–13.

12. Russell KF, Liang Y, O'Gorman K, *et al.* Glucocorticoids in croup. *Cochrane Review.* 2011. <http://onlinelibrary.wiley.com/doi/10.1002/14651858.CD001955.pub3/pdf/standard>

13. NICE guidelines: Feverish Illness in Children (2007) <http://www.nice.org.uk/nicemedia/live/11010/30523/30523.pdf>

14. Salour M. The steeple sign. *Radiology* 2000; 216:428–429.

15. Klassen TP, Craig WR, Moher D, *et al.* Nebulized budesonide and oral dexamethasone for treatment of croup: a randomized controlled trial. *JAMA* 1998; 279:1629–32.

16. Geelhoed GC, Macdonald WB. Oral and inhaled steroids in croup: a randomized, placebo-controlled trial. *Pediatr Pulmonol* 1995; 20:355–61.

17. Geelhoed GC, Turner J, Macdonald WB. Efficacy of a small single dose of oral dexamethasone for outpatient croup: a double blind placebo controlled clinical trial. *BMJ* 1996; 313:140–2.

18. Geelhoed GC, Macdonald WB. Oral dexamethasone in the treatment of croup: 0.15 mg/kg versus 0.3 mg/kg versus 0.6 mg/kg. *Pediatr Pulmonol* 1995; 20:362–8.

19. Terregino CA, Nairn SJ, Chansky EM, *et al.* The effect of heliox on croup: a pilot study. *Acad Emerg Med* 1998; 5:s1130–3.

26 The collapsed marathon runner

Lisa Black

 Expert commentary Katherine Henderson

Case history

A previously fit and well 32-year-old man is brought into the ED by the ambulance service after collapsing at mile 21 of a city marathon. His running partners assure you that he has trained consistently for the race over the last few months and had taken on regular hypertonic fluids throughout the race until he collapsed. The marathon course has remained dry throughout the day with an ambient temperature of 24 °C.

The paramedic's feedback that his observations at the scene were: HR 133 bpi or beats per minute, BP 160/60 mmHg and O_2 saturations of 99 % on high-flow oxygen. His initial GCS of 3 has now improved en route to 7 (E1, V1, M5). A temperature reading was not initially possible with the portable tympanic thermometer, however the paramedics report that the patient had felt 'very hot'.

While you prepare for his arrival you consider the specific potential causes of collapse in a marathon runner. See Box 26.1.

Box 26.1 Clinical summary of the collapsed marathon runner

Every marathon a number of runners will collapse and require medical treatment. The majority can be treated in the pre-hospital setting but some will need immediate intensive treatment and hospitalization. Exercise-associated collapse (EAC) is due to a number of factors including dehydration, fluid and electrolyte depletion, lactic acidosis, vasovagal-type syncope, and hyperthermia or hypothermia.

The majority of patients with EAC can be managed conservatively but it is important to be aware of more serious indicators of potentially serious outcomes. Presenting symptoms may include fatigue, muscle cramps, dizziness, vomiting, diarrhoea, abdominal pains, and feeling hot or cold. The serious conditions to consider are exertional heat stroke and hyponatraemia.

😮 **Learning point** Differential diagnosis of the collapsed marathon runner (See Table 26.1).

Table 26.1 Differential diagnosis of the collapsed marathon runner

1. Exercise-associated collapse	The participant is unable to walk or stand unaided
	Conscious level is unaffected. Temperature and biochemical markers may be abnormal initially but will normalise quickly
	Treat with oral hydration and nursing in the Trendelenberg position
2. Exertional heat-related illness	See Learning point

(continued)

3. Exertional hyponatraemia	Hyponatraemia ([Na⁺] <135 mmol/L) occurring during or up to 24 hours after strenuous physical activity
4. Hypoglycaemia	Common in pre-existing IDDM. Standard medical management required
5. Hypothermia	Common during unexpected changes of weather. Standard medical management required
6. Acute medical conditions	All collapsed marathon runners need to be considered for the usual range of differentials in any patient with 'collapsed query cause'—epilepsy, cardiac events (e.g. arrhythmias and cardiac arrest), and intra-cerebral events

Data from Chang TL, Shahin A, Scott C, *et al.* University of Nevada Sports Medicine Heat Illness Guideline. August 2010.

Strenuous prolonged activity such as long-distance running tests the body's ability to maintain thermoregulation and exposes the athlete to potential heat-related insults along with a plethora of electrolyte disturbances (see Table 26.2).[1] The London Marathon has experienced 10 deaths in 31 years with the majority being secondary to coronary heart disease; however, heat-related morbidity remains a significant presentation both immediately at the racecourse as well as in the ensuing days.

Table 26.2 Learning point Heat-related illnesses

Heat cramps	Body temperature is raised but usually < 40 °C with patients experiencing polydipsia, muscle cramps, and tachycardia. The body's ability to sweat and dissipate heat remains, however, and neurological function is preserved.
Exertional hyperthermia	Temperature remains <40 °C and overall neurological function remains; however, there are now symptoms such as headaches, nausea, irritability and mild confusion. Again, the body is still able to dissipate heat but due to these compensatory mechanisms, there is a profound tachycardia and orthostatic hypotension.
Heat stroke	Classified as exertional or non-exertional. The homeostatic mechanisms have now failed and temperatures rise > 40 °C.

Data from various sources (see references)

Clinical question: Is standard ED measurement of body temperature by tympanic thermometer adequate in the collapsed marathon runner?

Temperature is an essential ED observation parameter that should be performed in any unwell patient. It is common knowledge that extremes of temperature <36 °C degrees or >38 °C form a part of the SIRS criteria and thus impact upon potential morbidity. The methods of recording temperatures vary from department to department with a range of measuring techniques utilized. Commonly tympanic, axillary, or oral thermometers have been the mainstay of measurement; however, in the higher acuity patient, core temperatures via the rectal and oesophageal route can also be utilized. Although not commonly used within EDs, temporal artery temperature measurement can also be utilized as a non-invasive method (see Table 26.3).

Table 26.3 Analysis of temperature measuring in the ED

Author, date, and country	Patient group	Study type (level of evidence)	Outcomes	Key results	Study weaknesses
Ronneberg, 2008 USA[1]	60 collapsed marathon runners with potential for EHS	Prospective observational study	Temporal artery temperature compared to digital rectal temperature	Negative correlation coefficient (−0.142) in normothermic runners Poor correlation (0.37) in hyperthermia Temporal artery measurement only 0.12 sensitivity for detecting hyperthermia	Lack of blinding Different air temp across 2 races
Armstrong et al. 2007 USA[2]	N/A	Position Statement of the American College of Sports Medicine: Exertional Heat Illness During Training and Competition		Ear, oral, skin, temporal, and axillary temperature measurements should not be used to diagnose or distinguish EHS from exertional heat exhaustion	
Casa et al. 2007 USA[3]	25 athletic volunteers performing 180 min monitored exercise	Observational field study	Oral, axillary, aural, gastrointestinal, forehead and temporal measurements compared to criterion standard of rectal temp in all participants	Oral, axillary, aural, and temporal measurements invalid (mean bias > ±0.27°C) Forehead and GI measurements valid (mean bias < ±0.27°C)	Lack of blinding Subjects consuming food/fluids independently
Moran et al. 2002 Israel[4]	N/A	Review article	Review of accuracy of oral, axillary, tympanic, rectal, and oesophageal temperature measurements	Rectal temperature is the most accurate and available method for measuring temperature in thermal illness in sports activities	

Data from various sources (see references)

❝ Expert comment

In this clinical context a core temperature of over 40°C suggests exertional hyperthermia and, with CNS dysfunction, exertional heat stroke. Obtaining a core temperature is key to planning treatment, and any ED serving a large marathon should ensure a supply of rectal temperature probes is available.

An immediate sodium measurement will identify exertional hyponatraemia and prevent inappropriate use of IV fluids. Exertional hyponatraemia is potentially life-threatening and the ED physician should be strict that no fluid should be administered until a sodium level has been obtained. To facilitate this some marathon field teams have hand-held point-of-care sodium-monitoring devices for this purpose.

★ Learning point Exertional hyponatraemia

Fluid balance remains a constant challenge for the marathon runner.[13] Electrolyte balance after prolonged exercise is dependent upon multiple factors, and the volume and hypotonic status of ingested fluid is important to consider. The treating clinician must thus be alert to sodium levels and their rate of change.

Pathophysiology

Dilutional hyponatraemia—i.e. fluid consumption that exceeds urinary / sweat losses
Inappropriate vasopressin secretion
Not thought to be due to excess sodium losses

Risk factors

Excessive drinking during race
Female sex
Slow runners / longer race time
Drugs—NSAIDs, SSRIs, thiazide diuretics
Extremes of temperature

Clinical features

Generally, the relative decrease in Na+ is more significant than the absolute numerical value although significant effects are uncommon if levels are >130 mmol/L.

Mild symptoms:

- Bloating / oedema
- Nausea and vomiting
- Headache

Severe:

- Cerebral oedema / hyponatraemic encephalopathy, e.g. confusion, agitation, seizures, coma, death
- Respiratory distress secondary to pulmonary oedema

Asymptomatic patients

If hyponatraemia is found in asymptomatic patients, they should be advised to restrict oral fluid intake until they have passed urine. Giving patients salty crisps or stock cubes can facilitate this. They must not be given intravenous 'normal' saline or hypotonic fluids as this will increase dilution and exacerbate the problem.

Symptomatic patients

1. Confirm diagnosis with near-patient rapid testing or urgent laboratory measurement
2. Administer high-flow oxygen
3. Give an immediate intravenous bolus of 100 ml 2.7% NaCl

(continued)

4. Give up to 2 further 100 ml 2.7% NaCl boluses if there is no clinical improvement
5. Seizures should be treated with standard anti-convulsant medications although these may be ineffectual if hyponatraemia persists
6. Patients exhibiting signs of brainstem herniation (e.g. unilateral fixed pupil) should be intubated and ventilated to reduce intracranial pressure

Management of exertional hyponatraemia

The cautious approach employed in chronic hyponatraemia is unnecessary as there have been no reported cases of central pontine myelinolysis in exertional hyponatraemia.

Case progression

On arrival in the ED the patient is distressed and combative with an improved GCS of 11 (E4, V2, M5). Other observations are as follows: HR 137 bpm, BP 140/70mmHg, O_2 saturations 99 % on high-flow oxygen, rectal temperature 40.7 °C. Capillary blood glucose is 4.1mmol/L and the sodium on the venous blood gas is 148 mmol/L.

He has no significant medical history and had trained for 3 months appropriately for the event but subsequently had run faster than anticipated, eventually having to stop to walk at mile 21 before collapsing. In light of his clinical condition and his core temperature, you make the diagnosis of Exceptional Heat stroke (EHS) and proceed to cool the patient.

⭐ **Learning point** Exertional heat stroke

Definition

Life-threatening illness, induced by strenuous exercise, comprising core temperature > 40°C and central nervous system dysfunction.

Affects 1 in 10 000 marathon runners[5]

Pathogenesis involves[6]

Thermoregulatory failure and ineffective cooling
Exaggerated acute-phase response

Clinical features include:

Tachycardia +/- hypotension
Hyperventilation
Respiratory alkalosis and lactic acidosis
CNS derangement—altered behaviour, delirium, seizure, coma

Table 26.4 **Risk factors**

Extrinsic	Intrinsic
Hot humid conditions	Dehydration—>3 % weight loss during activity
Heavy clothing / costume	Effort unmatched to physical fitness—outrunning one's training
	High BMI
	Medications, e.g. antihistamines, ephedrine
	Any pre-existing illness

Management

Immediate cooling
Support of organ dysfunction

Clinical question: How should patients with EHS be cooled?

The most important predictor of outcome in EHS is the duration and the degree of hyperthermia[9] and therefore immediate whole-body cooling and a rapid reduction of core body temperature are essential. The aim is to achieve rapid cooling, ideally within 30–60 minutes of collapse, and prolonged pre-hospital times without cooling should be avoided (See Table 26.5).

Answer

Total-body immersion in ice-cold water is the quickest and most effective cooling method. Where this is unavailable, a combination of other techniques such as ice packs may be used.

Dantrolene has not been shown to be beneficial in the treatment of EHS. Active cooling should be stopped at 39 °C to avoid hypothermia but rectal temperature monitoring should continue to detect rebound hyperthermia.[12]

> **Expert comment**
>
> Many marathon medical teams have a 'cool first, transport second' policy. Rapid cooling in the field can be done using ice packs, ice water, and towels. Some teams use immersion in cold tubs or place the patient over a cold tub and ladle cold water over the skin. The key requirement is that as much of the body as possible is cooled. In hospital, soaking towels in buckets of water with added ice is more practical. The wet towels need to be rotated frequently and a fan will increase heat loss by evaporation. Once 39 °C is reached, active cooling is stopped but in our experience the patient should not be moved from the ED until it is clear the temperature is stable.

Case progression

The patient is given cold intravenous crystalloid via peripheral cannulae and is stripped and cooled using towels soaked in ice water.

Initial venous blood gas shows a compensated metabolic acidosis with pH 7.45, pCO2 3.36 mmHg, pO2 7.01 mmHg, BE −4.5 mmol/L, HCO3 17.3 mmHg, and lactate 9.3 mmol/L. Laboratory results reveal hypernatraemia with early renal impairment: sodium 148 mmol/L, potassium 4.3 mmol/L, urea 10.4 mmol/L and creatinine 186 mmol/L. The first CK is elevated at 889 IU/L.

After 60 minutes of cooling, and 3 litres of cold IV fluids, the patient's core temperature remains elevated at 39.3 °C. He remains agitated and is given a titrated dose of intravenous benzodiazepines and discussion is undertaken with the intensive care team regarding admission to the HDU.

> **Clinical tip** Cold IV fluids
>
> Extrapolation of evidence in therapeutic hypothermia in cardiac arrest patients suggests 'cold' IV fluid should in fact be 'ice-cold' and this is generally accepted to be 2–4 °C.[10] To avoid unnecessary delay in cooling fluids, they should be routinely stored in a refrigerator and therefore immediately available.[11]

> **Learning point** Complications of exercise-induced heat stroke
>
> Heat stroke can result in multi-organ failure, affecting any system:[6]
>
> - Neurological—cerebral oedema, encephalopathy, persistent neurological dysfunction
> - Cardiovascular—myocardial injury
>
> (continued)

Table 26.5 Cooling methods in the EHS

Author, date, and country	Patient group	Study type (level of evidence)	Outcomes	Key results	Study weaknesses
McDermott et al., 2009 USA[7]	68 subjects from 7 published articles 125 subjects from case reports / series	Systematic review	Comparison of cooling rates: Ice-water immersion Wet towel application Ice packs to neck, groin, axillae Ice packs to whole body Water splash and fanning Immersion hands / feet	Ice water or cold water immersion provides fastest cooling Continual dousing with fanning and rotation of cold, wet towels is viable alternative	All studies unblinded Included all exertional hyperthermia, not just EHS
Clements et al., 2002 USA[8]	17 distance runners competing in 19 km runs heat 3 separate runs each, 1 week apart Ambient temp 27±1°C	Randomized, crossover trial	Comparison of cooling rates: Ice-water (5°C) immersion Cold-water (14°C) immersion Mock (no water) immersion	Ice-water and cold-water immersion provide significantly faster cooling than mock immersion ($p<0.05$) No statistical difference between ice-water and cold-water immersion	No subjects had actual EHS Different ambient temperatures No detail on randomization process
Smith, 2005 UK[9]	109 subjects from 4 controlled trials and 187 subjects from 13 case reports / series Healthy volunteers and heat stroke patients	Systematic review	Comparison of cooling rates: Whole body immersion Evaporative cooling Immersion hands / forearms Ice packs in neck, groins, and axillae Dantrolene Invasive—iced gastric, bladder, or peritoneal lavage	Iced-water immersion is superior No evidence for use of dantrolene Combination of other techniques may be used if immersion unavailable	Many articles relating to classical heat stroke Predominantly data from case reports

Data from Henderson K. Guys & St Thomas' Trust Guidelines for Management of Marathon Related Medical Emergencies. 2011.

- Respiratory—acute respiratory distress syndrome
- Gastrointestinal—intestinal ischaemia / infarction, hepatocellular / pancreatic injury
- Renal—hyperkalaemia, acute renal failure
- Rhabdomyolysis
- Haematological—thrombocytopaenia, DIC
- Metabolic—hypocalcaemia, hyperphosphataemia

❝ Expert comment Initial blood results

In this case, early results demonstrated a sodium of 148 mmol/L, evidence of acute renal injury and a raised CK. These results suggest the patient is significantly volume-depleted and does require intravenous fluid replacement therapy. Assuming normal renal function before the race started, patients frequently show rapid improvement in their biochemistry once they have access to adequate hydration and the exercise has stopped.

The CK may well be in the thousands within the first few hours but comes down once normal renal function is restored. A very small number of patients have substantial CK rises to the tens of thousands leading to further renal impairment which may take weeks to resolve, especially if the initial heat insult has not been treated effectively.

Clinical question: What role does standard anti pyretic treatment play in the cooling of EHS patients?

Many clinicians will instinctively reach for antipyretics when faced with patients with a raised temperature. As applies to all patients in the ED, it is important to analyse what the actual underlying cause of their presentation is. The blind treatment of absolute numbers can be ineffectual or in some cases even detrimental. Paracetamol is the most commonly used antipyretic in the UK. It is recommended by the World Health Organisation for reducing fevers in all age ranges due to its antipyretic and analgesic properties without any significant anti-inflammatory effects.

No discrete trial data exist analysing the use of sole treatment of antipyretics in EHS. This is of course understandable considering the effectiveness of other cooling techniques. Bouchama *et al.* (2002) briefly consider the role of antipyretics in parallel with conventional treatments for EHS but found no conclusive benefits.

Examining the pharmacology of antipyretics including paracetamol, aspirin, and other NSAID agents explains why they play no role in the treatment of heatstroke, as antipyretics function by interrupting the change in the hypothalamic set point caused by pyrogens. They are not expected to work on a healthy hypothalamus that has been overloaded, as in the case of heat stroke.

Paradoxically antipyretics may actually be deleterious and potentially aggravate bleeding tendencies, especially in patients who develop hepatic, hematologic, or renal complications.

Answer

EHS is not intrinsically mediated via the hypothalamus so antipyretics have no role in its management. Antipyretics do not decrease core temperature in EHS as an increased thalamic set point is not the underlying aetiology in EHS.

Case outcome

The patient was admitted to the HDU and his temperature continued to settle without the need for paralysis and ventilation. Further blood tests show deranged liver function with ALT peaking on day 2 at 1600 iu/l with a bilirubin of 40 micromol/L but normal albumin and alkaline phosphatase. On day 3 an abnormal clotting is demonstrated with an INR of 1.7 and a CK peaking at 21000 iu/L. Intravenous fluid resuscitation is continued and all biochemical parameters return to normal and the patient is discharged after 5 days in the HDU.

Box 26.2 Future advances

Understanding exertion related heat illness is of major importance to the military, athletes, and organizations that deploy staff to work in hot environments. There is a focus on understanding the physiology and prevention of heat illnesses. Research into acclimatization has identified a preferred regime of 7–14 days with 2 hours of daily exertion to sweating. This has been shown to improve 'thermal comfort' and 'exercise performance'. Recreational runners intending to run in very hot and/or humid environments should be aware of this.

The military are also very interested in re-deployment as are runners who have suffered EHS and want to know whether they can run a marathon again. Having had EHS, victims are less resistant to heat stress. In one study it took 3–11.5 months[2] before the subjects had normal heat tolerance, the recommended state before resumption of potential heat stress exposing activities. Techniques for evaluating recovery and 'return to play' for an individual are a major research focus of sporting, military, and commercial organizations.

A Final Word from the Expert

Hyperthermic patients in the ED are extremely challenging and these patients can do badly or need prolonged hospitalisation if the condition is not recognized and managed promptly. Key to success is very rapid cooling, managing the airway if necessary – the priority is cooling so a patient who is very agitated may need a general anaesthetic to make this possible. Multi-organ failure can be minimized with rapid treatment and support.

References

1. Glazer JL. The Management of heatstroke and heat exhaustion. *Am Fam Physician* 2005 Jun 1; 71(11):2133–40.
2. Ronnebeg K, Roberts WO, McBean AD, *et al.* Temporal artery measurements do not detect hyperthermic marathon runners. *Medicine and Science in Sports and Exercise* 2008; 40(8):1373–5.
3. Armstrong LE, Casa DJ, Millard-Stafford M, *et al.* Exertional heat illness during training and competition. *Medicine and Science in Sports and Exercise* 2007; 39(3):556–72.
4. Casa DJ, Beckers SM, Ganio MS, *et al.* The validity of devices that assess body temperature during outdoor exercise in the heat. *J Athl Train* 2007; 42(3):333–42.
5. Moran DS, Mendal L. Core temp measurement: methods and current insights. *Sports Medicine* 2002; 32(14):879–85.

6. Henderson K. Guys & St Thomas' Trust Guidelines for Management of Marathon Related Medical Emergencies. 2011.
7. Bouchama A, Knochel JP. Medical progress: heat stroke. *N Engl J Med* 2002; 346(25):1978–88.
8. McDermott BP, Casa DJ, Ganio MS, *et al.* Acute whole-body cooling for exercise-induced hyperthermia: a systematic review. *J Athl Train* 2009; 44(1):84–93.
9. Clements JM, Casa DJ, Knight C, *et al.* Immersion and Cold-Water Immersion Provide Similar Cooling Rates in Runners With Exercise-Induced Hyperthermia. *J Athl Train* 2002; 37(2):146–50.
10. Smith JE. Cooling methods used in the treatment of exertional heat illness. *Br J Sports Med* 2005; 39:503–7.
11. Jacobshagen C, Pax A, Unsöld BW, *et al.* Effects of large volume, ice-cold intravenous fluid infusion on respiratory function in cardiac arrest survivors. *Resuscitation* 2009; (80):1223–8.
12. Kamel YM, Jefferson P, Ball DR. Cooling intravenous fluids by refrigeration: implications for therapeutic hypothermia. *Emerg Med J* 2009;609–10.
13. Chang TL, Shahin A, Scott C, *et al.* University of Nevada Sports Medicine Heat Illness Guideline. August 2010.
14. Hew-Butler T, Ayus JC, Kipps C, *et al.* Consensus Statement of the 2nd International Exercise-Associated Hyponatraemia Consensus Development Conference, New Zealand, 2007.

27 Haemorrhagic rashes in children

Harith Al-Rawi and Fleur Cantle

✚ **Expert commentary** Anne Frampton

Case history

A 2-year-old girl attends the paediatric ED at 5 p.m. with a 3-day history of fever, dry cough, and vomiting. She had been started on antibiotics the previous day by her GP. Her mother is concerned that she has noted a rash develop on her face and neck and when she applies a see-through glass bottle on the rash it does not blanch (see Figure 27.1). She is worried that this rash is a sign of meningitis.

The child has no medical history of note, is not on any medications, and is up to date with her immunizations. Her observations on arrival are as follows: HR 135/min, CRT<2 secs, O2 sats 99 % RA, RR 26/min and Temp 36.4. You note there are 2 petechiae <2 mm distributed on the chest above the nipples and a few petechiae beside each eye.

See Box 27.1 for a clinical summary of rashes in children.

Box 27.1 Clinical summary

- A non-blanching rash (with or without fever) is a common presentation in children with the major concern of parents and medical staff addressing these patients being the likelihood of meningococcal disease.

- Medical and public awareness of the signs and symptoms of meningococcal disease has increased following recent public campaigns.

- Approximately half of children presenting with meningococcal disease are missed at first presentation to a doctor.[1]

- Previous studies have found the incidence of meningococcal disease in children presenting with fever and petechiae to be between 0.5–15 %.[2-4]

- Excluding meningococcal disease is paramount as the mortality rate is between 3.7–17 %.[2,3]

Whilst excluding meningococcal disease is of paramount importance, there are a number of other diagnoses which need to be considered and excluded.

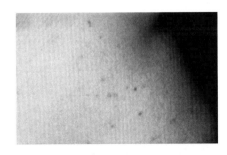

Figure 27.1 Petechial rash.
Reproduced from *British Medical Journal*, HE Nielsen *et al.*, 'Diagnostic assessment of haemorrhagic rash and fever', 85, 2, pp. 160–165, Copyright 2001, with permission from BMJ Publishing Group Ltd.

✚ **Clinical tip** definition

Petechia: Non-blanching spots on the skin <2 mm in diameter.[5]

Purpura: Non-blanching spots on the skins >2 mm in diameter.

Data from Wells LC, Smith JC, Weston V *et al*. The child with a non-blanching rash: How likely is meningococcal disease? *Arch Dis Child* 2001; 85(3) :218–22

> ☒ **Learning point** Causes of non-blanching rash
>
> See Table 27.1 for causes of non-blanching rash.
>
> **Table 27.1 Causes of a non-blanching rash**
>
> | Causes of non-blanching rash | Discriminating features |
> | --- | --- |
> | Sepsis (non-meningitis) e.g. Streptococcus pneumoniae | Fever. Signs of a focus of infection elsewhere |
> | Trauma, e.g NAI or post tourniquet for venepuncture | Characteristic pattern of petechia, e.g between fingers from slap. Distal to tourniquet post venepuncture |
> | Mechanical causes such as coughing and vomiting | History of cough/vomiting/screaming |
> | Viral infections | Non specific illness +/- fever |
> | Henoch Shonlein purpura | Palpable purpuric lesions over the buttocks and the extensor surfaces of the lower limbs |
> | Idiopathic thrombocytopenia purpura | Purpuric rash and mucous membrane bleeding, conjunctival haemorrhage, and GI bleeding. |
> | Acute leukaemias | Hepatomegaly, splenomegaly, and lymphadenopathy |

Case progression

Despite the child generally appearing well the mother states that she is very concerned about meningitis and requests the child is given intravenous antibiotics immediately to cover meningococcal disease.

Not all children require immediate antibiotics but if you are uncertain it is advisable to give antibiotics rather than delay for senior review or blood test results. The NICE guidance define criteria which, if met, antibiotics should be administered.

Clinical question: How likely is a rash distributed over the superior vena cava (SVC) territory to represent meningococcal disease?

> ⊕ **Clinical tip** NICE guidance management of the petechial rash
>
> Give intravenous ceftriaxone immediately to children and young people with a petechial rash if any of the following occur:[6]
>
> - Petechiae start to spread
> - Rash becomes purpuric
> - Signs of bacterial meningitis
> - Signs of meningococcal septicaemia
> - The young person appears to be ill to the healthcare professional.
>
> Data from The management of bacterial meningitis and meningococcal septicaemia in children and young people younger than 16 years in primary and secondary care Clinical guidelines, CG102 - Issued: June 2010. Available at: http://www.nice.org.uk/CG102

> ☒ **Learning point** Petechiae in the SVC distribution
>
> Petechiae in the SVC distribution (on the face and chest above the nipples) have been well described. They are probably caused by raised venous and capillary pressure resulting from coughing, vomiting, or crying.

> ✓ **Evidence base** Distribution of rash in meningococcal disease
>
> Wells *et al.* (2001)[5] conducted a prospective observational study for all children aged 15 years or less presenting with a non-blanching rash to their children's ED over a 12-month period. 233 patients were enrolled. 34% of these children had petechiae in the superior vena cava distribution. Most of these children were well and none of them had meningococcal infection. They also quote that there is a 95% chance that only 0–5% of children with such a rash will have meningococcal disease.
>
> Mandl *et al.* (1997)[7] conducted a prospective cohort study of children presenting with fever and petechiae. They enrolled consecutive infants and children presenting to the paediatric emergency department. 411 patients were enrolled over an 18 month period. None of the patients with petechiae found only above the nipple line (163 patients 39.7%) had a serious invasive bacteraemia.

Answer

A child that appears well with a petechial rash limited to the face and chest above the nipples is highly unlikely to have meningococcal disease.

❝ Expert comment

It is highly unlikely that significant bacteraemia is present if the child is well and the rash is localized to a SVC distribution with mechanical cause such as vomiting. However, it is worth remembering that in the early stages the rash may not be widespread and may be blanching.

One or two petechiae are common in well babies under 1 year of age. Although occurring less frequently, more than 2 petechiae can sometimes be present in well babies.

The presence of purpura (larger non-blanching spots >2 mm) makes meningococcal disease more likely (unless the clinical picture is suggestive of HSP).

Probably the most common cause of a non-blanching rash in a well child is a self-limiting viral infection, though this is often a diagnosis of exclusion. Clinicians should always be alert to less common pathologies such as ITP and acute leukaemia which are rare but important to recognize causes of this type of rash.

Case progression

You examine the child and find her to appear well. She is active and interacts well. Her cardiovascular, respiratory, and abdominal examinations are unremarkable. You note that her tonsils are mildly congested but no pus or exudate is seen. Her neurological exam is grossly normal, but you note there are a few more petechiae on her abdomen. You decide to do some blood tests.

Clinical question: How useful are blood tests in excluding meningococcal disease?

✔ Evidence base Using blood tests to exclude meningococcal disease

Nielson *et al.* (2001)[4] conducted a multicentre prospective study of children presenting with a haemorrhagic rash and fever. Five paediatric departments enrolled 264 consecutive patients over a period of 24 months. 39 patients (15%) had proven or probable meningococcal disease. They found that a neutrophil band form count >0.5×10^9/L and the CRP when elevated >68 mg/L both increased the likelihood of meningococcal disease (adjusted odds ratios of 38.3; 95% CI 3.8–385.1 and 12.4; 4.7–32.7 respectively).

Wells *et al.* (2001)[5] Conducted a prospective study in the ED recruiting 218 patients. This study found that children with meningococcal infection were more likely to have an abnormal neutrophil count (OR 2.7; 95% CI 1.1–6.5). They also found that clotting studies were more specific but lacked sensitivity. An abnormal INR was found in 58% of patients with meningococcal disease but only 5% of those without (OR 30; 95% CI 9.9–91.0). They did, however, find that no child with a CRP <6 mg/l had meningococcal disease. Their results showed that there was a 95% chance that only 0–4% of children with a normal CRP will have meningococcal disease.

Mandl *et al.* (1997)[7] Conducted a cohort study of 411 patients and found that an abnormal leukocyte count of <5000 or >15 000 was a good predictor of the seriousness of the illness; with a sensitivity of 1.0 (95% CI 0.53–1.0) and specificity of 0.64 (% CI 0.60–0.69). PT had a sensitivity of only 0.67 (95 CI 0.29–0.94) and a specificity of 0.97 (95% CI 0.96–0.99). They concluded that abnormal leucocyte count and coagulation profiles are predictive though not diagnostic of serious invasive bacteraemia.

Thompson *et al.* (2012)[8] A recent systematic review and validation of prediction rules for identifying children with serious infections which included the above studies pooled the results of 6 studies which looked at the diagnostic value of WCC in bacteraemia. The summary LR+ 2.04 (95% CI 1.51–2.75) and LR- was 0.54 (95% CI 0.40–0.73) and sensitivity was 62.71% (95% CI 52.6–71.81%) and specificity 69.27% (95% CI 62.71–75.13%). They concluded that WBC, absolute neutrophil `count, band count, or left shift demonstrated little diagnostic value for the outcome of serious infection.

⊕ Clinical tip NICE guidance[6]

If a child or young person has an unexplained petechial rash and a fever (or history of a fever), carry out the following investigations.

- Full blood count
- CRP
- Coagulation screen
- Blood culture
- Whole blood PCR for N menigitidis
- Blood glucose
- Blood gas

Data from The management of bacterial meningitis and meningococcal septicaemia in children and young people younger than 16 years in primary and secondary care Clinical guidelines, CG102 - Issued: June 2010. Available at: http://www.nice.org.uk/CG102

Answer

Blood tests are useful when taken into consideration with the clinical picture of the child; i.e. a child that appears well with a normal WBC and CRP is highly unlikely to have meningococcal disease.

> **✪ Learning point** Procalcitonin as an inflammatory marker in serious infection
>
> Procalcitonin (PCT) is a precursor of the hormone calcitonin that is seen to rise in infection and inflammation particularly of bacterial origin and does not rise significantly in viral infections. It has been shown that the level of calcitonin and the degree of increase correlates to the degree of sepsis,[9] It has also been shown that PCT may rise earlier in the infection process[10] when severe infection is challenging to detect clinically in young children. In a systematic review[11] of 8 studies (1883 patients) comparing test characteristics of procalcitonin, CRP, and leucocytosis for detection of serious bacterial infection in children presenting with fever without a source, it was found that overall sensitivity for procalcitonin was 0.83 (95% CI 0.70–0.91), for CRP was 0.74 (95% CI 0.65–0.82) and for leucocytosis was 0.58 (95% CI 0.49–0.67). It was concluded that that procalcitonin was the best performing marker in this population but was better for ruling out serious infection rather than ruling it in.

Case progression

The child remains in the observation unit whilst awaiting the blood results. She eats and drinks but remains quiet, coughs and retches a few times but does not vomit. The mother comes and informs you that there appear to be more petechiae on her face and neck. Her observations have remained within the normal range. Despite the blood results not being back you administer an intravenous dose of ceftriaxone 80 mg/kg.

Distinguishing those children who present with serious illness and those who present with a self-limiting problem can cause a diagnostic challenge to emergency physicians. Assessing children of different ages at different times of the day or night pre and post antipyretics can significantly affect the physician's perception of the severity of illness and this is often compounded by parental anxieties. Children who present early on in their illness may not display any 'red flag' signs for illness despite a serious infection. All these issues, together with the fact that physicians may have had limited exposure to sick children, can lead to a situation in which the subtle signs of ill health are missed. Recognition of these challenges has lead to the investigators to look for clinical features or laboratory tests which may be of diagnostic value and aid the formulation of clinical decision rules in order to try to standardize the assessment of these children.

The Thompson systematic review[8] highlighted 2 decision rules which were able to rule out meningitis and meningococcal disease. The first[12] was able to identify 35% who did not require a lumbar puncture despite signs of meningitis (see Table 27.2). This rule is for children aged 1 month to 15 years.[12] A score of >8.5 indicates the need for a lumbar puncture.

Table 27.2 The Oostenbrink clinical decision rule for predicting bacterial meningitis risk in children with meningeal signs

Risk factor	Points
History	
Duration of main problem in patient history	1.0 per day
History of vomiting	2.0

(continued)

Risk factor	Points
Physical examination findings:	
Cyanosis	6.5
Disturbed consciousness	8.0
Meningeal irritation	7.5
Petechiae	4.0
Laboratory tests:	
Serum C-reactive protein per 10 mg/l^{-1}	0.1

Reproduced from Oostenbrink R et al., 'Prediction of bacterial meningitis in children with meningeal signs: reduction of lumbar punctures', *Acta Paediatrica*, 90, 6, pp. 611–617, © 2007, John Wiley and Sons

Practically it is rare for ED physicians to make the final decision about whether a lumbar puncture is required and often antibiotics are administered before this occurs as it may lead to a delay in treatment. The challenge in the ED is the early recognition of ill health. In one prospective study[4] of 264 infants with fever and skin haemorrhages, 5 clinical variables were found to distinguish between meningococcal disease and other condition (see Table 27.3 and Figure 27.2).[4]

Table 27.3 Factors found to be predictive of meningococcal disease

Skin haemorrhages of characteristic appearance
Universal distribution of skin haemorrhages
Maximum diameter of one or more skin haemorrhages greater than 2 mm
Poor general condition (structured observation scheme)
Nuchal rigidity

Data from Nielsen HE, Andersen EA, Andersen J *et al.* Diagnostic assessment of haemorrhagic rash and fever. *Arch Dis Child* 2001; 85(2):160–5.

The presence of two or more features gives a 97 % probability of identifying a patient with meningococcal disease and a false positive rate of 12 %. Whilst this suggests that large, widely distributed lesions are of greatest concern, any petechial rash must be considered to be a potential marker of serious infection.

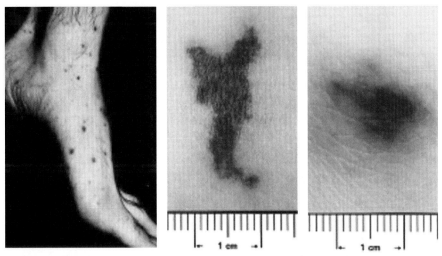

Figure 27.2 Characteristic appearances of skin haemorrhages in meningococcal disease.
Reproduced from *British Medical Journal*, HE Nielsen *et al.*, 'Diagnostic assessment of haemorrhagic rash and fever', 85, 2, pp. 160–165, Copyright 2001, with permission from BMJ Publishing Group Ltd.

> ✪ **Learning point** Antibiotics prior to diagnosis of meningitis
>
> It is not uncommon for children to present to the ED with a possible serious infection who have been given antibiotics in the community. In such cases it is difficult to decipher retrospectively if these children were misdiagnosed or had a coexisting infection or an infection which progressed to meningitis. The prior use of antibiotics poses a number of diagnostic challenges as it may affect the way in which a child presents and/or the results of investigations.
>
> The fever interval (time from onset of fever to the diagnosis of meningitis) is thought to vary between causative organisms. In a sample of 288 children aged 3–36 months *S. pneumonia* was found to have the longest duration of fever[13] interval. The longer the duration of fever preceding diagnosis, the higher the probability that a child would have made contact with a clinician and antibiotics commenced. In this study it was found that there was no significant difference in complication rate (death, or neurological, or audiological sequelae) between children who had received antibiotic pre-treatment and those who had not (OR 0.59, 95% CI, 0.27–1.3, $p=0.19$). It was also suggested that when the causative organism was *S. Pneumonia*, pre-treatment with antibiotics conferred some benefit.
>
> Doctors should also be aware that pre-treated children may present differently or more subtly than those who have not received prior antibiotics. In 1 retrospective case[14] series of 258 children aged 24 months or younger significantly less fever >38.3 °C and altered mental status were found in the pre-treated group however there was no difference found in overall mortality rates between the groups. It is important therefore that prior antibiotic use be sought in the history.
>
> The literature suggests that the administration of antibiotics prior to diagnosis does not significantly affect the CSF findings.[15]

> ⓘ **Expert comment**
>
> Well children who have received antibiotics prior to arrival in the ED can prove a real challenge for emergency physicians. On the one hand, the course of the disease may be tempered by the antibiotic administration and therefore the child demonstrates less features of severe disease; on the other, admission and further antibiotics may be unnecessary if in fact the child does not have serious bacterial infection.
>
> Whilst blood tests are still of use in these children, it is often the case that if they remain well then a more prolonged period of observation may be required, with or without antibiotics. If there is any doubt a senior paediatric review should be obtained and any child discharged must have adequate safety netting advice which may include a face-to-face review within 24 hours to ensure they remain well.

Case progression

The child's blood results return and the white cell count and inflammatory markers are normal. In view of the progressing rash the child is referred to the paediatric team for admission and observation. The paediatric team state they are reassured by the blood results and the distribution of the rash and advise the patient be observed in the clinical decision unit.

Clinical question: How long should the child be observed for before discharge?

> ✔ **Evidence base** Duration of observation in a child with a petechiae rash
>
> Klinkhammer *et al.* (2008)[3] conducted a literature review on children presenting with fever and petechiae. They recommend for children who present with petechiae below the nipple line and who otherwise appear well, bloods should be taken for cultures, FBC, and CRP, and to proceed with fever
>
> (continued)

evaluation based on the patient's age, and giving antibiotics and observing the child. If the CRP is normal and the child appears well after a 4-hour observation period, he/she could be discharged home with close follow-up, whereas children with CRP values greater than 6 mg/L or clinical deterioration should be admitted.

Brogan et al. (2000)[16] conducted a retrospective and prospective audit of 55 children presenting with fever and petechiae to a paediatric assessment unit. Their aim was to identify risk factors predicative of significant bacterial sepsis. They proposed the ILL criteria (irritability, lethargy, and low capillary refill) and suggested that children with fever and petechiae who have none of the ILL criteria and normal WBC and CRP should be observed for a minimum of 4 hours. If no deterioration occurred then outpatient or ambulatory care was recommended.

Answer

A period of 4-hours' observation seems appropriate with the proviso that once the child is considered to be well and discharged, close follow-up should be pre-arranged, and parents given strict guidance to re attend should their children appear ill.

ⓘ Expert comment

Observation of 4 hours is recommended in all cases where diagnosis is uncertain. This gives a reasonable length of time to observe the child's behaviour, interaction and to assess whether the clinical condition is rapidly progressing.

N.B. no child should be discharged from the ED if there is any doubt about his/her clinical condition simply to meet the 4-hour target. It may be the case that these children are best observed on a paediatric assessment unit or ED clinical decision unit to ensure that an adequate period of observation has occurred.

Always wake a child to assess him/her fully so you are confident that he/she is well and watch him/her play and interact. It is not possible to assess fully a sleeping child.

✚ Clinical tip Safety netting

If a child is to be discharged from the ED it is important to empower parents to feel that they can seek additional medical help if they feel their child is deteriorating. It is important to not behave in a manner which may deter parents from re-presenting. The NICE guidance on Feverish illness in children[16] makes the following recommendations about the provision of discharge information.

The safety net should be one or more of the following:

- Provide the parent with verbal and/or written information on warning signs on how further healthcare can be accessed.
- Arrange a follow up appointment at a certain time or place.
- Liaise with other healthcare professionals, including out-of-hours providers, to ensure the parent/ carer has direct access to further assessment for their child.

A Final Word from the Expert

Petechial rashes in children can be frightening both for parents and clinicians. It is important to remember that although they may indicate serious illness, often they are simply a feature of more mild, self-limiting conditions.

Always take a good look at the child you see in front of you and consider are the well or ill. If in doubt, treat.

In well children you can afford to take a little longer to assess and observe, but always be prepared to step in rapidly if the child deteriorates.

Many departments have a written advice sheet when discharging children with fever or rash and parents should always be advised what features to look for to prompt them to seek further medical attention.

References

1. Thompson MJ, Ninis N, Perera R, *et al.* Clinical recognition of meningococcal disease in children and adolescents. *Lancet* 2006; 367(9508):397–403.
2. Van Nguyen Q, Nguyen EA, Weiner LB. Incidence of invasive bacterial disease in children with fever and petechiae. *Pediatrics* 1984; 74(1):77–80.
3. Klinkhammer M, Colletti J. Pediatric Myth: fever and petechiae. *CJEM* 2008; 10(5):479–82.
4. Nielsen HE, Andersen EA, Andersen J, *et al.* Diagnostic assessment of haemorrhagic rash and fever. *Arch Dis Child* 2001; 85(2):160–5.
5. Wells LC, Smith JC, Weston V, *et al.* The child with a non-blanching rash: How likely is meningococcal disease? *Arch Dis Child* 2001; 85(3):218–22.
6. The management of bacterial meningitis and meningococcal septicaemia in children and young people younger than 16 years in primary and secondary care Clinical guidelines, CG102 - Issued: June 2010. <http://www.nice.org.uk/CG102>
7. Mandl KD, Stack AM, Fleisher GR. Incidence of bacteraemia in infants and children with fever and petechiae. *J Pediatr* 1997; 131(3):393–404.
8. Thompson M, Van den Bruel A, Verbakel J, *et al.* Systematic review and validation of predictaion rules for identifying children with serious infections in emergency departments and urgent access primary care. *Health Technology Assessment* 2012; 16(15):ISSN 1366–5278.
9. Meisner M, Tschaikowsky K, Palmaers T, *et al.* Comparison of procalcitonin (PCT) and C-reactive protein (CRP) plasma concentrations at different SOFA scores during the course of sepsis and MODS. *Crit Care* 1999; 3(1):45–50.
10. Luaces-Cubells C, Mintegi S, García-García JJ, *et al.* Procalcitonin to detect invasive bacterial infection in non-toxic-appearing infants with fever without apparent source in the emergency department. *Pediatr Infect Dis J* 2012; 31(6):645–7.
11. Yo CH, Hsieh PS, Lee SH, *et al.* Comparison of the test characteristics of procalcitonin to C-reactive protein and leukocytosis for the detection of serious bacterial infections in children presenting with fever without source: a systematic review and meta-analysis. *Ann Emerg Med* 2012; 60(5):591–600.
12. Oostenbrink R, Moons KG, Donders AR, *et al.* Prediction of bacterial meningitis in children with meningeal signs: reduction of lumbar punctures. *Acta Paediatr* 2001 Jun; 90(6):611–7.
13. Bonsu, B. Harper M. Fever interval before diagnosis, prior antibiotic treatment, and clinical outcomes for young children with bacterial meningitis. *Clin infect Dis* 2001; 32(4):566–72.
14. Rothrock S, Green SM, Wren J, *et al.* Pediatric bacterial meningitis: Is prior antibiotic therapy associated with an altered clinical presentation? *Ann of Emerg Med* (1992); 21(2):146–52.
15. Jarvis C, Saxena K. Does prior antibiotics treatment hamper the diagnosis of acute bacterial meningitis? An analysis of a series of 135 childhood cases. *Clin Pediatr (Phila)* 1972; 11(4):201–4.
16. Brogan P, Raffles A. The management of fever and petechiae: making sense of rash decisions. *Arch Dis Child* 2000; 83(6):506–7.
17. Feverish illness in children: Assessment and initial management in children younger than 5 years. CG160. May 2013. <http://publications.nice.org.uk/feverish-illness-in-children-cg160>

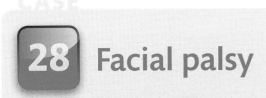

28 Facial palsy

Anna Forrest-Hay

🔾 **Expert commentary** Colin A Graham

Case history

A 48-year-old female attends the ED with her husband who is concerned that she has had a stroke. Two days ago she complained of vague earache on the right side of her head that subsided, but today her husband has noticed her face looks odd. She reports that she has been dribbling from the right side of her mouth and has found it hard to blink for a couple of days.

She is taking warfarin for a deep vein thrombosis (DVT) in her left calf that she acquired on a long-haul flight around a month ago. Her INR has been checked regularly and is stable and within the therapeutic range. She takes no other medicines. She says that she is penicillin-allergic. She has no other past medical history of note, but has a family history of hypertension.

Her observations on arrival are as follows: HR 82/min, BP 155 / 85 mmHg, SaO_2 99 %, RR 12/min and temp. 37.4 °C.

The triage nurse asks the doctor to see the patient as a priority as she has performed the FAST test and identified that the patient has abnormal facial movement, and thinks that her speech is also affected. She wants to know if she should request an immediate CT brain and ask the acute stroke team to see her urgently.

See Box 28.1 for a clinical summary of Bell's palsy.

Box 28.1 Clinical summary of Bell's palsy

- Bell's palsy is the most common cause of unilateral facial paralysis, accounting for 60–70 % of cases.[1]
- The other name for Bell's palsy is idiopathic facial paralysis (IFP) as the aetiology is not fully understood. Inflammation, ischaemia, oedema, autoimmune, and infectious causes have all been suggested with a focus on Herpes simplex type I and Herpes zoster virus reactivation.
- Bell's palsy is a diagnosis of exclusion and can only be applied to patients with paralysis or paresis of all muscle groups on one side of the face, with no other cranial nerves affected and no long tract signs.
- The right side is affected 63 % of the time.[3]
- Very few cases are observed over the summer months.[3]
- It affects people mainly between the ages of 14–45 years.[4]
- It is more common in females, and pregnancy[5] and diabetes[2] predispose to it. Pregnant women have 3.3× the chance of developing a facial nerve palsy and it occurs most often in the third trimester.
- The onset is fairly rapid (<72 hours) with the peripheral lower motor neuron lesion of the 7th cranial nerve often preceded by an ache beneath the ipsilateral ear.
- It may be accompanied by decreased taste sensation, decreased lacrimation, and hyperacusis.
- A family history of Bell's palsy is reported in 4 % of cases, so it is thought that it might be autosomal dominant with low penetration.[6]
- It can also be recurrent with such cases recovering less well.[7]
- 75 % of patients with Bell's palsy resolve completely within three weeks.[1]

---

⑥ Expert comment

Facial palsy is acutely concerning to patients and may occur from a multitude of causes. Rapid early assessment to identify reversible pathology such as acute ischaemic stroke is critical. It is very important for the first emergency care provider to find out and document the time that the patient was last completely normal, and the suddenness of onset of any neurological deficit, as this will help the emergency physician and the stroke team to determine the likelihood of stroke and the appropriateness of acute treatment. It is also important to perform a detailed history and examination of the patient to ensure that subtle, sinister pathologies are not missed. A confident diagnosis is critical as prognosis can be time-dependent and can be improved by the early initiation of treatment.[8]

Case progression

After speaking to the patient you are not suspicious of a new stroke within the last 4.5 hours as the onset of symptoms has been gradual over the last 48 hours. Without the need for immediate stroke team activation, you embark on a detailed history and examination.

On review, you find a female patient who is able to mobilize and fully alert and orientated. On examination, the cardiovascular and respiratory systems are normal. Paralysis of the upper and lower face on the right side is noted. The right eye cannot be closed and the patient is unable to elevate her right eyebrow. The mouth is drooping and the movements of the mouth are paralysed with drawing up of the lips on the left.

The tongue is seen to deviate towards the left side. Her face is fully sensate to light touch. On drinking, she complains of altered taste, but her cough reflex is intact. ENT examination is normal. Eye movements are full in all directions and the retina appears normal with no signs of papilloedema. There is no neck stiffness and power, tone, sensation are normal in the upper and lower limbs with symmetrical reflexes. No rashes are seen (e.g. erythema chronicum migrans).

⊕ **Clinical tip** ENT examination

Examination of the ears is essential to exclude Herpes zoster infection. Vesicles in the external auditory meatus or on the pinna suggest the diagnosis of Ramsey-Hunt syndrome. Infection within the geniculate ganglion causes loss of taste to the anterior two-thirds of the tongue on the affected side. The mouth should be inspected to detect lesions of the fauces and palate. Ramsay-Hunt syndrome is theoretically a contraindication to steroid therapy, although this is very controversial and rational guidance on treatment is impossible due to the lack of evidence.[10,11]

The clinician should look specifically for a cholesteatoma, which is associated with recurrent discharge, deafness, and dizziness. Hyperacusis is associated with paralysis of the facial nerve. A bluish red nodule on the earlobe or nose may represent Borrelial lymphocytoma which is associated with Lyme disease, an important cause of facial palsy.[12]

✪ **Learning point** Other clues in the clinical examination

- The bilateral innervation of the frontalis muscle is a helpful discriminator between lower and upper motor neurone pathology. If the forehead is unaffected and the paralysis is present on voluntary but not involuntary movements of expression, then it suggests an upper motor neurone lesion.

(continued)

- Sometimes, having examined the patient in detail, you may suspect other cranial nerve involvement, but it is important to know about the following findings in keeping with the diagnosis of Bell's palsy:
  - Bell's phenomenon is where the eyeball is seen to turn up on attempted closure.
  - Deviation of the tongue is frequently observed in patients with facial nerve palsy but does not represent additional involvement of the hypoglossal nerve. A unilateral lower motor neurone lesion of the 12th cranial nerve would make the tongue curve to that side and would have wasting and possible fasciculation.[13]

Clinical question: Should we be prescribing steroid therapy for facial palsy and if so, when and how much?

See Table 28.1. The aetiology of Bell's palsy is thought to arise from oedema secondary to viral infection of the facial nerve, or from ischaemia as it passes through the confines of the temporal bone. The early prescription of steroids should help to reverse the swelling and lead to more rapid and complete recovery. This has been highly controversial until recently. Steroids are relatively contraindicated in pregnancy, diabetes, patients with hypertension or pulmonary TB, a history of peptic ulcer disease, and those with middle ear infections; a careful risk–benefit assessment should be performed.

Table 28.1 Evidence for steroid therapy in facial palsy

Author and date	Patient group Study type Outcome	Key results
Salinas RA, Alvarez G, Daly F, Ferreira J 2010[14]	1507 patients in 7 trials Cochrane database systematic review Meta-analysis of recovery of facial motor function at 6 months and motor synkinesis. Cosmetically disabling sequelae were looked at.	The available evidence from RCTs shows significant benefit from treating Bell's palsy with corticosteroids
Sullivan FM, Swan I, Donnan P 2007[8]	496 patients. Double-blind, placebo-controlled, randomized, factorial trial involving patients with Bell's palsy recruited within 72 hours. Recovery of facial function as rated on the House-Brackmann scale. Secondary outcome was quality of life, appearance and pain	At 3 months 83.0% in the prednisolone group had recovered facial function compared with 63.6% among patients who did not receive prednisolone. Early treatment with prednisolone significantly improves the chance of complete recovery at 3 and 9 months. This paper is a major contributor to the Cochrane review by Salinas *et al.*
Engström M *et al.* 2008[15]	829 patients. Double-blind, placebo-controlled, randomized, factorial trial involving patients with Bell's palsy recruited within 72 hours. Primary outcome was time to complete recovery of facial function, assessed with Sunnybrook scale score of 100 points.	Time to recovery was significantly shorter in the 416 patients who received prednisolone compared with the 413 patients who did not (hazard ratio 1·40, 95% CI 1·18–1·64; $p<0.0001$). This paper is a major contributor to the Cochrane review by Salinas *et al.*
Sherbino J 2010[16]	Review	Supports RCT findings by Sullivan *et al.*

Data from various sources (see references)

Answer

The use of steroids to limit facial nerve damage in the acute phase is now accepted as beneficial. It improves outcome in complete paralysis, but has no effect on time of recovery. It should be prescribed within the first 3 days and works best if given within 24 hours. Typical trial doses of prednisolone were 50–60 mg daily (in single or divided doses) for 5 days, then reducing by 10 mg per day over 5–6 days.

> **❻ Expert comment**
>
> The evidence supporting early use of steroids for Bell's palsy, and in particular high-dose oral prednisolone, is now compelling. Two major randomized controlled trials, each with more than 500 randomized patients, showed that early prednisolone treatment improved the proportion of patients who recovered within 9–12 months. Crucially, both of these trials recruited patients who presented within 72 hours of onset, thus making initiation of this therapy an important decision for the emergency physician. The subsequent Cochrane review[14] and an evidence-based emergency medicine review[16] supported early high-dose prednisolone therapy based mostly on these 2 landmark studies. This should now be the standard of care for patients with Bell's palsy presenting to the ED within 72 hours of onset.

In the majority of cases, thorough history and clinical examination will negate the need for extensive investigations in the ED. The House-Brackman grading system[17] is an accepted scheme to describe the degree of facial paralysis and it is the standard method of assessing response in facial palsy trials.

The blood glucose, blood pressure, and temperature should be checked in all patients as gross abnormalities in these may suggest an alternative diagnosis. Lacrimation can be assessed by performing Schirmers test; a small strip of filter paper is placed in the lower conjunctival fold, the eye is closed and the length of wet filter paper is measured after 5 minutes. A young person would be expected to moisten 15 mm of filter paper. If there was any uncertainty regarding the diagnosis of Bell's palsy, further investigations may be required. In this case, an early CT of the brain is important, as the patient is taking Warfarin and has a family history of hypertension, and facial paralysis was preceded by a vague headache. A CT would be helpful here to exclude an intracranial or subarachnoid haemorrhage.

Clinical question: Is treatment with antiviral agents (acyclovir or valacyclovir) indicated in Bell's palsy?

See Table 28.2. Many emergency physicians prescribe antiviral agents, commonly Acyclovir, in addition to corticosteroids in the treatment of Bell's palsy if the patient presents within 72 hours of onset. The theory behind this is that Bell's palsy may be associated with Herpes simplex infection, although a causal link has never been definitively established.

Table 28.2 Evidence for antivirals in facial palsy

Author and date	Patient group Study type Outcome	Key results
Numthavaj et al. 2011[18]	1805 patients with Bell's palsy aged 18 years or over Meta-analysis of 6 RCTs Recovery rate within 3 months	Pooled odds ratio failed to meet the accepted criteria for statistical significance. For acyclovir plus prednisolone OR 1.24 (with 95% confidence interval: 0.79–1.94) vs 1.02 (95% CI: 0.73 to 1.42) for valacyclovir plus prednisolone vs prednisolone alone
Quant et al. 2009[19]	1145 patients with Bell's palsy excluding children and pregnant women. Meta-analysis of 6 RCTs. 574 patients received steroids alone and 571 patients received steroids and antivirals Facial muscle recovery	Pooled odds ratio for facial muscle recovery showed that antivirals provided no added benefit to steroids alone (OR 1.50, 95% confidence interval 0.83–2.69; $p=0.18$)
Mattar S 2012[20]	Short cut review of 4 systematic reviews and 2 small studies	There is insufficient evidence to recommend an antiviral agent in addition to prednisolone in the treatment of Bell's palsy.
Van der Veen EL, Roves MM 2012[21]	Literature search of 250 original research articles, 6 randomized trials.	Complete functional facial nerve recovery 75% with prednisolone and 83% when antiviral added, but 95% CI –1.0–15; NNT 14 Antivirals for Bell's palsy are precluded by lack of evidence, but it should be discussed with the patient
Worster A, Keim SM, Sahsi R 2010[22]	1500 adult patients with paroxysmal, unilateral paresis of cranial nerve VII. Review of 3 multicentre randomized controlled trials Recovery using validated measures of facial nerve function.	Prednisolone is inexpensive, readily available and is effective for this common condition. There is no statistically significant difference observed with acyclovir
de Almeida JR 2009[23]	2786 patients with Bell's palsy. Statistical analysis of 18 different papers Risk of unsatisfactory recovery ≥4 months	P values were statistically significant, but heterogeneity makes comparison of data unreliable
Goudakos JK 2009[24]	738 patients with unilateral facial nerve weakness of no identifiable cause Systematic review of 5 papers Treatment with either steroids or steroids with any antiviral agent	No significant improvement in complete recovery at 3 months in combined therapy

Data from various sources (see references)

Answer

Acyclovir does not make any statistically significant difference to the recovery of patients with Bell's palsy and should not be routinely prescribed, except as part of a controlled clinical trial. It is not justified at the present time to treat patients with Bell's palsy with antiviral agents in addition to corticosteroids; it remains to be shown whether antivirals may be beneficial in treating patients with severe or complete facial paralysis.

> **❝ Expert comment**
>
> The question of routine antiviral therapy for Bell's palsy has been a controversial topic for decades and there is still no definitive answer to the question. Studies have been hampered by poor design, inadequate numbers, lack of standardized end points, and heterogeneity. Some studies do suggest marginal benefit when compared to placebo, but now that prednisolone therapy is accepted as the cornerstone of acute treatment in Bell's palsy, the real question is: what is the incremental benefit of adding an antiviral agent to high-dose prednisolone? Outcomes need to be standardized and the timing of the primary outcome needs to be long enough to show any possible benefit of an antiviral agent, probably 12 months. Finally, the bioavailability of valacyclovir is greater than that of acyclovir, so there may be improved outcomes with valacyclovir; however, previous studies using both agents have not shown any difference in efficacy or outcomes. Future studies should compare valacyclovir with prednisolone against prednisolone alone. There is no further place for trials of antivirals as monotherapy given the demonstrated efficacy of steroids in Bell's palsy.

Case progress

The diagnosis and likely prognosis is explained to the patient. The patient is most distressed about her inability to close her eye; you therefore consider what management options there are and what advice to provide.

Clinical question: How can potential hazards to the eye be reduced?

See Table 28.3. As the surface of the eye is insensate and the eyelid does not fully close, it is vulnerable to trauma which might go undetected. On discharging the patient, most emergency physicians provide some advice on this, explaining that at the first signs of trauma(e.g. an injected sclera or blurred vision) the patient should attend an ED to have the affected eye assessed. What evidence is there for effectiveness of any interventions offered at the time of diagnosis?

There are no specific studies which have considered ocular interventions in Bells palsy, therefore conclusions must be inferred from studies which have looked at other disorders.

Table 28.3 Evidence for treatment for ocular issues in facial palsy

Author and date	Patient group	Study type	Outcome	Key results
Alsuhaibani AH April 2010[25]	Patients with facial palsy	Systematic review of papers regarding eye comfort and cosmesis in facial nerve palsy	Consensus agreement is best level evidence	Ocular lubrication and eye protection is recommended

Data from various sources (see references)

Answer

Artificial tears should be used during the daytime to provide topical ocular lubrication. At night, lubricating ophthalmic ointment can be applied to prevent exposure keratopathy. An eye pad can be applied at night. The eyelids can be closed with tape at night as an alternative to padding.

75 % of cases of Bell's palsy recover within 3 weeks. Follow-up at an ENT clinic should be at around 2 weeks after diagnosis. Full paralysis indicates nerve

degeneration at a point along its pathway. Regeneration is slow and after 6–12 months, 10–15 % of patients have incomplete recovery. A common complaint amongst this cohort of patients is lacrimation when they eat or other synkinesias. These patients need follow-up with a maxillofacial or plastic surgery specialist to consider further treatment. The GP can ensure ongoing treatment is provided in the interim. Coordinating patient management via the GP will also enable the other consequences of this condition to be treated, such as any psychological sequelae and any side effects from medication.

A Final Word from the Expert

It is not unusual for patients with Bell's palsy to present to the ED as it usually comes on fairly rapidly and it is commonly perceived as a possible acute stroke. It is therefore imperative that emergency physicians remain skilled at detailed neurological examination, especially when looking for the subtle signs of cranial nerve pathology so they do not confuse Bell's palsy with more sinister pathology. The experienced emergency physician should find making the diagnosis of Bell's palsy straightforward but failure to recognize infection or vascular abnormalities may result in adverse patient outcomes.

Important differentials include Ramsey-Hunt syndrome, meningitis, Guillain-Barre syndrome, or Lyme disease. An occult neoplasm is always a concern, but pointers in the history like slowly progressive paralysis, headache, or other cranial nerve abnormalities would suggest more sinister pathology. Follow-up within 2 weeks with an ENT specialist or the patient's GP will reduce the risk of any missed diagnosis masquerading as Bell's palsy.

An adequately powered, definitive, double-blind randomized clinical trial is required to rationalize antiviral therapy for Bell's palsy. The early administration of high-dose oral steroids is now the standard of care for acute Bell's palsy.

References

1. Kennedy PG. Herpes simplex virus type 1 and Bell's palsy-a current assessment of the controversy. *J Neurovirol* 2010 Feb; 16(1):1–5.
2. Adour K. Prevalence of concurrent diabetes mellitus and idiopathic facial paralysis (Bell's palsy). *Diabetes* May 1975;24950;449–51.
3. Katusic SK. Incidence, clinical features, and prognosis in Bell's palsy, Rochester, Minnesota, 1968-1982. *Ann Neurol* Nov 1986; 20(5):622–7.
4. Holland NJ. Recent developments in Bell 's palsy. *BMJ* 2004; 329:553–7.
5. Taylor DC, Khoromi A, Zachariah SB. Bell Palsy. Medscape Reference: < http://emedicine. medscape.com/article/1146903-overview >
6. Yanagihara N. Familial Bell's Palsy: analysis of 25 families. *Ann Otol Rhino Laryngol Suppl* Nov-Dec 1988; 137:8–10.
7. Peitersen E. Bell's Palsy: the spontaneous course of 2,500 peripheral facial nerve palsies of different etiologies. *Acta Otolaryngol Suppl* 2002; 549:4–30.
8. Sullivan FM, Swan I, Donnan PT, *et al.* Early treatment with prednisolone or acyclovir in Bell's palsy. *N Engl J Med* 2007; 357(16):1598–607.
9. Aik Kah T, Hanom Annuar F. A Systemic Approach to Facial Nerve Paralysis. *Webmed Central Ophthalmology* 2011;2(4):WMC001856. < http://www.webmedcentral.com/ article_view/1856 >

10. Uscategui T, Doree C, Chamberlain IJ, *et al.* Corticosteroids as adjuvant to antiviral treatment in Ramsay Hunt syndrome (herpes zoster oticus with facial palsy) in adults. *Cochrane Database of Systematic Reviews* 2008, Issue 3. Art. No.: CD006852. DOI:10.1002/14651858.CD006852.pub2.

11. de Ru JA, van Benthen PP. Combination therapy preferable for patients with Ramsey Hunt Syndrome. *Otol Neurotol* 2011 Jul; 32(5):852–5.

12. Sharma S, Kaushal R. *Rapid Review of Clinical Medicine for MRCP Part 2.* Second Edition. Manson Publishing, 2006.

13. Ryder REJ, Mir MA, Freeman EA. *An Aid to the MRCP Short Cases.* Second Edition. Wiley-Blackwell, 1998.

14. Salinas RA. Corticosteroids for Bell's plasy (idiopathic facial paralysis). *Cochrane Database Syst Rev* 2010 Mar 17; (3):CD001942

15. Engström M, Berg T, Stjernquist-Desatnik A, *et al.* Prednisolone and valaciclovir in Bell's palsy: a randomised, double-blind, placebo-controlled, multicentre trial. *Lancet Neurol* 2008 Nov; 7(11):993–1000.

16. Sherbino J. Evidence-based emergency medicine: clinical synopsis. Do antiviral medications improve recovery in patients with Bell's palsy? *Ann Emerg Med* 2010 May; 55(5):475–6.

17. House JW, Brackmann DE. Facial nerve grading system. *Otolaryngol Head Neck Surg* 1985; 93:146–7.

18. Numthavaj P. Corticosteroids and antiviral therapy for Bell's Palsy: a network meta-analysis. *BMC Neurology* 2011; 11:1.

19. Quant EC, Jeste SS, Muni RH, *et al.* The benefits of steroids versus steroids plus antivirals for treatment of Bell's palsy: a meta-analysis. *BMJ* 2009 Sep 7: 339:b33542009

20. Mattar S. Treatment of Bell's palsy: should antiviral agents be added to prednisolone? *Emerg Med J* 2012; 29:340–2.

21. van der Veen EL, Roves MM, de Ru JA. A small effect of adding antiviral agents in treating patients with severe Bell's palsy. *Otolaryngol Head Neck Surg* 2012 Mar; 146(3):353–7.

22. Worster A. Do either corticosteroids or antiviral agents reduce the risk of long-term facial paresis in patients with new-onset Bell's palsy? *J Emerg Med* 2010 May;38(4): 518-23. Epub 2009 Oct 21

23. De Almeida. Combined corticosteroids and antiviral treatment for Bell's Palsy. *JAMA* 2009; 302:985–93.

24. Goudakos JK. Corticosteroids versus corticosteroids plus antiviral agents in the treatment of Bell's Palsy. *Arch Otolaryngol Head Neck Surg* 2009; 135:558–64.

25. Alsuhaibani AH. Facial nerve palsy: Providing eye comfort and cosmesis. *Middle East Afr J Ophthalmol* 2010; 17:142–7. <http://www.meajo.org/text.asp?2010/17/2/142/63078>

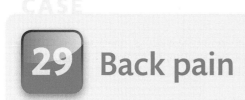

29 Back pain

Andrew Neill

✪ **Expert commentary** T. J. Lasoye

Case history

A 40-year-old builder attends the ED at 8 p.m. with an 8-hour history of low back pain after lifting a 25 kg box at work. He had initially attempted to continue working but within minutes realised that he would need to stop. He has taken the remainder of the day off work but now has had to call an ambulance to attend the ED as the pain has increased despite over the counter anti-inflammatory tablets. He is still able to weight bear but is in pain and has an obvious limp.

On questioning, the pain is solely localized to the paravertebral lumbar region. It has been increasing through the day and is not improving with simple analgesia. He has opened his bowels as normal earlier in the day and has reported no difficulties with passing urine. There was no leg weakness or sensory disturbance on examination but he complains of occasional shooting pains down the back of his right leg.

See Box 29.1 for a clinical summary of back pain.

Box 29.1 Clinical summary Back pain

Acute back pain is an extremely common presentation to the ED with 85% of us experiencing an episode of low back pain (LBP) at some point in our lives.[1]

Presentations of back pain make up 1.9% of all ED visits[2]

The vast majority of low-back pain is benign and will resolve spontaneously.

Classification can be acute (<6 weeks), sub-acute (6–12 weeks) or chronic (>12 weeks)

It remains a significant cause of lost work days with the demographic now shifting from manual labourers to office / desk workers.

Recurrence is common within the next one year[2]

See Table 29.1.

Table 29.1 Differential diagnoses of LBP

Diagnosis	Features
Abdominal aortic aneurysm	Shock, abdominal pain/mass, absence of back tenderness
Renal colic	Hyperacute, haematuria, flank tenderness
Cauda equina syndrome	Sciatica (often bilateral), sphincter disturbance (incomplete voiding a useful sign), motor weakness
Malignancy ± spinal cord compression	History of or signs suggesting malignancy, gradual onset
Spinal epidural abscess/osteomyelitis	Fever, IV drug use, immunosuppression
Unstable fracture	History of trauma
Inflammatory arthritis	Insidious onset, distal involvement (i.e. other joints or bowel or eye involvement)

Although the majority of back pain seen in the ED and in primary care is benign, it is important to be aware of the features that require the clinician to suspect a more potentially sinister diagnosis and to investigate further (Table 29.2).

Table 29.2 'Red Flag' low back pain

Historical features of cancer	Examination findings
Unexplained weight loss	Loss of sphincter tone, urinary retention
Immunosuppression	Focal lower extremity weakness
Intravenous drug use	Focal back pain with fever
Prolonged use of steroids	
Age >70	
Fever	
Recent trauma	

Case progression

The patient scores his pain as a 9 out of 10 despite the paracetamol previously given at triage. His initial observations are however still normal and he declines any further analgesia until he 'gets an X-ray to find out what's wrong'. As per your usual practice, you explain that you do not feel that a fracture is likely in his case and that an X-ray will not diagnose any other significant pathology. The patient nonetheless remains adamant, stating that both he and his colleagues have previously been given X-rays after identical accidents, and that his work will demand proof of the injury sustained.

> ### ⊕ Clinical tip Sciatica
>
> Sciatica is a commonly used lay term for any pain radiating into the buttock, knee, calf, and heel. 90% of cases are caused by nerve root compression by a herniated disc however canal stenosis and malignancy can also cause sciatica. Approximately 5–10% of patients with LBP develop sciatica. Risk factors for this include increasing height, age between 45–64 years, smoking, and occupations with strenuous activities of lifting and twisting.[3]
>
> Clinical examination to differentiate simple LBP and sciatica involves looking for a history of leg pain that is worse than back pain, radiating pain to toes, and straight leg raises causing worsening pain. Lasegue's straight leg raise test has been shown to have a sensitivity of 91% but a specificity of only 26%. A crossed straight leg test where the contralateral leg is raised and pain is elicited in the affected leg is shown to have a higher specificity of 88% but a sensitivity of 29%.[3]
>
> Bed rest is no longer advised and activities of daily living should be continued.

Clinical question: Is there a role for plain film imaging in any-age patient with acute low back pain?

Public perception still remains that all forms of back pain necessitates plain film imaging in the first instance. This may hold true for direct trauma or specifically axial compression trauma; however, atraumatic back pain must be considered as a distinct clinical presentation. An important aspect to consider is the radiation dose delivered and the exposure to the patient's gonads with the ionizing dose being significantly high at 2.4 millisieverts (msv) or the equivalent of 120 chest X-rays.

NICE guidelines have examined the contentious topic of imaging in back pain and now suggest the avoidance of plain film radiography for LBP.[4] Chou *et al.* reinforced this conclusion having performed a large systematic review and meta-analysis that considered the role of early imaging in acute LBP. They found no improvement in any clinical outcomes with the use of any form of early imaging.[5] Both the NICE guidelines and the paper by Chou *et al.* excluded patients with what are known as 'red flags'. These are symptoms suggestive of a potentially serious cause of LBP (such as malignancy, infection, and spinal cord compression) and first came into widespread use and acceptance with the publication of the America Healthcare Centre for Policy Research guidelines in 1994.[6]

With the exception of acute traumatic fractures, it is unlikely that a plain X-ray of the lower back will be of any use in diagnosing any of the emergent pathologies suggested by the presence of a red flag. There are numerous studies [7-13] (see Table 29.3) investigating the usage of plain X-rays, both in primary care and in the ED, and none have been able to conclude a benefit to the use of plain films of the lower back. In a patient with worrying features, more advanced imaging like CT or MRI is more likely to be beneficial in diagnosing any of the important differentials suggested by red flag symptoms.

⊘ **Evidence base** Plain X-rays in low back pain

Chou *et al.* (2009)[5] conducted a large, well conducted, systematic review of imaging for early management of LBP without 'red-flags'. Half of the patients included in the review were in studies assessing plain X-rays. They found no benefit of early imaging in 1804 patients.

Van den Boschh *et al.* (2004)[7] assessed 2100 referrals and radiology reports for lumbar spine x-ray. Only 0.5 % had signs suggestive of infection on X-ray, all of which were false positives. 15/2100 (0.7 %) had signs suggestive of malignancy, 7 of which were false positive and the others were all known to have disseminated malignancy prior to the X-ray.

Reinus *et al.* (1998)[8] collected prospective data on ED patients receiving lumbar spine X-ray. Excluded major trauma. All of the fractures detected in those over 60 were either old or osteoporotic. All of the malignancies detected were known prior to X-ray.

Espeland *et al.* (1998)[9] 3 radiologists separately evaluated 200 X-rays of the lumbar spine. Excluding vertebral fractures and spondylolisthesis there was poor agreement on X-ray findings.

Table 29.3 RCTS studying use of plain films in LBP (red flags excluded)

Author and setting	n =	Intervention	Outcomes	Difference between groups	Serious pathology in either group
Djais and Kalim (2005)[10] Rheumatology OPD, Indonesia	101	L-spine X-ray v usual care	Pain	None	None
			Back specific function	None	
			Quality of life	None	
Kerry *et al.* (2002)[11-12] Primary Care, UK	153	L-spine X-ray v usual care	Pain	None	None
			Quality of life	None	
			Mental health	None	
Kendrick *et al.* (2001)[13] Primary Care, UK	421	L-spine v usual care	Pain	None	None
			Back specific function	Worse	
			Patient satisfaction	None	

Data from various sources (see references)

Answer

In a patient presenting with atraumatic LBP but no red flags there is no indication for plain film imaging.

> **❝ Expert comment**
>
> It is not uncommon for patients to expect to have an X-ray for their back pain, which they perceive to be serious because of the intensity of the pain. However, once their pain has been effectively dealt with, it is often possible to make these patients understand that X-rays don't add any value to the management of their condition and may carry a small risk because of radiation. Clinicians should avoid requesting unnecessary X-rays to satisfy the patient as this may reinforce the patient's misconception about the role of X-rays during future benign episodes.

Case progression

The patient explains that he has had similar pains in the past after long periods of strenuous labouring work and has had to attend an ED on two previous occasions. He is not confrontational but is confused as to why he was investigated and treated differently on those episodes. He has not been able to pass a urine sample for you as of yet but is unable to stand and not happy to attempt to use a bottle.

When he last attended the ED 2 years ago he states that he was effectively treated with intravenous opiates and oral benzodiazepines and requests for a small dose of these previously successful medications. You are concerned whether this treatment rational is too heavy-handed and wonder if other milder medications would suffice.

Clinical question: Is there a treatment hierarchy between simple analgesics, NSAIDs, muscle relaxants, and opiates in the treatment of lower back pain?

The significant pain that many patients with LBP appear to be in is often the main reason why strong analgesics are prescribed. Experience will tell us, however, that prescribing large amounts of opiates does not guarantee immediate resolution of symptoms.

Despite guideline recommendations that paracetamol be used as a first-line treatment in acute LBP, there is remarkably limited evidence for its use. The first placebo controlled, randomized controlled trial for paracetamol in acute back pain is currently underway.[13] Of course, absence of evidence is not evidence of absence when it comes to effect and it is still reasonable to try an inexpensive, well-tolerated medicine like paracetamol as a first-line medication in acute LBP. If the patient remains in pain despite adequate doses of paracetamol, then what medicine should the clinician consider next? See Table 29.4.

Roelofs *et al.* (2008)[15] conducted a large well executed systematic review for the Cochrane collaboration that looked at a total of 65 trials. Their analysis of NSAIDs v placebo in 745 patients resulted in a 8.4 mm [CI = 12.6, 4.1] reduction in pain in a visual analogue scale.

Table 29.4 Systematic reviews of pharmacological management of LBP

Author	Intervention	Study type	Outcomes	Key results	Weaknesses
Roelofs *et al.* (2008)	NSAID	Cochrane review	Reduction in pain on visual analogue scale (VAS) at 3 weeks	8.4 mm [12.6, 4.1] reduction in pain	Variety of NSAIDs in included studies
Van Tulder *et al.* (2003)	Muscle relaxants	Cochrane review	Risk of being in pain 2–4 days following intervention	Risk ratio 0.58 [0.45, 0.67]	Limited availability of muscle relaxants in the UK
Deshpande *et al.* (2007)	Opioids (mainly tramadol)	Cochrane review	Reduction in pain	Standard mean difference −0.71 [−0.84, −0.57]	Studies only included chronic LBP

Data from various sources (see references)

Van Tulder *et al.* (2003)[16] looked at 30 trials involving a variety of muscle relaxants including diazepam and cyclobenzaprine. They found moderate benefit for cyclobenzaprine in acute LBP but as it is not available in the UK this is unlikely to help our patient. They found only one small trial ($n = 50$) looking at benzodiazepines in acute LBP and found only limited evidence of efficacy.

Deshpande *et al.* (2007)[17] studied opioids (mainly tramadol) for *chronic* LBP as there was a paucity of evidence for their use in acute LBP. They found a small benefit in 908 patients from the use of opiates; standard mean difference −0.71 [−0.84, −0.57].

Despite the lack of evidence, paracetamol is still probably the best choice of initial analgesic given its tolerability. If this is insufficient then the bulk of the evidence for acute LBP suggests that NSAIDs are the next best choice if tolerated. Although common practice, there is little evidence at present to support the use of drugs like diazepam or even opiates for *acute* LBP.

It should be noted that the effect size for all these interventions is small to moderate and even the best studied (NSAIDs) was shown to only improve pain scores by 8 mm, below the often quoted 'minimal clinically significant threshold of 13 mm.[18] In other words, while there may be *statistical* difference between placebo and treatment groups it may not be *clinically* significant. Thankfully, the natural history of the vast majority of back pain is to improve over time without any intervention.

Answer

Acute LBP should be treated with paracetamol and NSAIDs initially. There is no definitive evidence that benzodiazepines and strong opiates improve pain more clinically significantly.

❝ Expert comment

NSAIDs such as diclofenac 100 mg rectally or ketorolac 30 mg IM/IV are usually effective at bringing the back pain to tolerable levels; this enables the patients to mobilize reasonably. It is easy for the clinician to assume that morphine will be the panacea for all presentations of back pain, however as the evidence base demonstrates, a methodical use of the pain ladder should be adhered to. Most patients can have an early trial of mobilization in the department and then be discharged on oral NSAIDs and paracetamol rather than opiates.

Case progression

You review a second patient with lower back pain for your junior doctor. This 30-year-old male with no previous medical history had sudden onset lower back pain whilst lifting today and has been in your minor injuries area for over 3 hours and he is still unable to stand up unaided, as his pain is unremitting despite rectal NSAIDs and morphine.

You are now concerned that he has only passed urine once since the accident 11 hours ago and that he is complaining of sustained motor weakness and some patchy peri anal sensory loss.

His observations remain stable though his pain score has only marginally improved to 7 out of 10. Routine bloods had been performed but demonstrated a normal white cell count, inflammatory markers, and bone and renal function.

Your department protocol suggests that if any patient has the potential for a Cauda equina syndrome (CES) they should have an MRI scan and emergent discussion with the neurosurgical team. It is now, however, out of hours and your hospital MRI scanners are only operational during working hours.

> ⊕ **Clinical tip** Distinguishing Conus Medullaris syndrome
>
> The anatomy of the spine is such that the spinal cord ends at the level of L1 to L2 with the distal portion known as the Conus Medullaris, though the upper border is poorly defined. It is from here that the filum terminale extend down into the sacrum and form the cauda equina.
>
> Conus Medullaris lesions classically present with:
>
> - Predominantly upper motor neurone signs and thus hyertonicity and hyper reflexia
> - Positive Babinski's reflex
> - Mostly bilateral symptoms and signs
> - No loss of anal tone
> - Commonly urinary retention rather than incontinence
> - Constipation

Clinical question: If cauda equina is suspected can an MRI be ordered as an urgent outpatient test?

In the UK the majority of EDs will not have immediate access to MRI scanning. CES is of course recognized as a surgical emergency and as such radiology departments will strive to provide as comprehensive a service as possible; however, service limitations currently continue to exist. ED clinicians are faced with the conundrum of whether to admit patients under their own care and await MRIs (potentially overnight) or to refer acutely to neurosurgeons on the clinical basis of presentations.

> ⊕ **Learning point** Cauda equina syndrome
>
> CES is one of the most important conditions to consider when assessing a patient in the ED with low back pain. Although rare (incidence estimated at 0.04 % of all back pain attending primary care settings[19] and 2–3 % of all lumbar disc operations),[20] it commonly leads to irreversible loss of bladder function.
>
> (continued)

CES most commonly results from a large, midline herniation of a lumbar intervertebral disc, resulting in pressure on the cauda equina of the spinal cord resulting in a varied presentation of sciatica, motor weakness, and sphincter disturbance.

The spinal cord proper terminates at the lower border of the L1 vertebrae and continues as a series of spinal nerve rootlets that lie in the spinal canal until they exit the spinal column below their corresponding vertebra. The distinct anatomic nature of the cauda equina results in the varied, confusing and non-segmental distribution of symptoms as seen in Figure 29.1.

CES is regarded as a surgical emergency and if suspected, emergent MRI is required to help confirm the diagnosis. If a diagnosis of CES is made, emergent surgical intervention has been traditionally advocated. While MRI is less commonly available than CT, some centres have instituted out of hours access to MRI to facilitate rapid diagnosis and management of CES.

While MRI is our most useful test in confirming a clinical suspicion of CES, it should be noted that the diagnosis is not straightforward. MRI scans of the lower back are often abnormal in patients with no symptoms.[22] One study showed that 80 % of patients referred to a neurosurgical centre with a suspicion of CES who receive an MRI scan will not have a diagnostic lesion demonstrated.[23]

Crocker *et al.*[21] examined all patients at their neurosurgical referral centre who had an MRI scan performed outside the hours of 8 a.m. to 5 p.m. They were than able to identify which ones had been transferred and had an MRI scan for query CES. They report on 82 patients who had an emergency out-of-hours MRI scan. 55 (67 %) had no or non-surgical pathology. Of 27 patients undergoing surgery, 15 (56 %) were operated on the next available daytime list, 6 (22 %) were operated on more than 24 hrs following the scan, and 5 (19 %) went on to have emergency surgery. Put another way, only 5 of 82 (6 %) of those referred to have emergency MRI went on to have emergency surgery. Unfortunately the report does not detail the diagnoses requiring surgery so we do not know if this represents a specific

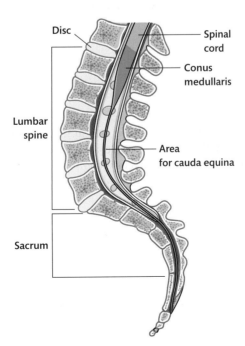

Figure 29.1 Spinal cord anatomy.

This figure was published in *Gray's Anatomy*, Henry Gray, Figure 661, Copyright 1918, with permission from Elsevier.

cohort of CES patients or whether it also included malignant or infective spinal cord compression.

There have been no studies showing that *emergent* MRI is beneficial to outcomes so we must answer the question of whether emergent or outpatient MRI is appropriate by first looking at whether or not emergent surgery improves outcomes. If emergent surgery improves outcomes then the onus is on the emergency physician to make the diagnosis as quickly as possible. If emergent surgery does not improve clinical outcomes then deferring the investigation until the next available slot may be appropriate.

Despite the traditional concept of CES as a spinal emergency, there has been controversy in the neurosurgical literature as to whether there is benefit to emergent decompression of CES.[20,24] Tables 29.5 and 29.6 summarize the evidence for and against emergent intervention in CES.

There are multiple facets to the debate but central to this is the lack of a clear definition of CES. Kostuik, in a frequently cited review article,[25] defined CES as a complex set of symptoms and signs consisting of low back pain, unilateral or bilateral sciatica, motor weakness in the extremities, sensory disturbance in the saddle area, and loss of visceral function. While descriptive, this definition is not specific enough to allow clear diagnoses. For example, are all components required or only the sphincter disturbance and back pain?

Table 29.5 Evidence AGAINST early surgery in CES

Author	Study type	Outcomes	Key results	Weaknesses
Ahn et al. 2000	Meta-analysis	Correlation of timing of surgery and various post-op outcomes	Found no benefit for surgery within 24 hrs v within 48 hrs	Literature search unsystematic Studies included mostly retrospective Data not appropriate to meta-analyse Study was actually a logistic regression not a meta-analysis
Qureshi et al. 2007	Prospective cohort of CES pts	Multiple including pain and disability at follow-up following surgery	No correlation between timing of surgery (<24 hrs; 24–48 hrs; >48 hrs) and outcomes	Selected pts only included Uncontrolled data Small numbers ($n = 33$)
Gleave et al. 1990	Retrospective cohort data	Recovery of bladder function	No correlation between timing of surgery (<48 hrs v >48 hrs) and outcomes	Selected pts only included Uncontrolled data Small numbers ($n = 33$)

Data from various sources (see references)

Table 29.6 Evidence FOR early surgery in CES

Author	Study type	Outcomes	Key results	Weaknesses
Todd 2005	Meta-analysis	Recovery of normal bladder functions	Early surgery (comparing either < 24 hrs v >24 hrs or <48 hrs v >48 hrs) results in improved outcome	Literature search unsystematic Studies included mostly retrospective Small numbers ($n = 141$)
Kennedy et al. 1999	Retrospective cohort data	Functional outcome at 2 years	Patients operated on early (within 24 hrs of full CES) did better than those operated on earlier	Retrospective No clear definition of CES

Data from various sources (see references)

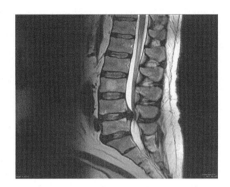

Figure 29.2 MRI T2 weighted image of cauda equina syndrome.

Reproduced with kind permission from Frank Gaillard at Radiopaedia.

Gleave proposed that CES be thought of in two forms, complete and incomplete, based largely on bladder symptoms. A patient with altered urinary function would have an incomplete CES (CESi) and a patient with painless urinary retention and overflow incontinence would be regarded as a complete CES. Gleave argued that only the CESi patients would benefit from early surgery and patients with a complete lesion (who make up the majority of presentations) could be operated on in a less emergent basis. This was reinforced by a poorly done meta-analysis of surgical outcomes that showed no benefit of surgery within 24 hours versus surgery within 48 hours.[26] There is as yet, little convincing evidence to back up the concept of incomplete CES, or any clear way to distinguish the two without resorting to urodynamic studies[27] and even these have yet to be validated.

There is currently no robust data to either support or refute the use of early surgery in CES and in lieu of such evidence, it would seem prudent for the emergency physician to pursue the diagnosis emergently and allow the surgeon to decide on timing of surgery (see Tables 29.5 and 29.6).

Answer

Although service provision limitations mean that MRI scans are often not performed immediately, there is not conclusive evidence to delay imaging as currently emergent treatment is still performed where possible.

Case outcome

An out-of-hours MRI scan was performed revealing a prolapsed disc and evolving cauda equina syndrome as seen in Figure 29.2. The patient was transferred to the care of the neurosurgical team and decompressive surgery was performed 6 hours later. The patient went on to make a full recovery and returned to active work within 6 months.

A Final Word from the Expert

The increasing incidence of back pain means that it will continue to remain a common and challenging presentation to the ED. Early pain scoring and early analgesia are simple but imperative measures.

The use of plain film radiograph imaging in the younger patient is rarely indicated in the atraumatic scenario. Those patients that have a clinical diagnosis of spinal cord pathology do however still require definitive imaging in the modality of MRI and thus early discussion with spinal or neurosurgical teams is needed.

For the emergency clinician, the emphasis should be on diligent and thorough clinical assessment and early detection of red flags followed by prompt referral of red flag cases to the spinal surgical teams.

As with many conditions, an early multidisciplinary approach may also aid early discharge for patients with non-specific muscular back pain. Emergency physicians pain teams, physiotherapists, orthopaedic and neurosurgical teams could all work together to deliver an expedited back pain service.

References

1. Cassidy JD, Carroll LJ, Côté P. The Saskatchewan health and back pain survey. The prevalence of low back pain and related disability in Saskatchewan adults. *Spine* 1998 1 Sep; 23(17):1860–6; discussion 1867.
2. Lovegrove MT, Jelinek GA, Gibson NP, et al. Analysis of 22,655 presentations with back pain to Perth emergency departments over five years. *Int J Emerg Med* 2011; 4:59.
3. Koes BW, Van Tulder MW, Peul WC. Diagnosis and treatment of Sciatica. *BMJ* 2007 June 23; 334(7607):1313–1317.
4. National Collaborating Centre for Primary Care. Low back pain: early management of persistent non-specific low back pain. *Royal College of General Practitioners* 2009; May:1–240.
5. Chou R, Fu R, Carrino JA, et al. Imaging strategies for low-back pain: systematic review and meta-analysis. *Lancet* 2009 7 Feb; 373(9662):463–72.
6. Bigos S, Bowyer R, Braen R. Clinical Practice Guideline 14. Acute Low Back Problems in Adults. US Department of Health and Human Services, Public Health Service, Agency for Health Care Policy and Research (AHCPR).
7. Van den Bosch MAAJ, Hollingworth W, Kinmonth AL, et al. Evidence against the use of lumbar spine radiography for low back pain. *Clin Radiol* 2004 Jan; 59(1):69–76.
8. Reinus WR, Strome G, Zwemer FL. Use of lumbosacral spine radiographs in a level II emergency department. *AJR Am J Roentgenol* 1998 Feb; 170(2):443–7.
9. Espeland A, Korsbrekke K, Albrektsen G, et al. Observer variation in plain radiography of the lumbosacral spine. *Br J Radiol* 1998 Apr; 71(844):366–75.
10. Djais N, Kalim H. The role of lumbar spine radiography in the outcomes of patients with simple acute low back pain. *APLAR Journal of Rheumatology*. Wiley Online Library 2005; 8(1):45–50.
11. Kerry S, Hilton S, Dundas D, et al. Radiography for low back pain: a randomised controlled trial and observational study in primary care. *Br J Gen Pract* 2002 Jun; 52(479):469–74.
12. Kerry S, Hilton S, Patel S, et al. Routine referral for radiography of patients presenting with low back pain: is patients' outcome influenced by GPs' referral for plain radiography? *Health Technol Assess* 2000; 4(20):i–iv, 1–119.
13. Kendrick D, Fielding K, Bentley E, et al. Radiography of the lumbar spine in primary care patients with low back pain: randomised controlled trial. *BMJ* 2001 Feb 17; 322(7283):400–5.

14. Williams CM, Latimer J, Maher CG, et al. PACE--the first placebo controlled trial of paracetamol for acute low back pain: design of a randomised controlled trial. *BMC Musculoskelet Disord* 2010; 11:169.

15. Roelofs PD, Deyo RA, Koes BW, et al. Non-steroidal anti-inflammatory drugs for low back pain. *Cochrane Database Syst Rev* 2008; (1):CD000396.

16. Van Tulder MW, Touray T, Furlan AD, et al. Muscle relaxants for non-specific low back pain. *Cochrane Database Syst Rev* 2003; (2):CD004252.

17. Deshpande A, Furlan A, Mailis-Gagnon A, et al. Opioids for chronic low-back pain. *Cochrane Database Syst Rev* 2007; (3):CD004959.

18. Todd KH, Funk KG, Funk JP, et al. Clinical significance of reported changes in pain severity. *Ann Emerg Med* 1996 Apr; 27(4):485–9.

19. Deyo RA, Rainville J, Kent DL. What can the history and physical examination tell us about low back pain? *JAMA* 1992 12 Aug; 268(6):760–5.

20. Gleave JRW, Macfarlane R. Cauda equina syndrome: what is the relationship between timing of surgery and outcome? *Br J Neurosurg* 2002 Aug; 16(4):325–8.

21. Crocker M, Fraser G, Boyd E, et al. The value of interhospital transfer and emergency MRI for suspected cauda equina syndrome: a 2-year retrospective study. *Ann R Coll Surg Engl* 2008 Sep; 90(6):513–6.

22. Jensen MC, Brant-Zawadzki MN, Obuchowski N, et al. Magnetic resonance imaging of the lumbar spine in people without back pain. *N Engl J Med* 1994 14 Jul; 331(2):69–73.

23. Bell DA, Collie D, Statham PF. Cauda equina syndrome–What is the correlation between clinical assessment and MRI scanning? *Br J Neurosurg* 2007 Jan; 21(2):201–3.

24. Todd NV. Cauda equina syndrome: The timing of surgery probably does influence outcome. *Br J Neurosurg* 2005 Jan; 19(4):301–6.

25. Kostuik J. Controversies in cauda equina syndrome and lumbar disc herniation. *Current Opin Orthopaed* 1993; 4(2):125–8.

26. Ahn UM, Ahn NU, Buchowski JM, et al. Cauda equina syndrome secondary to lumbar disc herniation: a meta-analysis of surgical outcomes. *Spine* 2000 15 Jun; 25(12):1515–22.

27. Nielsen B, de Nully M, Schmidt K, et al. A urodynamic study of cauda equina syndrome due to lumbar disc herniation. *Urol Int* 1980; 35(3):167–70.

INDEX